Mosby's manual of neurological care

Mosby's manual of neurological care

GORDON VOGT, R.N., M.S.N.

Associate Chief, Nursing Service for Education,
Fort Lyon VA Medical Center,
Fort Lyon, Colorado

MARGARET MILLER, R.N., M.S.Ed.

Coordinator, Department of Continuing Education,
Creighton University School of Nursing,
Omaha, Nebraska

MYRNA ESLUER, R.N., C., B.S.N.

Coordinator, Evening and Night Shifts,
Immanuel Medical Center,
Omaha, Nebraska

with 190 illustrations

The C. V. Mosby Company

ST. LOUIS • TORONTO • PRINCETON 1985

MOSBY

A TRADITION OF PUBLISHING EXCELLENCE

Editor: Barbara Ellen Norwitz
Developmental editor: Sally Adkisson
Manuscript editor: Jessica Bender
Book design: Jeanne Genz
Cover design: Tilford Smith
Production: Barbara Merritt, Kathleen L. Teal, Mary Stueck

Printed in the United States of America

The C.V. Mosby Company
11830 Westline Industrial Drive, St. Louis, Missouri 63146

Library of Congress Cataloging in Publication Data

Vogt, Gordon.
Mosby's manual of neurological care.

Includes bibliographies and index.
1. Neurological nursing—Handbooks, manuals, etc.
I. Miller, Margaret, R.N. II. Esluer, Myrna. III. Title.
IV. Title: Manual of neurological care. [DNLM: 1. Nervous System Diseases—nursing—handbooks. WY 39 V886m]
RC350.5.V64 1985 610.73′68 84-16675
ISBN 0-8016-5255-3

AC/VH/VH 9 8 7 6 5 4 3 2 1 03/C/305

Contributing author

KAREN ANDREASEN-SMITH, R.N., M.S.N.

Maternity Facilitator,
College of Saint Mary, Nursing Division,
Omaha, Nebraska

To all our clients, who deserve
the highest quality care we can give

Gordon Vogt

To Don, Therese, and Kelly

Margaret Miller

In appreciation to Mom, Dad, Duey, and all
my friends and colleagues for your continued love,
understanding, and support to make this manual possible

Myrna Esluer

Preface

Until now a single reference for care of the neurologically dysfunctional patient has not been available. Yet these patients are seen in a variety of health care settings as well as in special neurological units. *Mosby's Manual of Neurological Care* is intended to be used as a quick clinical reference by nursing students and professional nurses. Nurses practicing in a variety of clinical settings as well as home health care will find this manual beneficial in providing total patient care. Following an explanation of neurological assessment and diagnostic studies, the nursing process is applied to patients with neurological dysfunctions inclusive of all age groups.

This manual is divided into 14 chapters. Chapter 1 focuses on history taking and neurological assessment. Chapter 2 discusses common diagnostic studies; normal and abnormal findings are correlated with potential and actual causes of neurological dysfunction. Nursing responsibilities related to diagnostic studies, including patient preparation and posttest care, are discussed. Subsequent chapters focus on specific neurological dysfunctions. The format includes etiology, pathophysiology, and classifications of various neurological dysfunctions. Using the nursing process, the nurse can make comprehensive assessments, analyze the subjective and objective data to determine a nursing diagnosis, and plan and implement care. Each nursing diagnosis is correlated with dependent and independent nursing interventions and specific expected patient and family care outcomes. This reference manual is intended to provide general guidelines from which patient care can be individualized.

We wish to acknowledge the following persons who helped make this manual possible:

Our families for their understanding and continued support during the completion of this project.

Our typists: Terri Faga, Lorraine Bagstad, and Janis Marco.

Companies who provided illustrations: Span-America, Inc., Greenville, S.C., and Kinetic Concepts, San Antonio, Tex.

Our primary illustrator, Gaye Mayhew, and the C.V. Mosby personnel.

Gordon Vogt
Margaret Miller
Myrna Esluer

Contents

CHAPTER 1 Neurological assessment

Obtaining data relevant to an individual's neurological condition is an ongoing process. This process can be very complex because the nervous system is highly integrated. It is also quite dependent upon the proper functioning of the other bodily systems. Adding to the complexity of the process, in the infant the central nervous system is not fully mature, resulting in findings that differ from those of a child, adolescent, or adult.

The nurse must utilize proper skills to distinguish abnormal findings from normal as the patient's condition may be in constant flux, requiring continuous monitoring by the nurse to recognize, interpret, record, and report significant changes in the patient's neurological status. This requires using appropriate questioning techniques, conducting pertinent testing procedures, and making astute observations to gather data from a variety of sources including the patient, family, and other significant people. This puts the nurse in the position to acquire relevent information that will:

1. Assist the health team in correctly diagnosing the disorder.
2. Assist the health team in determining the severity and progression of the disorder.
3. Assist the nursing staff in identifying an actual or potential problem and in making an appropriate nursing diagnosis.
4. Aid the nursing staff in utilizing individualized and therapeutic interventions relevant to the patient's actual or potential problems.

A comprehensive neurological assessment contains an evaluation of the patient's relevant neurological history, vital signs, skull examination in the infant, cerebral function, cranial nerves, cerebellar function, sensory and motor systems, and deep tendon reflexes. The nurse may need to assess all of these areas or to emphasize one or two aspects of the assessment, depending on the patient's condition and the reason for evaluation.

THE PATIENT'S HISTORY

It is important to obtain a complete neurological history of the patient. The following topics should be included:

1. Description of present illness
   a. Onset: date, initial symptoms, sudden or gradual beginning, precipitating or predisposing factors
   b. Characteristics: location and type of symptoms, quality, quantity, intensity,

incidence, and duration (for example, memory or personality changes; disturbances of sleep, speech, hearing, sight, or writing; pain)
   c. Therapy: what kind, starting date, any effects
2. Description of past illnesses
   a. Any previous neurological disorders (for example, seizures, vertigo, head trauma, unconsciousness)
   b. Any other medical diseases that can complicate a neurological history (for example, vascular, metabolic, infectious diseases)
   c. Allergies
3. Birth and developmental data
   a. Birth: any hypoxia, signs of increased intracranial pressure, congenital syphilis, infectious process
   b. Developmental: types of delays, learning disabilities, detailed description of school progress (A developmental history should *always* be obtained in infants, children, and adolescents. This includes information regarding a person's performance of developmental tasks within a particular stage of the life cycle. Two tools that when used together will accomplish this assessment are the Erickson's developmental framework and the Denver Developmental Screening Test [DDST].)
4. Education and vocation
   a. Highest level of education attained and grade
   b. Vocation and how well patient functions in that position
5. Social data
   a. Unusual stressful events
   b. Present job: any working hazards
   c. Drinking habits, drug use, tobacco use
   d. Hobbies such as boxing, sky diving
   e. Foreign travel (for unusual diseases)
   f. The patient's ability to maintain normal activities of daily living and any recent changes
6. Family data
   a. Familial diseases
   b. Neurological disorders of family members

CEREBRAL FUNCTIONING—MENTAL STATUS

In evaluating cerebral functioning the patient's level of consciousness, behavior, and intellectual performance should be assessed.

Level of consciousness

In determining a patient's level of consciousness (LOC) the nurse is assessing the person's ability to relate to himself and to the environment. Terms such as alert, stuporous, lethargic, and comatose are commonly used to describe a patient's LOC but their meanings vary from one nurse to another and they should not be used unless a working definition is consistently used by all members of the health care team. One

Table 1-1 Glasgow Coma Scale

Area tested	Best response	Points
Eyes	Open spontaneously	4
	Open to speech	3
	Open to painful stimuli	2
	No response	1
Speech*	Oriented to person, place, and time	5
	Converses but not fully oriented	4
	Converses in disorganized manner	3
	Vocalizes no recognizable words	2
	No response	1
Motor	Obeys simple commands	6
	Does recognize local pain, but does not obey commands	5
	Withdraws from painful stimuli by arm flexion	4
	Decorticate rigidity†	3
	Decerebrate rigidity†	2
	No response	1

*Omit if aphasic or intubated.
†Described in section on motor testing.

simple, objective, reliable tool that is used to describe and standardize observations is the Glasgow Coma Scale. It consists of evaluating eye opening and best verbal and motor responses. The scale assigns numerical values to each response. These are added and yield a sum indicative of the level of consciousness. Scores of 7 or less are commonly accepted as meaning coma. A normal person would score 15 (Table 1-1).

Behavioral components

1. General appearance
   a. Age, weight, height, and body build
   b. Physical appearance in relation to chronological age
   c. Eye contact
   d. Body posture and position (for example, weakness or paralysis of extremities)
2. Behavioral activity
   a. General activity level
   b. Appropriateness (for example, unusual gestures)
3. Motor activity
   a. Coordination
   b. Unusual activities (for example, twitches, tics, grimaces)
4. Personal grooming
   a. General state of cleanliness (for example, condition of skin, hair, nails)
   b. Condition of teeth and gums
   c. Style, condition, and cleanliness of clothing
   d. Application and appearance of cosmetics

5. Mood and affective responses
   a. Cooperativeness and attitude during assessment (for example, depressed, hostile, apathetic)
   b. Inappropriate emotional responses
   c. Fluctuations in mood (for example, swings from joy to sadness)
   d. Expressed feelings inconsistent with behavior
   e. Speech (for example, rapid versus slow)
6. Thought content
   a. Evidence of delusions or hallucinations
   b. Stream of thought (for example, spontaneous and clear, changes of subject in the middle of a sentence)
   c. Distortions or bizarre associations
   d. Distractibility of patient
   e. Incoherence, confusion, undue preoccupations, patient's insight into his confusion

Intellectual performance

1. Immediate, recent, and remote memory
   a. Immediate (short-term): Have the patient repeat a sequence of numbers after you say them (for example, 6, 2, 5, 4, 1) or have the patient repeat them backwards.
   b. Recent: Question the patient about events that occurred earlier in the day.
   c. Remote (long-term): Question the patient about his earlier life and about past events. (For example, ask who were the last five presidents of the United States)
2. Ability to perform simple calculations
   a. Add two digits (for example, $2 + 4 = 6$)
   b. Count backwards from 100 by threes.
3. Fund of general information: Question the patient about current events.

SPECIFIC DYSFUNCTIONS OF THE CEREBRUM

Language dysfunctions

Aphasia is the inability of a person to understand and express himself in written or spoken language. The two main types of aphasia are expressive (Broca's, motor) and receptive (Wernicke's, sensory). In expressive aphasia the patient understands the spoken language but is unable to express himself. This results from a lesion in Broca's area of the frontal lobe. In receptive aphasia the patient is unable to understand or comprehend spoken language. This results from a lesion in Wernicke's area of the temporal lobe (Fig. 1-1). The patient with aphasia may have both expressive and receptive problems rather than strictly one form. Having both forms is called global aphasia. For any type of aphasia the nurse should assess the person's word usage, flow of speech, response to simple commands, and ability to identify familiar objects.

Dysfunctions in skilled motor activity

Apraxia is the inability to perform purposeful acts in the absence of paralysis. This may result from a lesion in the parietal lobe. To evaluate such dysfunctions it is necessary to assess the patient's ability to perform activities of daily living (for example; washing

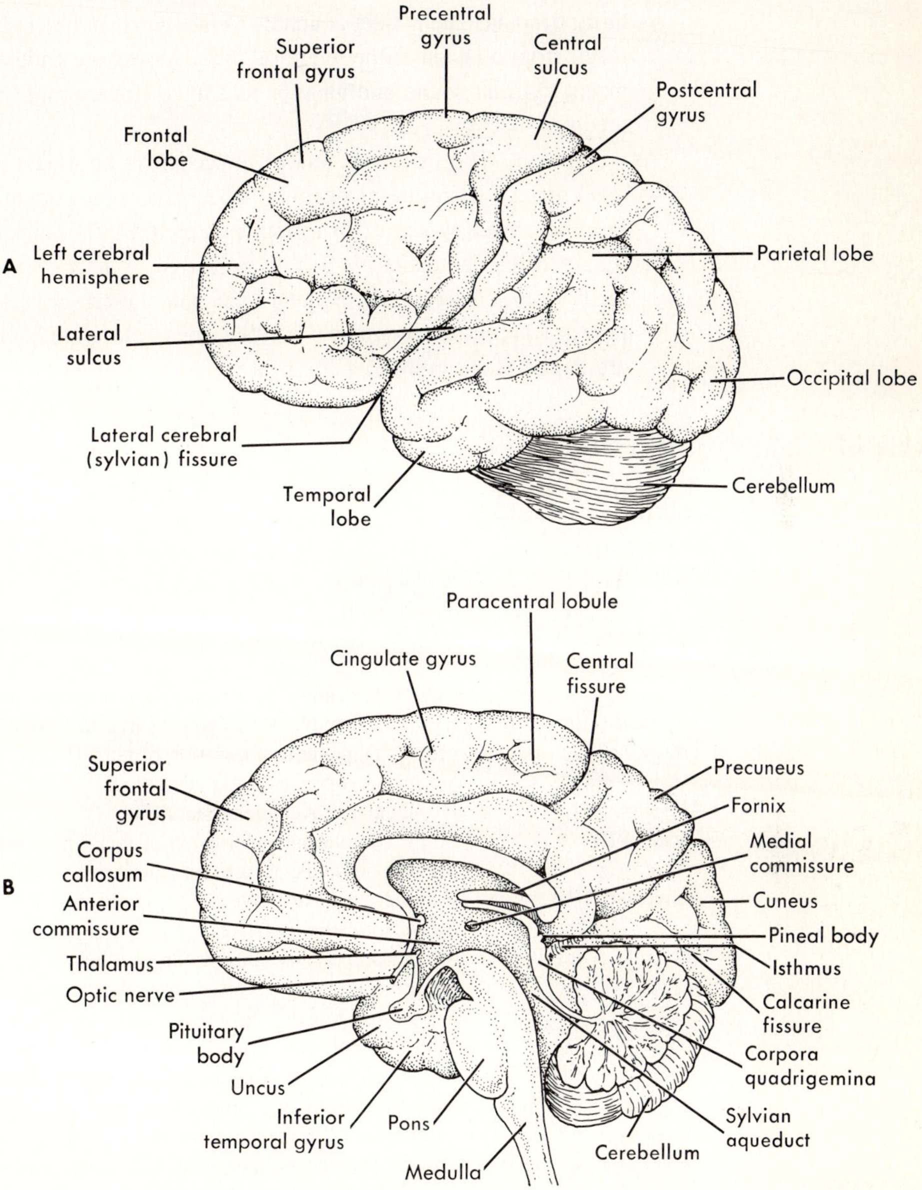

Fig. 1-1 Cerebral cortex. **A,** Lateral view. **B,** Medial view. (From Budassi, S.A., and Barber, J.M.: Emergency nursing: principles and practice, St. Louis, 1981, The C.V. Mosby Co.)

the face, combing hair) and to imitate familiar actions (for example, blowing out a match).

Sensory dysfunctions

Agnosia is the inability to recognize objects by sensory stimulation. Three common agnosias are auditory, visual, and tactile.

Auditory agnosia: The patient is unable to recognize an object by sound. This may result from a lesion in the temporal lobe. Assess the patient's ability to recognize a familiar sound and identify its source (for example, glass breaking, cat meow).

Visual agnosia: The patient is unable to recognize an object by sight. This may result from a lesion in the occipital lobe. Assess the patient's ability to name a familiar object by sight (for example, a picture of a house).

Tactile agnosia: The patient is unable to recognize an object by touch. This may result from a lesion in the parietal lobe, spinal cord, or cerebellum. Assess the patient's ability to recognize a familiar object placed in his hand while his eyes are closed (for example, a comb, a pen).

Table 1-2 Cranial nerves

Nerve	Functions
Olfactory (I)	Smell
Optic (II)	Visual acuity Visual fields
Oculomotor (III)	Pupillary constriction Upper eyelid elevation Extraocular movements (upward, downward, and medially)
Trochlear (IV)	Extraocular movements (downward and medially)
Trigeminal (V)	Motor component: innervation of temporal and masseter muscles Sensory component: facial sensation
Abducens (VI)	Extraocular movements (laterally)
Facial (VII)	Motor component: innervation of facial muscles Sensory component: taste on anterior two thirds of tongue
Acoustic (VIII)	Hearing: cochlear nerve Balance: vestibular nerve
Glossopharyngeal (IX)	Motor components: innervation of pharynx and parotid gland Sensory components: taste on posterior third of tongue; mucosa of pharynx, tonsils, and larynx; and carotid sinus
Vagus (X)	Motor components: innervation of pharynx and larynx; parasympathetic effects of thoracic and abdominal viscera Sensory components: mucosa of respiratory tract (pharynx, larynx, trachea, etc.); digestive tract
Spinal accessory (XI)	Motor components: innervates sternocleidomastoid (turns head), trapezius (shrugs shoulders), and pharyngeal muscles; thoracic and abdominal viscera
Hypoglossal (XII)	Motor component: innervates tongue

CRANIAL NERVES
(Table 1-2, Fig. 1-2)
Olfactory nerve (I)

The sensory receptor cells for smell are located in the roof of the nasal cavity and upper third of the septum. Grouped as fibers they become the olfactory nerve tract, which transmits neural impulses to the olfactory bulb located in the temporal lobe of the brain.

In infancy and early childhood the sense of smell is usually not tested. For the adolescent and adult, testing procedures are the same. As the adult gets older, there may be a diminished sense of smell because of atrophy and a decrease in the number of olfactory nerve fibers.

Testing procedure

1. Check the nasal passages for obstruction.
2. Have the patient close the eyes and occlude one nostril with an index finger.
3. Place a substance with a familiar odor under the open nostril. Have the patient describe the odor.
4. Test the other nostril using a source with a different odor. When testing, use substances that have a familiar odor such as coffee, oranges, cloves, or soap. Do

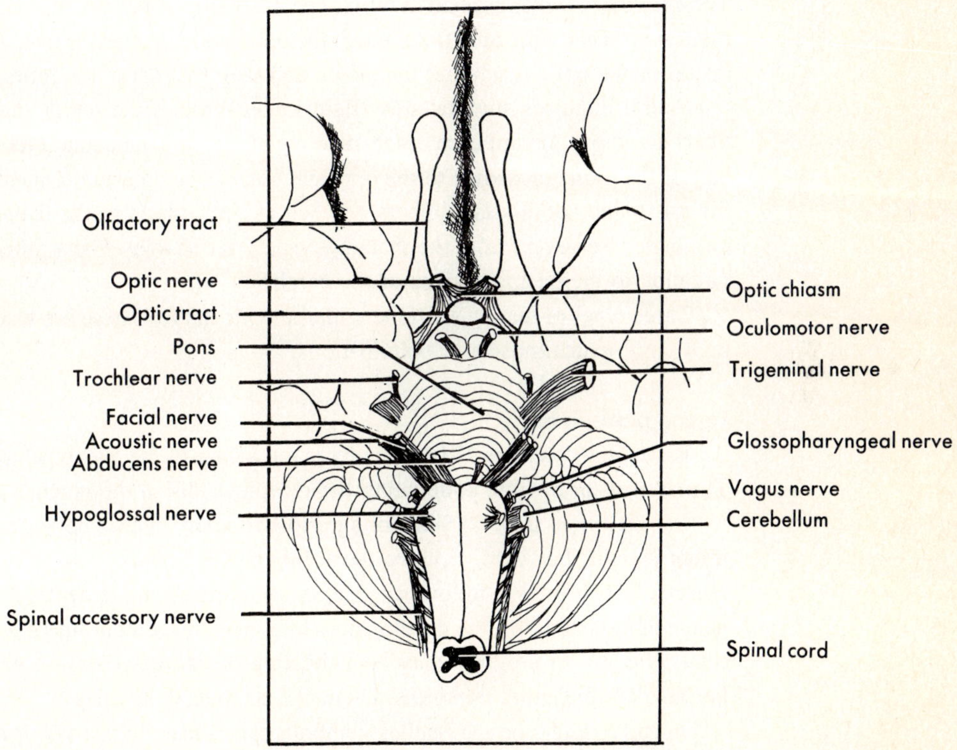

Fig. 1-2 Attachment of cranial nerves in the brain.

not use a substance that has a pungent odor such as ammonia. These are very irritating to the nasal mucosa and a false positive result may be obtained because pungent odors are detected through the oral mucosa.

Anosmia is the absence of the sense of smell. Hyposmia is the decreased ability to smell. Factors that may affect the sense of smell are:

Inflammations of the mucous membranes
Excessive cigarette smoking
Neoplasms of the nerve tract (resulting in a unilateral loss of smell)
Allergic rhinitis
Polyps
Lesions of the sinuses

Optic nerve (II)

The sensory receptor cells for vision are located in the retina. The images formed on the retina are reversed right to left and are also upside down; thus an object in the lower nasal field of vision is formed on the upper temporal quadrant of the retina. Within the retina are several specialized structures. The *macula* is an oval yellowish spot located near the midline of the lateral aspect of the retina. In the center of the macula is a funnel-shaped formation called the *fovea,* which is the area where vision is most acute. The *optic disc,* which is about 3 mm to the inner side of the macula, is referred to as the blind spot. This is the area from which the optic nerve leaves the eye. Also, through the center of the optic disc enter the artery and vein that serve the retina.

Neural impulses stimulated by light travel through the retina and the optic nerve fibers and move toward each other, meeting at the optic chiasma. Fibers from the inner half of the retina crossover to the opposite side in the chiasma. Outer fibers remain on the same side. Both sets of fibers proceed as optic tracts to the thalamus where most terminate. However, from the thalamus a new set of relay fibers proceed via the optic radiation to the occipital lobes of the cerebrum.

Three types of testing are done with the optic nerve. These are visual acuity, visual field, and ophthalmoscopic examinations.

Testing procedures

Visual acuity testing. Visual acuity is the ability of the eye to perceive visual detail. This is a result of light stimulating the receptor cells in the macula and fovea.

For the infant under 3 years of age, visual acuity cannot be accurately tested. The infant should, however, achieve the following behaviors: 2 to 4 weeks, fixation on objects; 5 to 6 weeks, follows objects in coordinated movements; 3 months, convergence of eyes and then the development of eye and hand coordination and the ability to focus. Failure to progress may be indicative of decreased vision or a loss of vision because of congenital blindness, cataracts, or mental slowness.

In early childhood the Snellen symbol chart is used to test visual acuity (Fig. 1-3). During adolescence and adulthood the Snellen letter chart is the appropriate testing tool (Fig. 1-3). Disturbances of visual acuity may indicate a decrease in the clarity of the

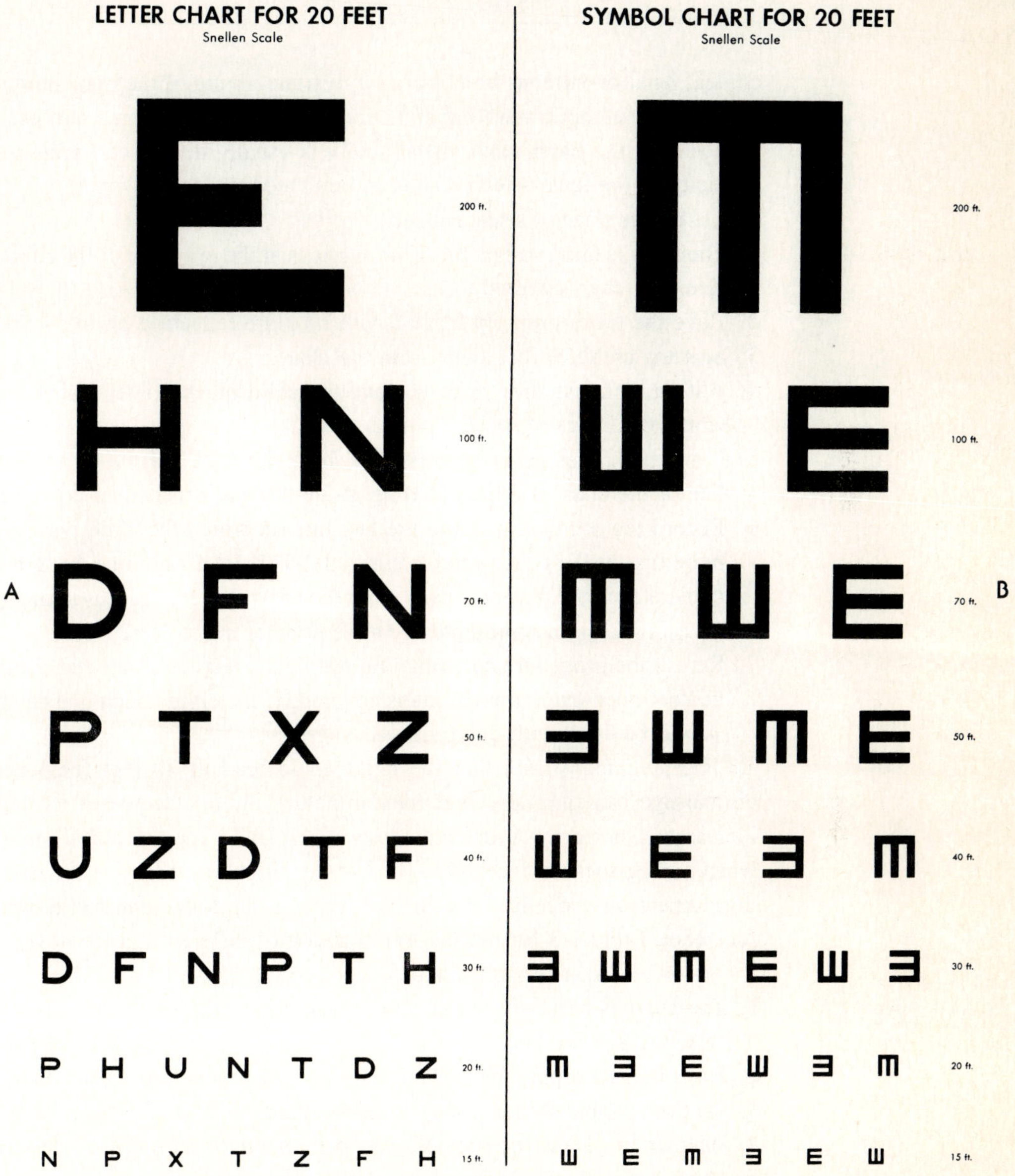

Fig. 1-3 Snellen chart. **A,** Letter chart for 20 feet. **B,** Symbol chart for 20 feet. (Courtesy of National Society to Prevent Blindness, Inc., New York. Member of National Health Council.)

Table 1-3 **Normal visual acuity**

Age (years)	Acuity
2	20/40
3-4	20/30
5-older	20/20

cornea, lens, or vitreous humor and/or dysfunctioning of the optic nerve tracts. Common causes of optic nerve dysfunction include head trauma, tumors, and multiple sclerosis. In the older adult visual acuity is usually decreased because of the loss of elasticity of the lens, which results in farsightedness (presbyopia).

USE OF THE SNELLEN SYMBOL CHART

1. The chart is hung so that the 30-foot line is at the eye level of the child when seated. Keep the chart covered.
2. Have the room properly lighted with no glare reflecting on the chart.
3. Seat the child 20 feet away from the chart.
4. With a demonstration E card, have the child practice identifying the direction in which the "legs of the E" point.
5. Using both eyes have the child describe "the legs" of the symbols. Uncover one line of the chart at a time starting at the top and proceeding downward.
6. Record the number opposite the last line on which the child was able to describe more than half of the symbols correctly. This is recorded as the denominator. The numerator is the distance away from the chart that the child is sitting (20 feet). The resulting fraction represents visual acuity (for example, 20/40).
7. Repeat the procedure covering one eye. Then test the other eye. Both eyes should be kept open even though one is covered. If the child wears glasses, the procedure should be done with them on.

Interpretation shows that the child could read at 20 feet (numerator) what the normal eye can read at *y* feet (denominator). Acuity decreases as the denominator increases. During the procedure observe the child for nonverbal signs of difficulty when testing such as excessive eye rubbing, blinking, tilting of the head, and squinting. Repeat the procedure if abnormal readings are found and make appropriate referrals. (See Table 1-3 for normal visual acuity of different age groups.)

USE OF THE SNELLEN LETTER CHART

1. The chart is hung so that the 30-foot line is at the eye level of the patient when seated. Keep the chart covered.
2. Have the room properly lighted with no glare reflecting on the chart.
3. Seat the patient 20 feet away from the chart.
4. Instruct the patient to keep both eyes open but to cover one eye. Uncover the chart.
5. Have the patient read the chart starting at the top.
6. The number opposite the last line on which the patient was able to read more than half of the letters correctly is recorded as the denominator.

7. The numerator is the distance away from the chart (20 feet). The resulting fraction is the visual acuity for the tested eye.
8. Repeat the procedure on the other eye. If the patient wears glasses, the procedure should be done with them on.

Interpretation and observations are the same as that of the Snellen symbol chart used for early childhood.

Determination of visual fields. Visual fields are assessed to inspect peripheral vision, which results from light stimulating the receptor cells of the retina outside the macula. Fields of vision are not formally tested in the infant. However, the infant's eye movements should be observed when an object such as a toy is brought into the field of vision.

For all other age groups the testing procedure is the same. The nurse should observe for gross defects such as hemianopsia, scotoma, and blindness. *Hemianopsia* is blindness in half of a visual field. *Scotoma* is an area of decreased vision that is encircled by normal vision. Common diseases that affect the visual field include diabetes, glaucoma, retinal detachments, cataracts, and vascular diseases (strokes). In the older adult peripheral vision is sometimes decreased.

1. Seat the patient and instruct him to cover his right eye with his hand.
2. The patient then focuses the eye being tested on a stationary object directly ahead.
3. While standing directly behind the patient, bring a test object such as your finger or a pencil from the periphery to the central vision area (Fig. 1-4). Vibrate the object rather than holding it static since the eye perceives a moving object more clearly.
4. The patient indicates when he first sees the object. Check all four quadrants of the visual field.
5. Repeat the procedure on the left eye.

Visual fields normally extend 130 degrees vertically, 100 degrees temporally, and 60 degrees to the nasal side. This procedure will detect a gross defect. Any gross defects of visual fields will need to be assessed through a more thorough examination using a tangent and perimeter screen. Patients with such defects should be referred to an ophthalmologist. (See Table 1-4 for common visual field disturbances.)

Ophthalmoscopic assessment. The ophthalmoscopic assessment is the same for all age groups. It may be difficult to do with children because children may be uncooperative. Having the parent hold the child or play a game with the child may help to get the child's cooperation.

1. Darken the room slightly to dilate the pupils. Keep enough illumination so that the patient can focus straight ahead on a distant, stationary object.
2. Stand facing the patient.
3. Turn the ophthalmoscope on with the dial set at zero.
4. Hold the ophthalmoscope in front of your eye. When examining the right eye hold the ophthalmoscope in your right hand and use your right eye. Use your

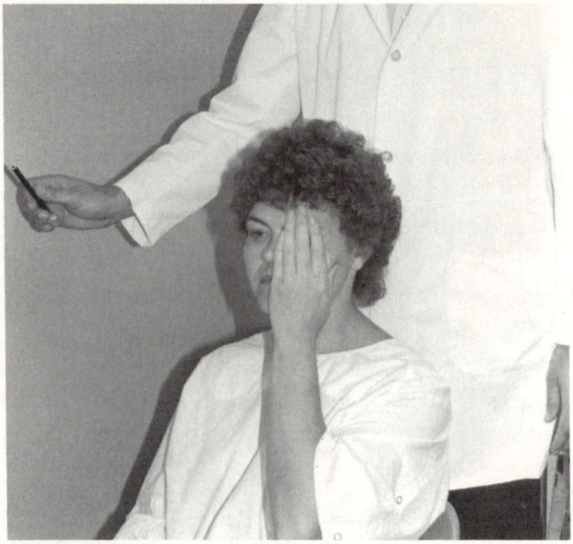

Fig. 1-4 Determination of visual fields. Optic nerve.

Table 1-4 Common visual field disturbances

Type	Description	Lesion
Blind left eye	Loss of vision in left eye	The retina; the optic nerve anterior to the chiasma
Bitemporal hemianopsia	Loss of vision in both temporal fields	Optic chiasma (only in the fibers crossing over)
Left homonymous hemianopsia	Loss of vision in temporal field of left eye and nasal field of right eye	Right optic trait posterior to the optic chiasma; right optic radiation (complete interruption)
Right homonymous hemianopsia	Loss of vision in temporal field of right eye and nasal field of left eye	Left optic tract posterior to the optic chiasma; left optic radiation (complete interruption)
Homonymous right upper quadrant defect	Loss of vision in right upper temporal quadrant of right eye and right upper nasal quadrant of left eye	Portion of fibers in left optic radiation (incomplete interruption)

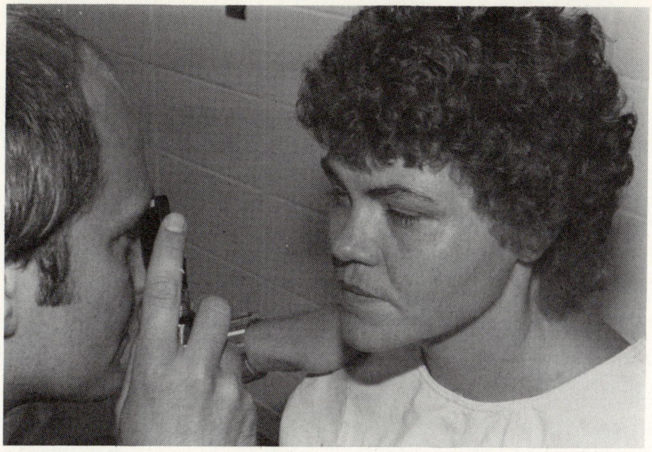

Fig. 1-5 Ophthalmoscopic assessment. Optic nerve.

other hand and eye when examining the left eye. Use your index finger holding the ophthalmoscope to focus the lens disk. You may need to use the higher black or plus numbers for the farsighted patient and the more negative or red numbers for the nearsighted patient.

5. Direct the light beam toward the patient. Keep both eyes open.
6. Move closer to the patient with the light focused on the pupil. At a position of approximately 6 inches in front of the patient you should be able to see the red reflex.
7. Moving in closer you should be able to visualize the structures of the retina (Fig. 1-5).
8. Repeat the procedure with the other eye.

NORMAL OPHTHALMOSCOPIC FINDINGS

Infants	**Children, adolescents, and adults**
Light red reflex	Bright red reflex
Pale round macula	Pink round macula
Absent fovea light reflection	Fovea light reflection (glistening)
Pale oval or round optic disc	Pink oval optic disc
Poorly developed peripheral blood vessels	Well-defined red blood vessels

ABNORMAL OPHTHALMOSCOPIC FINDINGS. Papilledema or swelling of the optic nerve head results in a blurred optic disc. This is a sign of increased intraocular pressure, possibly caused by malignant hypertension, hematoma, a brain tumor, or eclampsia. Increased cupping (bulging) of the disc may result from the increased intraocular pressure created by glaucoma. A late sign of increased intraocular pressure is pallor of the disc, which is indicative of optic atrophy.

A decrease in the diameter of the arterioles, which normally are three fourths the diameter of intraocular veins, may be indicative of hypertension. Sclerotic changes in the blood arterioles may cause them to lose their red color, resulting in opaque, lighter-colored vessels.

Mild retinal hemorrhages are sometimes seen in infants. However, if severe or seen in adults, hemorrhages are abnormal. Hemorrhages may be indicative of anoxia, subdural hematoma, diabetes mellitus, or hypertension. An abnormal (dull) red reflex may be indicative of retinal detachment, chorioretinitis, or retinoblastoma.

Oculomotor nerve (III)

A light shining on the eye stimulates the direct light reflex, causing constriction of the pupil. The eye not being tested also constricts. This is called the consensual light reflex. This phenomenon occurs because the optic nerve, when stimulated by light, carries the sensorineural impulses to the midbrain. In the midbrain a series of synapses transports the impulses to the oculomotor nerve, and this results in the constriction of both pupils.

The oculomotor nerve has three other motor responsibilities: accommodation, eyelid innervation, and extraocular eye movements. Accommodation enables the eyes to maintain a clear visual image of an object as it travels from a distant point to a point very close to the eye. The response in normal accommodation includes pupillary constriction, convergence of the eyes, and thickening of the lens. Innervation of the eyelid is important because the eyelid is responsible for the protection and lubrication of the eye. The extraocular eye movements controlled by the oculomotor nerve enable an individual to gaze upward, downward, and medially. These movements occur because the oculomotor nerve innervates the interior, superior, and medial rectus eye muscles and also the inferior oblique muscle. Extraocular eye movements are discussed in further detail in the sections on the trochlear and abducens nerves since extraocular eye movements are controlled by all three cranial nerves and the nerves are tested together in the neurological examination.

Testing procedures

Direct and consensual light reflexes. The testing procedure for direct and consensual light reflexes are the same for all age groups.

1. Slightly darken the room to dilate the pupils.
2. To test direct light reflexes shine a light in one eye. Observe the size, shape, and rate of constriction (Fig. 1-6).
3. Repeat the procedure on the other eye.
4. For testing consensuality, place the lateral aspect of your hand on the bridge of the patient's nose. Shine the light in one eye and observe the pupillary constriction of the other eye.
5. Repeat the procedure on the other eye.

Normal pupils are round, clear, and equal. They constrict briskly when stimulated

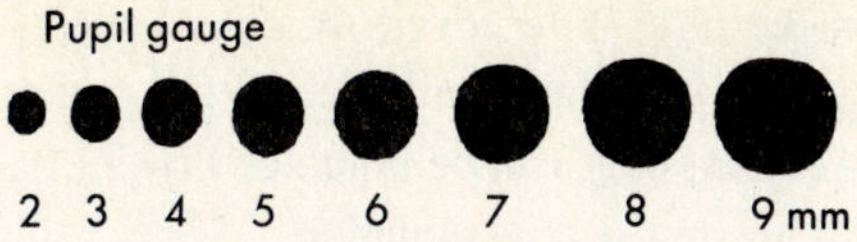

Fig. 1-6 Pupil gauge.

Table 1-5 Examples of abnormal pupillary findings

Response	Possible causative factors
Blind eye: no direct light reflex in affected eye; normal eye has direct and consensual light reflexes	Retinal or optic nerve damage
One dilated pupil: no light reflexes in the eye; downward and outward turning of eye with ptosis	Oculomotor nerve paralysis
Bilaterally small and irregularly shaped pupils; no light reflexes; accommodation reaction remains (Argyll-Robertson pupil)	Associated with syphilis of the central nervous system
Bilateral enlargement of pupils (mydriasis)	Acute glaucoma, local trauma, parasympatholytic or sympathomimetic drugs, and mydriatics
Unilaterally enlarged and fixed pupils	Head trauma resulting in increased intracranial pressure, local injury to eye
Bilaterally enlarged and fixed pupils	Central nervous system damage, deep anesthesia, death.
Constriction of pupils (miosis)	Miotics (pilocarpine), inflammation of iris, sleep, morphine.

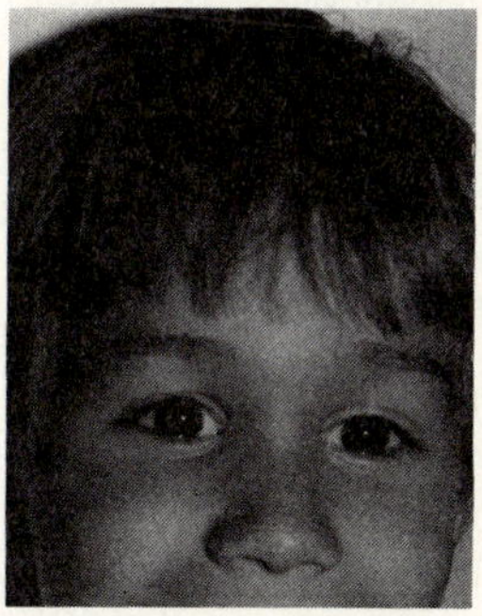

Fig. 1-7 Innervation of the eyelid. Oculomotor nerve.

by light and dilate when the light is removed. In consensuality the pupil without the light stimulus constricts when the other pupil does. When testing the light reflexes and accommodation, normal functioning can be noted as PERRLA, which means "pupils equal, round, react to light, and accommodation." (See Table 1-5 for examples of abnormal pupillary findings.) In the older adult visual perception may be reduced as a result of decreased pupillary size. Many older adults will have a slower adaptation to light and have some degree of decreased visual acuity.

Innervation of the eyelid. The testing procedure for the innervation of the eyelid is the same for all ages. Observe placement and movement of the upper eyelid (Fig. 1-7). When the eye is open, the upper eyelid should be between the upper iris and pupil. When closed, the eye should be completely covered. A drooping of the upper eyelid to the pupil is called ptosis. This may be indicative of a congenital condition or of oculomotor nerve paresis caused by infection, tumor, aneurysm, trauma, muscular dystrophy, or myasthenia gravis.

Accommodation. In the infant accommodation cannot be accurately tested. However, the convergence of the eyes can be observed when a toy is brought close to the child. Eye convergence develops at approximately 3 months of age. The development of eye-hand coordination and the ability to focus follows. For all other age groups the testing procedure for accommodation is the same. Improper accommodation is indicative of oculomotor, trochlear, or abducens nerve damage.

1. Slightly darken the room to dilate pupils.
2. Hold a pencil 2 feet away from the patient's eyes.
3. Have the patient focus on the pencil as it is moved closer to the face. There should be pupillary constriction and convergence of both eyes. Normal convergence should break at about 2 cm from the face. When convergence is broken, the pupils will dilate.

Trochlear nerve (IV)

The motor fibers of the trochlear nerve originate in the midbrain. These fibers extend to the superior oblique muscles of the eye, enabling the extraocular movements of looking downward and medially. The trochlear nerve is tested as a unit with the oculomotor and abducens nerves.

Trigeminal nerve (V)

The trigeminal nerve has both motor and sensory fibers. The motor fibers originate in the pons, and neural impulses travel via the mandibular branch of the nerve to the temporal and masseter muscles, which control chewing and jaw movement. The sensory receptors are located in the skin and mucosa of the head and the teeth. Neural impulses travel via the ophthalmic, maxillary, and mandibular branches to the pons.

Testing procedures

Motor component. The motor component of the trigeminal nerve is tested in the infant by observing facial expressions. This nerve is easier to assess when the child is old enough to eat solid foods. For all other age groups the testing procedure is as follows:

1. Place your fingers on the patient's mandible (use both hands). Have the patient bite down tightly (Fig. 1-8).
2. Place your fingers on the patient's temples (use both hands). Have the patient bite down slightly. Assess size, strength, and symmetry of the masseter and temporal muscles.
3. With the palms of your hands on the patient's mandible, have the patient open his mouth slightly and move the mandible laterally. Assess any weakness.

The masseter and temporal muscles should be equally strong bilaterally. Diseases that affect the motor component of the trigeminal nerve include amyotrophic lateral sclerosis, myasthenia gravis, and tetanus.

Sensory component. The sensory component of the trigeminal nerve in the infant is usually not tested. If there is a question concerning the infant's facial sensations, a pin may be used to touch different areas of the face. This should elicit a withdrawal response and a cry.

For young children tell the patients what you are going to do and that you will not hurt them. This will keep a child from becoming too scared and will also help to obtain

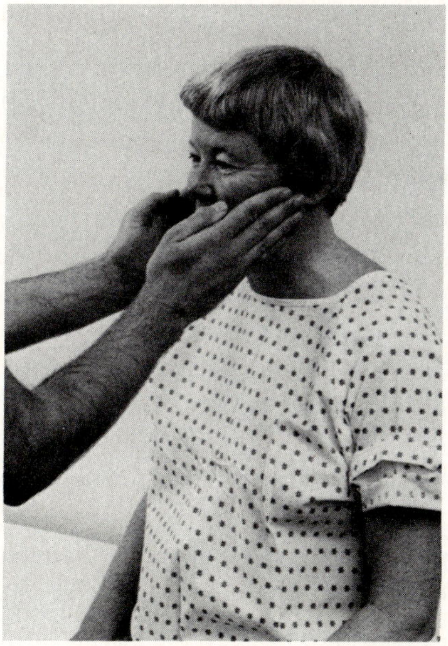

Fig. 1-8 Masseter muscle innervation. Trigeminal nerve.

cooperation from the patient, which is very important in this procedure. The procedure should be done as follows:

1. Have the child close his eyes.
2. Use cotton to lightly touch different areas of face. Have the child tell you when he is being touched.
3. The corneal reflex is usually not tested.

The testing procedure for all other age groups should include the following:

1. Have the patient close the eyes.
2. Touch different areas of the face randomly with cotton or a pin. Have the patient tell you where he is being touched and whether it is by a soft or sharp object.
3. Touch various areas of the oral mucosa with a wooden applicator. Have the patient tell you where he is being touched.
4. To assess the corneal reflex, lightly touch the lateral aspect of the cornea of the eye with a wisp of cotton. Normally there should be a rapid blink of the eye.

Observe and note areas where there is a loss of feeling that may be indicative of anesthesia or paralysis. Diseases that affect the sensory component of the trigeminal nerve include trigeminal neuralgia (tic douloureux) and herpes zoster.

Abducens nerve (VI)

The motor fibers of the abducens nerve originate in the pons. These fibers extend to the lateral rectus muscles of the eye, enabling the extraocular movement of looking laterally. The abducens nerve is tested as a unit with the oculomotor and trochlear nerves.

Testing procedures. At 5 to 6 weeks of age the infant should start to follow objects in coordinated movements. Searching nystagmus (an involuntary rhythmic oscillation of the eyeball when searching around) is common in the first days after birth. It may indicate blindness if it does not disappear after a few days. Intermittent alternating strabismus (crossing of the eyes) is normal in the first 6 months of life. It is abnormal, however, when the strabismus movements are unilateral or divergent. Doll's eyes are normal during the first 7 to 10 days of life. Assess for doll's eyes by turning the infant's head to the side; the eyes will deviate in the direction away from the head movement.

During early childhood utilize the Hirschberg and cover tests to assess age movements. The following guidelines should be used:

Hirschberg test

1. Hold a light so that it shines from the middle of your forehead to the bridge of the child's nose.
2. Have the child watch it. The eyes should be held fixed in the midline.
3. Turn the child's head to the right and left. Observe changes in the reflection pattern.

Cover test

1. Hold a light so that it shines from the middle of your forehead to the bridge of the child's nose.

2. Place one hand on top of the child's head with your thumb in front of one eye. Observe the other eye for movement.
3. Remove your thumb and observe both eyes for movement. Movement in either or both eyes is indicative of a strabismus.

For all other age groups the assessment includes range-of-motion test (Fig. 1-9).

Range-of-motion test

1. Have the patient cover one eye with a card or his hand.
2. Hold your finger 18 to 24 inches from the patient's face.
3. Have the patient follow your finger as you move it in all directions of gaze.
4. Repeat the procedure on the other eye.
5. Repeat the procedure with the patient using both eyes.

Observe for the following abnormal eye movements that may be caused by a weakness or paralysis of one or more of the extraocular muscles or a deficit in one of the nerves innervating the muscles.

Esotropia: one eye deviates inward.
Exotropia: one eye deviates outward.
Amblyopia exanopsia ("lazy eye"): reduced vision in one eye because of disease.
Strabismus: uncoordinated eye movements; the eyes do not always point in the same direction.
Nystagmus: involuntary, rapid eye movements that usually appear to be jerky.

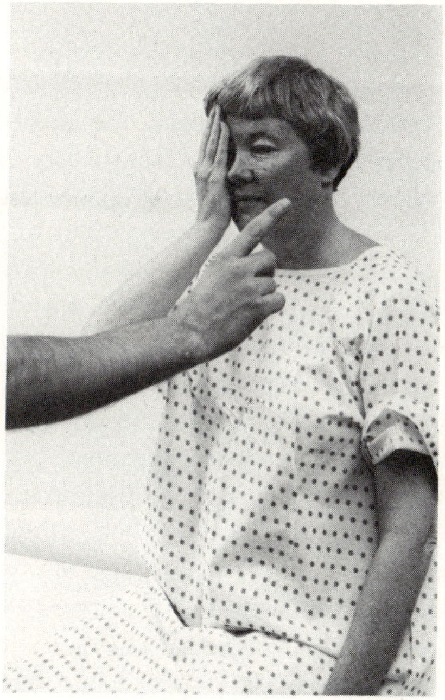

Fig. 1-9 Range of motion test. Oculomotor, trochlear, and abducens nerves.

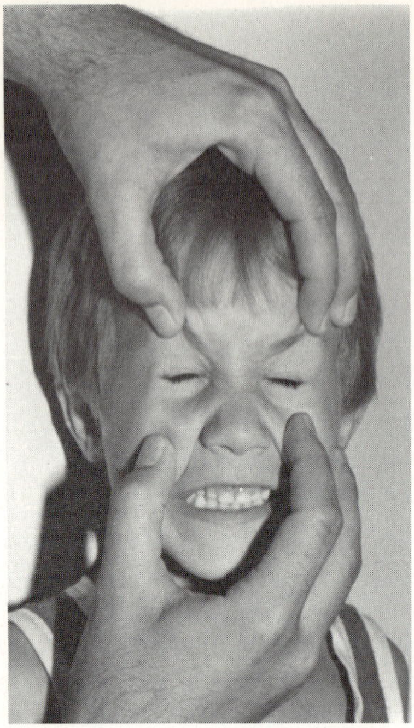

Fig. 1-10 Motor testing. Facial nerve.

Facial nerve (VII)

The facial nerve has both motor and sensory fibers. The motor fibers originate in the pons and form several branches extending to the submaxillary and sublingual muscles of the scalp and face. The sensory receptors are located in the taste buds on the anterior two thirds of the tongue.

Testing procedures

Motor component. Assessment of the motor component of the facial nerve is the same for all age groups; however, strength is usually not tested in the infant.

1. Have the patient smile, raise the eyebrows, frown, wrinkle the forehead, and puff out the cheeks. Observe the facial expressions.
2. Have the patient try to keep his eyes closed while you try to open them (Fig. 1-10).

During the motor assessments, observe for any sign of asymmetry. This may be indicative of facial nerve paralysis. Bell's palsy is a neuropathy of the facial nerve that is usually unilateral; it causes paralysis of the muscles on one side of the face.

Sensory component. Assessment of the sensory component of the facial nerve is usually not tested in the infant and in early childhood. The following guidelines should be used for older children and adults:

1. Have the patient protrude the tongue.
2. With a cotton swab, place a little saltwater on a small portion of the anterior two thirds of the tongue. The tongue should remain protruded as the patient identifies the substance.
3. Have the patient rinse the mouth out with water.
4. Repeat the procedure using different tasting substances such as sweet (sugar solution) and sour (lemon juice). The older adult may require concentrations of substances one to three times stronger than for children or younger adults because of weakened sensory perception.

Ageusia is the absence or partial loss of the sense of taste, which may be caused by lesions of the facial nerve tract. The loss of taste may be unilateral or bilateral. The individual who has ageusia needs more detailed testing to determine the location of the lesion.

Acoustic (vestibulocochlear) nerve (VIII)

The acoustic nerve has two parts or divisions. These are the cochlear and the vestibular nerves, both of which are sensory in nature. The cochlear nerve is responsible for hearing, while the vestibular nerve is responsible for the sense of balance. The sensory receptors of the cochlear nerve are located in the organ of Corti in the cochlea and they send impulses to the temporal lobe of the cerebrum. The sensory receptors of the vestibular nerve are located in the semicircular canals and they send impulses to the cerebellum.

Testing procedures. The following procedures are only used to determine if the patient may have a hearing loss. They do not distinguish between sensorineural and conductive losses, unless that is as indicated.

Cochlear nerve. The following observations should be made in assessing the intactness of the cochlear nerve during infancy and early childhood. The infant will respond to a loud noise such as a clap of the hands by crying, blinking the eyes, abducting the arms, and flexing the elbows. This is the startle reflex that will disappear at about 4 months of age. Its absence is indicative of a hearing loss. At 4 to 24 months of age the infant will turn the head toward a sound and progressively become more aware of the exact source of the noise. In early childhood the child should respond to commands and be able to vary voice tones, name objects, and identify objects on command.

For all other age groups the following test procedures and guidelines should be used.

VOICE TEST

1. Have the patient occlude one ear with the index finger.
2. Stand 1 to 2 feet away from patient's unoccluded ear in a position where the patient cannot read your lips.
3. Softly whisper numbers and have the patient repeat them. If necessary, speak at different intensities (loud, medium) and have the patient repeat your message after each change of tone.

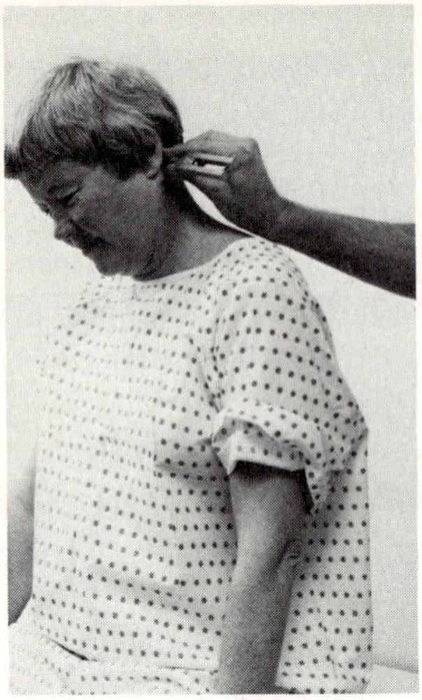

Fig. 1-11 Rinne test. Acoustic nerve.

WATCH TICK

1. Place a ticking watch next to the patient's ear.
2. Move the watch away from the ear until the patient no longer hears it.
3. Move the watch back into the range of hearing. Determine the point where the patient can just barely hear the tick.
4. Test the other ear.
5. Compare with yourself or another person.

RINNE TEST (AIR AND BONE CONDUCTION)

1. Place a vibrating tuning fork on the patient's mastoid process (Fig. 1-11).
2. When the patient can no longer hear the tuning fork, place it immediately next to the ear. The sound should again be heard. (The sound should be heard twice as long by air conduction as by bone conduction.) If no sound is heard by air conduction, then the deafness or hearing loss is the result of a conductive problem.

WEBER TEST (LATERALIZATION)

1. Place a vibrating tuning fork on the vertex of the skull.
2. Ask the patient whether the sound is equal in both ears or whether it is louder in one ear. If there is a conductive hearing loss, the sound will be referred to the deafer ear. If there is a sensorineural hearing loss, the sound will be louder in the better ear.

Hearing losses may be conductive or sensorineural or mixed. Conductive hearing losses result from disorders of the outer and middle ear. Potential causes are excessive cerumen, tympanic membrane perforation, pus in the middle-ear, otosclerosis and chronic ear infections. Sensorineural hearing losses are caused by disorders of the inner ear, the acoustic nerve, or the brain.

Hearing loss is very common in the older adult. Two common causes of hearing loss are otosclerosis and presbycusis. In otosclerosis there is an abnormal growth of bone tissue around the footplate of the stapes of the middle ear, which causes fixation of the footplates. This usually occurs unequally but bilaterally. In presbycusis there is degeneration and atrophy of the cochlear or acoustic nerve of the inner ear, resulting in a hearing loss that is greater at high frequencies.

Vestibular nerve. The vestibular nerve is tested by observing the patient for any loss of equilibrium or the presence of vertigo. Meniere's disease is one disorder that affects the vestibular nerve. It is a result of increased fluid pressure within the vestibular labyrinth in the inner ear. Further testing of the cochlear and vestibular nerves will have to be done by the physician. These include the audiometric, caloric, and electronystagmographic procedures.

Glossopharyngeal nerve (IX)

The glossopharyngeal nerve has both motor and sensory fibers. The motor fibers originate in the medulla and extend to the pharynx and parotid gland. The sensory receptors are located in the posterior one third of the tongue and in the soft palate, pharynx, tonsils, larynx, and carotid sinus. The glossopharnygeal nerve is tested together with the vagus nerve because they innervate many of the same areas.

Vagus nerve (X)

The vagus nerve has both motor and sensory fibers. The motor fibers originate in the medulla and extend to the pharynx and larynx muscles and also to the thoracic and abdominal viscera. The sensory receptors are located in the respiratory tract (including the pharynx, larynx, and trachea), and also in the digestive tract.

Testing procedures. The glossopharyngeal and vagus nerves are tested together because many structures are innervated by both nerves and it is difficult to distinguish between the two.

Motor components. During infancy the following observations are made concerning the proper functioning of the motor components of the glossopharyngeal and vagus nerves.

1. Gag reflex: Stimulation of the pharynx causes the infant to gag. This reflex is present throughout life.
2. Sucking reflex: Stimulation of circumoral area creates sucking movements (Fig. 1-12). This reflex is also seen during sleep.
3. Cries, differentiation of type:
   a. High-pitched or shrill: indicative of increased intracranial pressure.
   b. Hoarse: may be caused by vocal cord paralysis as a result of a vagus nerve lesion or hypocalcemic tetany.
   c. Absent cry: may be the result of severe illness, mental retardation, or cretinism.
4. Yawn reflex: This is an involuntary response to oxygen deficiency. The reflex lasts throughout life.

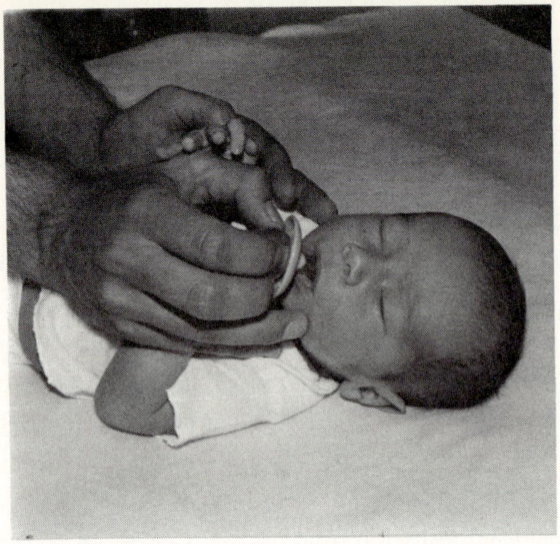

Fig. 1-12 Test of sucking reflex: infant. Glossopharyngeal and vagus nerves.

5. Cough reflex: Response to a respiratory tract irritation. This reflex lasts throughout life.

For all other age groups the following test procedures should be used.

1. Have the patient open the mouth and say "ah." Observe the symmetrical rise of the palate and uvula.
2. Touch the posterior aspect of the pharynx with an applicator. The gag reflex should be elicited.
3. Observe the patient swallowing a small amount of water. Dysphagia is difficulty in swallowing. This may result from a lesion of the glossopharyngeal and/or vagus nerves.
4. Listen to the patient's speech. Hoarseness may indicate a vagus nerve lesion.

Sensory component. Testing of the sensory components of the glossopharyngeal and vagus nerve is not done on infants. For all other age groups the procedure is as follows:

1. Stimulate the pharynx to elicit the gag reflex.
2. Test taste on the posterior third of the tongue. Repeat the procedure used for testing taste on the anterior two thirds of the tongue (see Facial nerve).

Cerebrovascular accidents are the most common cause of glossopharyngeal and vagus nerve malfunction. The swallowing and gag reflexes may be very weak or absent after cerebrovascular accidents.

Spinal accessory nerve (XI)

The spinal accessory nerve originates in the lower aspect of the medulla and also in the first five or six cervical segments of the spinal cord. It is a motor nerve innervating the sternocleidomastoid and trapezius muscles (Fig. 1-13).

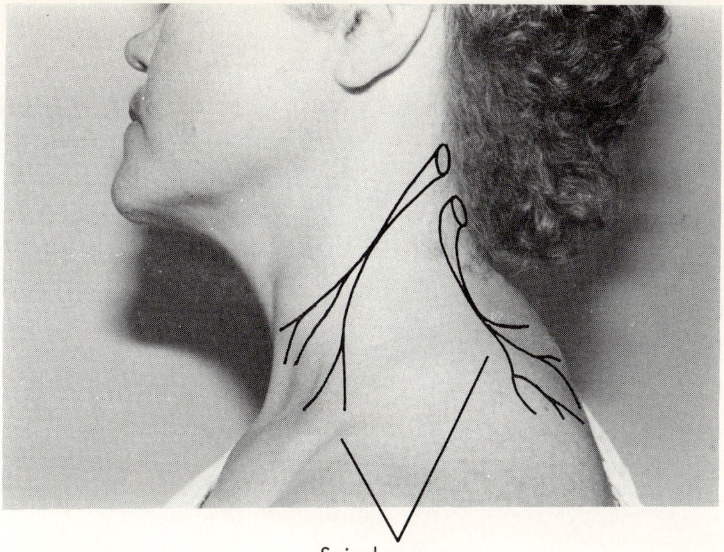

Fig. 1-13 Spinal accessory nerves. Innervation of sternocleidomastoid and trapezius muscles.

Testing procedures

Sternocleidomastoid muscle. The sternocleidomastoid muscle enables an individual to turn the head from side to side. This muscle is never tested in a trauma victim unless it is certain that the patient has no cervical injuries. Infants' head movements are observed in response to reflexes, such as the startle reflex, and for symmetry of movements. For all other age groups the following testing procedure is used:

1. Place your hand on the side of the patient's head.
2. Against your resistance, have the patient try to turn his head.
3. Repeat the procedure on the other side of the head. Observe the size, strength, and symmetry of each contralateral sternocleidomastoid muscle.

Trapezius muscle. The trapezius muscle enables an individual to shrug the shoulders. This muscle is not tested during infancy. For all other age groups the following test procedure is used:

1. Place your hands on the patient's shoulders.
2. Against your resistance, have the patient shrug the shoulders. Observe the size, strength, and symmetry of the trapezius muscles.

Cerebrovascular accidents and neck and head trauma are very common causes of spinal accessory nerve malfunction. The muscles innervated may be weak unilaterally or bilaterally or they may be atrophied or paralyzed.

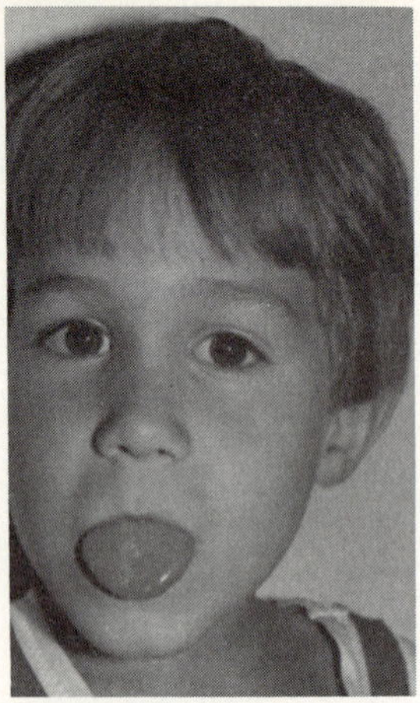

Fig. 1-14 Testing hypoglossal nerve.

Hypoglossal nerve (XII)

The hypoglossal nerve originates in the medulla. It is a motor nerve innervating the muscles of the tongue.

Testing procedures. To assess the hypoglossal nerve during infancy observe for extrusion of the tongue. An infant will stick out the tongue to force out an object when the tongue is touched. This response disappears by 4 months of age. If the tongue protrudes constantly, it is highly indicative of Down's syndrome. For all other age groups the following test procedures are used:

1. Have the patient protrude the tongue. It should fall in the midline. Observe the tongue for signs of atrophy, symmetry, abnormal movements such as fasciculations, and deviations (Fig. 1-14).
2. With the patient's tongue back in the mouth, place your hand on his cheek. Have the patient push against your hand with his tongue. Repeat the procedure on the other side. The tongue should be equally strong on both sides.

A partially paralyzed tongue will deviate toward the unaffected side. Lower motor neuron diseases will result in atrophy and fasciculations of the tongue.

CEREBELLAR FUNCTION

Neural impulses traveling to and from the cerebellum connect it with other structures of the central nervous system. These structures include the medulla, pons, thalamus, spinal cord, and the motor areas of the cerebral cortex. The cerebellum's influence on these structures allow movements to be smooth, steady, and coordinated. The cerebellum is also important in maintaining equilibrium and posture.

Testing procedures

In infancy and early childhood it is very difficult to assess cerebellar functions. The nurse may adopt some of the tests used for the other age groups and observe for

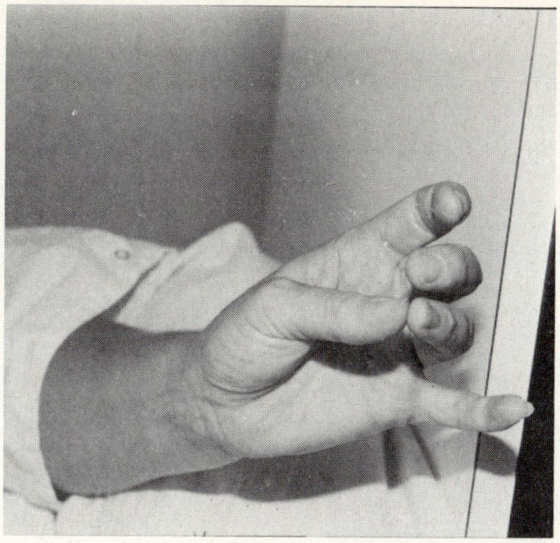

Fig. 1-15 Thumb-to-fingers test. Cerebellar function.

movements that are awkward and uncoordinated. For all other age groups the following testing procedures and guidelines are used:

Finger-to-nose test

1. Have the patient touch his nose with an index finger while his eyes are open.
2. Repeat the procedure with the other hand.
3. Repeat the procedure with the eyes closed.
4. With his eyes open, have the patient touch his nose with an index finger and then touch your finger as you move it around.
5. Have the patient increase the speed of his actions as you move your finger.

Thumb-to-fingers test

1. With his eyes open, have the patient touch his fingers to the thumb of the same hand (Fig. 1-15).
2. Repeat the procedure with the other hand.

Supination and pronation of hands

1. With his eyes open, have the patient rapidly pat his leg, alternating supination and pronation of his hands.

Heel-down-shin test

1. With the patient sitting, have him run his heel down the opposite leg's shin (Fig. 1-16).
2. Repeat the procedure with the other heel.

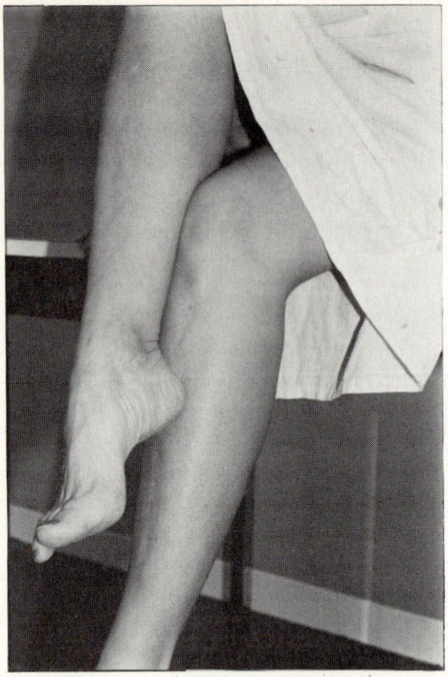

Fig. 1-16 Heel-down-shin test. Cerebellar function.

Romberg test

1. Have the patient stand erect with feet together for 30 seconds with his eyes open.
2. Have the patient remain standing and close his eyes for 30 seconds. A small amount of swaying is normal. An excessive amount of swaying or falling to one side is abnormal. (Be prepared to protect the patient from falling.)

Walking

1. Observe the patient's walk. Each arm should swing with the opposite leg.
2. Have the patient walk heel-to-toe in a straight line.

Abnormal findings

The following are abnormal findings that the nurse may see when there is a dysfunction of the cerebellum.

Intention tremor: there are rhythmic, involuntary movements of voluntary muscles that increase when doing voluntary activities.

Vertigo: the patient has feelings of dizziness. There is a sensation of rotation or of movement of the patient's self (subjective) or of his surroundings (objective).

Cerebellar ataxia: the patient may have a positive Romberg test with eyes open and closed. The legs have to be wide apart in order for the patient to stand, and the gait is unsteady.

Cerebellar nystagmus: there are abnormal rhythmic movements of the eye. These may be in any plane (vertical, horizontal, or rotary)

Adiadochokinesia: the patient is unable to perform fine, rapidly repeated, coordinated movements, such as rapid supination and pronation of the hands.

Dysarthria: the patient has slurred or broken speech. This occurs because speech requires fine muscle coordination.

SENSORY SYSTEM

Sensory receptors are nerve endings located throughout the body (skin, muscles) that respond to various forms of stimuli such as touch, temperature, and pain. The impulses received from the receptors then travel via peripheral nerves to specific spinal cord segments. The cutaneous areas of the body in which the receptors are located are called dermatomes. Each dermatome corresponds to the specific spinal cord segment that its peripheral nerve enters.

Once the impulses enter the spinal cord, they travel to the brain via special tracts. Two of these important tracts are the lateral spinothalamic and the medial lemniscal. Although there are other tracts, for our purposes we shall deal only with these two. Both of these tracts are crossed (as are the other tracts of the spinal cord). This means that each side of the brain registers sensations from the opposite side of the body. The lateral spinothalamic tract cross in the spinal cord to the opposite side immediately when the tract fibers enter the cord from an extremity. The medial lemniscal tract crosses in the spinal cord when the tract fibers reach the medulla. From the medulla both tracts travel to the thalamus and then to the cerebral cortex (Fig. 1-17).

Functions of the lateral spinothalamic tract are to relay simple touch, pain, and temperature sensations to the cerebral cortex. The medial lemniscal tracts function in the discriminating touch and pressure sensations, including stereognosis (which is the awareness of an object's size, shape, end texture), two-point discrimination, and the sense of vibrations. These tracts also function in kinesthesia (which is the knowledge of the movement and position of body parts) and in the extinction phenomenon affecting sensations to the cerebral cortex.

Testing procedures

During infancy and early childhood the peripheral sensory system is difficult to assess because perceptions of touch, pain, and temperature are not as strong as in the adult. Also, the infants cannot describe the special sense. The following testing procedures are used for infants and young children:

1. Gently rub an extremity. This should evoke a withdrawal from the stimulus. The facial expression may also change.
2. Pin prick: Slightly depress the skin area several times with a pin. The infant should change his facial expression, withdraw from the pin, and possibly cry.
   a. If there is no removal of the extremity but the infant cries or changes facial expression, the nurse should suspect a motor dysfunction.
   b. If there is removal of the extremity but no cry or changes in facial expression, the nurse should suspect a sensory dysfunction.
3. Rooting reflex: Lightly rub the side of the infant's mouth. The mouth will open and the infant will turn the head in that direction (Fig. 1-18). This reflex disappears at 3 to 4 months of age. Absence is indicative of central nervous system disease.

For all other age groups the following general guidelines and testing procedures are

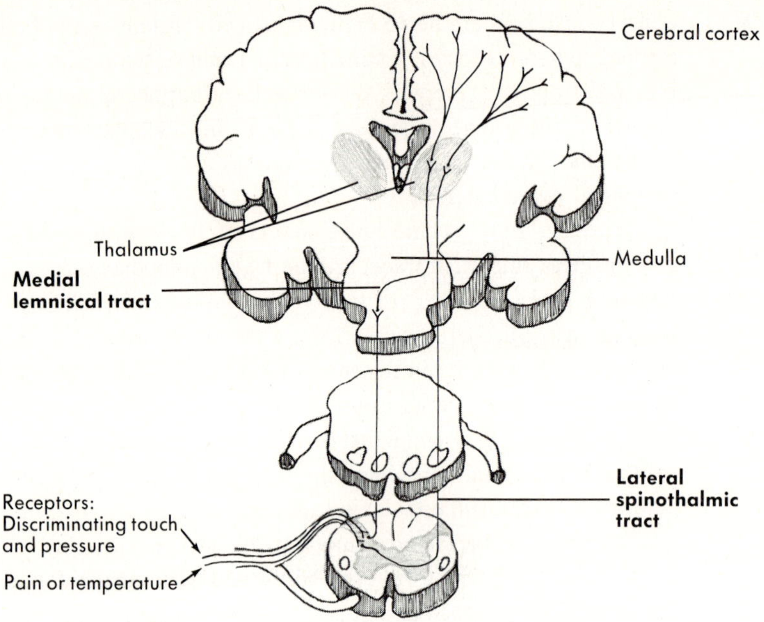

Fig. 1-17 Lateral spinothalamic and medial lemniscal neural tracts.

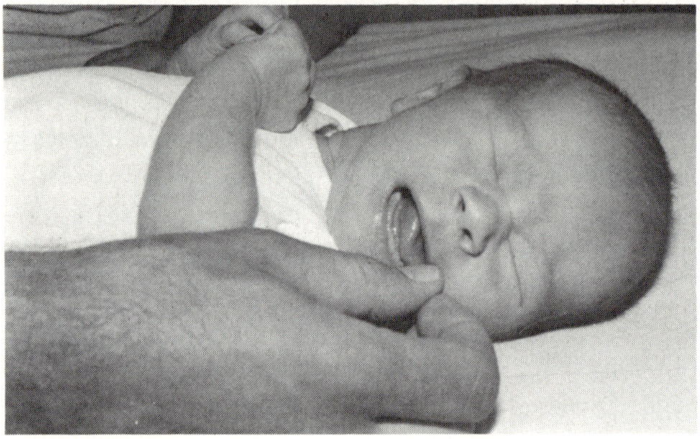

Fig. 1-18 Testing rooting reflex: infant.

used. Note that in the older adult tactile sense may be decreased because of decreased vascularity of the spinal cord, changes in nerve fibers, and an increase in synapse delay. This is normal and necessitates the use of stronger clues.

General guidelines for all sensory testing procedures

1. The patient's eyes are closed in all sensory tests.
2. The patient's cooperation is very important. The patient must understand that you are testing sensations felt on different parts of the body and you will not hurt him.
3. Adapt instructions to the patient's level of consciousness.
4. Compare both sides of the trunk.
5. Compare areas of corresponding extremities.
6. Compare the distal and proximal portions of each extremity.
7. Map out areas of sensory changes.

Simple touch

1. With a wisp of cotton, touch and compare the different areas of the patient's body.
2. Have the patient tell you when he feels the sensation and his interpretation of the stimulus.

Pain

1. Using a pin depress the skin slightly without hurting the patient. Randomize your movements using the sharp and dull ends and compare the different areas of the patient's body (Fig. 1-19).
2. Have the patient tell you whether the sharp or dull end of the pin is felt.

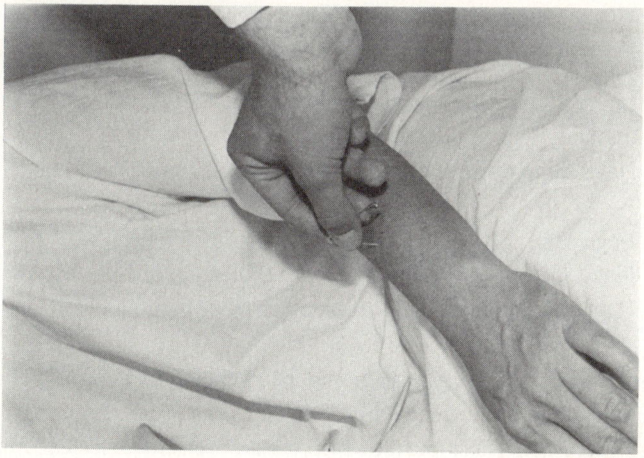

Fig. 1-19 Testing pain perception: adult.

Temperature

1. Using the same procedure as with testing pain, touch the various parts of the body with test tubes of hot and cold water.
2. Temperature is usually not tested if pain perception is normal.

Vibration sense

1. Hold a vibrating tuning fork on the bony prominences (such as the knee and elbow)
2. Have the patient tell you when the vibrations start and stop. Compare corresponding extremities and also their distal and proximal portions.

Kinesthetic sense

1. Grasp the sides of the patient's fingers between your index finger and thumb.
2. Passively move each separate finger (upward or downward). Do not apply excessive pressure on the skin as this may be a clue to the patient.
3. Have the patient tell you the direction of each movement.
4. Repeat this procedure with the other digits.

Two-point discrimination

1. Simultaneously touch two pins to the body surface.
2. Have the patient tell you whether he is being touched by one or two points. The following have been determined to be the average distances at which normal individuals can distinguish one from two points on various skin areas.

Fingertips	2 to 3 mm
Toe tips	3 to 8 mm
Palms	8 to 12 mm
Chest and forearms	40 mm
Back	40 to 70 mm
Upper arms and thighs	75 mm

Extinction phenomenon

1. Lightly touch the patient simultaneously on two points that are on opposite sides of the body and in corresponding areas.
2. Have the patient tell you whether he was touched on one side or both sides.

Stereognosis

1. Place a familiar object, such as a coin or comb, in the patient's hand.
2. Have the patient identify the object. Test both hands.

Abnormal findings

The peripheral sensory system may be assaulted by a variety of neurological disorders including tumors, degeneration, inflammations, and trauma. Where the sensory system is affected will determine the distribution of sensory loss. The following are examples:

1. A sensory cortex tumor usually results in the loss of discriminating touch and pressure sensations (stereognosis, two-point discrimination, sense of vibrations) and of kinesthesia and extinction on the side of the body opposite the tumor.

2. A posterior spinal cord tumor results in the loss of discriminating touch and pressure sensations on the same side of the body in the area below the level of the tumor.
3. A central spinal cord tumor results in the loss of pain and temperature sensations in one or more dermatomes below the level of the tumor.
4. Transection of one half of the spinal cord results in the loss of discriminating touch and pressure sensations on the same side of the body and loss of pain and temperature sensations on the side opposite the transection (Brown-Séquard syndrome).
5. Complete transection of the spinal cord results the loss of all sensations below the transection.
6. Peripheral nerve injury results in the loss of all sensations distal to the injury.

MOTOR SYSTEM

The motor system is composed of neurons that carry impulses from the cerebrum to the skeletal muscles. There are two motor tracts, the pyramidal and extrapyramidal.

The pyramidal (corticospinal) tracts are motor neuron fibers that come together in the medulla. In the medulla approximately three fourths of these fibers cross over from one side to the other, thereby enabling the left side of the cerebrum to control the right side of the body and vice versa. The other one fourth do not cross over. Both sets of fibers then extend down the spinal cord and synapse with the anterior horn motor neurons. The impulses traveling down these fibers result in the stimulation of individual muscles.

The extrapyramidal (reticulospinal) tracts are the motor neuron fibers that have not formed together to create the pyramidal tracts. These fibers also extend down the spinal cord and synapse with interneurons, which in turn synapse with anterior horn motor neurons. The impulses traveling down these fibers result in the stimulation of groups of muscles, bringing about larger, more automatic movements than movements resulting from pyramidal tract stimulation.

The portions of the pyramidal and extrapyramidal tracts from the cerebrum up to but not including the anterior horn motor neurons are called the upper motor neuron tracts. The portions from the anterior horn motor neurons to the skeletal muscles are considered lower motor neuron tracts.

Testing procedures

In the infant the following testing procedures are used when assessing the motor system.

Muscle tone

1. Put each joint through its range of motion. Observe for signs of spasticity, flaccidity, or paralysis.

Palmar grasp reflex

1. Place one of your fingers in the infant's palm. The infant should involuntarily grasp the finger tightly (Fig. 1-20).

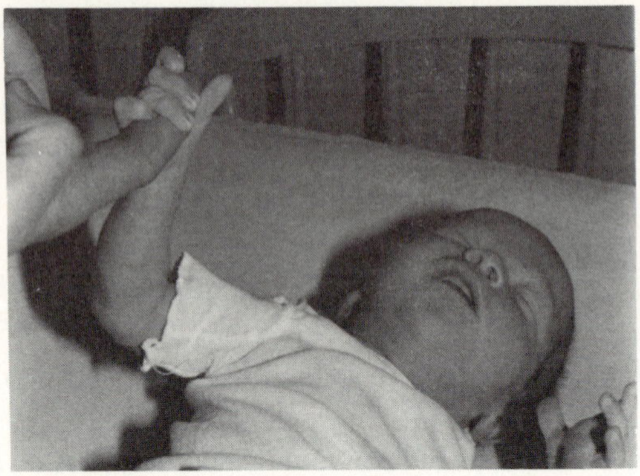

Fig. 1-20 Testing palmar grasp reflex: infant.

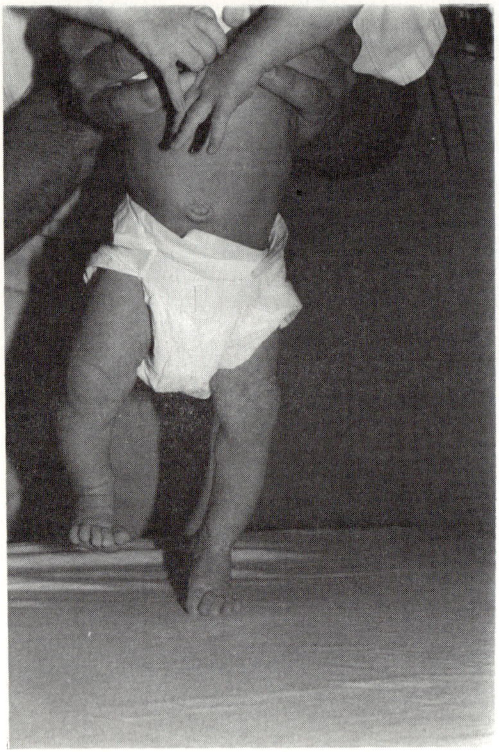

Fig. 1-21 Testing stepping response: infant.

2. Compare the hands. Asymmetry may be indicative of paralysis.
3. This reflex disappears at 3 to 4 months of age. If it is persistent, the nurse can suspect cerebral dysfunction.

Moro reflex

1. Place the infant supine on an examining table.
2. Make a loud noise such as by striking the table or clapping the hands. The infant should rapidly abduct and extend all extremities and then bring them back close to the trunk. Asymmetry may be indicative of paralysis or possible bone fractures.
3. The Moro reflex disappears after 6 months of age. If it is persistent, it may indicate cerebral damage.

Perez reflex

1. Hold the infant prone in the palm of your hand.
2. Move the thumb of your other hand firmly along the infant's spine starting at the sacrum and proceeding up to the neck. Observe for elevation of the buttocks and head and for flexion of the arms and legs. The infant will cry and urinate. Asymmetry or absence may be indicative of paralysis or bone fractures.
3. The Perez reflex disappears after 3 to 4 months of age. If it is persistent, it may indicate cerebral damage.

Tonic neck reflex

1. Place the infant supine on an examining table.
2. Turn the head to one side. The arm and leg on that side should extend, while the other arm and leg should flex.
3. Test the other side.
4. The tonic neck reflex disappears after 3 to 4 months of age. If it is persistent, it is highly indicative of cerebral damage.

Trunk incurvature (Galant) reflex

1. Hold the infant prone in the palm of your hand.
2. Rub the lateral side of the infant's trunk with your thumb. The buttocks and shoulders should move toward the stimulated side. Absence is indicative of a spinal cord lesion.
3. Test the other side of the trunk.
4. Trunk incurvature disappears at 1 to 2 months of age.

Stepping response

1. Hold the infant vertically in both hands so that the bottom of one foot touches a hard surface. The leg should flex and then extend. If the infant's feet alternate in touching the surface, a simulated walking movement is elicited (Fig. 1-21).
2. The stepping response disappears after 1 month of age.

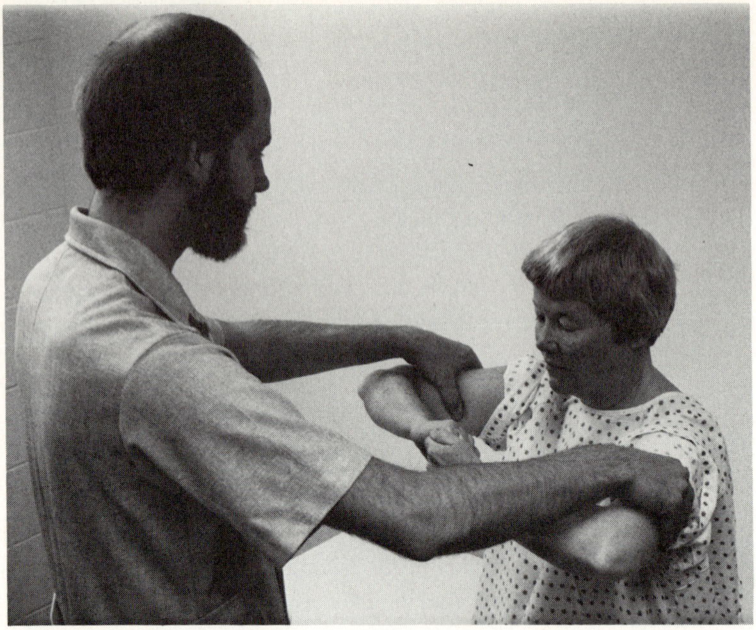

Fig. 1-22 Testing muscle strength.

Muscle size

1. With a tape measure compare the size of corresponding body parts.
2. Inspect for atrophy and asymmetry.

Muscle tone

1. Palpate the muscles at rest and their resistance to passive movements.
2. Inspect for rigidity or flaccidity and spasms.

Muscle strength

1. Examine flexion and extension of the major joints without resistance.
2. Examine with resistance (Fig. 1-22).
3. Compare the corresponding muscles. They should be equally strong.

Abnormal findings When there is an injury to the motor system, the specific signs and symptoms found depend upon whether the dysfunction is an upper or lower motor neuron tract disturbance.

Upper motor neuron symptoms	Lower motor neuron symptoms
Hyperreflexia below level of the disturbance	Reflexes absent below level of the disturbance
Pathological reflexes represent	No pathological reflexes present
Hypertonicity of a large group of muscles	Hypotonicity confined to a specific group of muscles
No fasciculations	Fasciculations present
Mild muscle wasting (atrophy)	Severe muscle wasting (atrophy)

Abnormal involuntary muscle movements that the nurse may encounter when there is damage to the motor system include the following:

Fasciculations: fine, spontaneous contractions of resting muscles, which are often present with muscle atrophy. They are a sign of lower motor neuron disease.

Resting tremors: nonpurposeful, involuntary, rhythmical contractions of a limb at rest. These occur as a slow and regular movement in parkinsonism.

Chorea: rapid, involuntary, jerky, irregular contractions of the trunk, limbs, or face. These are a sign of upper motor neuron disease. They may be seen in Huntington's chorea.

Athetosis: contractions similar to chorea contractions but slower and having writhing and twisting action. Athetosis is a sign of upper motor neuron disease resulting from basal ganglia dysfunction. Athetosis occurs frequently in cerebral palsy.

Hemiballismus: violent motor movements of large muscle groups. The movements are confined to one half of the body and may occur in upper motor neuron disease.

Myoclonus: involuntary, nonpurposeful, unpredictable, quick, and forceful jerking contractions of large groups of muscles. Myoclonus occurs as a normal part of falling asleep and is also involved in myoclonic epilepsy. It may be a sign of either upper or lower motor neuron diseases.

Observe for the following abnormal gaits and postures that reflect upper or lower motor neuron disease.

Spastic hemiparesis: arm of affected side is flexed and immobile. Affected leg is stiff and is moved forward in a semicircular motion with the ball of the foot dragging. This can be caused by a unilateral upper motor neuron disease, such as a stroke.

Scissor gait: slow, short steps with leg movements that tend to cross at the knees. This is caused by paresis that has affected the legs bilaterally. It is indicative of upper motor neuron disease and is seen in multiple sclerosis and cerebral palsy.

Steppage gait: patient appears to be walking up a flight of stairs. With each step the knee is flexed and the foot is lifted high and is then brought down to the floor with a slap. It is the gait of footdrop and is indicative of lower motor neuron disease.

Sensory ataxia: patient has a decreased sense of position in the legs. The legs are not steady and the patient walks with the feet far apart. With each step the foot is lifted high and is then brought down to the floor with a slap. The Romberg test may be positive with the eyes open.

Parkinsonian gait: short, shuffling steps with a rigid posture and flexion of the elbows, neck, hips, and knees. This is the result of a basal ganglia disorder.

Decorticate posturing: flexion of fingers, wrists, and arms with adduction of the arms. Legs are rigidly extended and internally rotated. Feet are plantar flexed. The patient may have unilateral or bilateral involvement. This is indicative of a lesion in the area of the pons.

Decerebrate posturing: arms are extended and hyperpronated. Legs are rigidly extended and the feet are plantar flexed. The jaw is clenched tightly shut. This may be indicative of a lesion in the midbrain or in the upper brainstem.

Upper motor neuron tract disorders include infections, demyelinating diseases (multiple sclerosis, amyotrophic lateral sclerosis), trauma, neoplasms, and vascular diseases (cerebrovascular accidents). Lower motor neuron tract disorders include peripheral nerve damage (trauma), poliomyelitis, and neoplasms.

REFLEXES

When assessing any reflex, one is eliciting an involuntary response to a stimulus. A reflex involves both a sensory and motor component. Three types of reflexes may be tested: (1) deep tendon, (2) superficial, and (3) pathological.

A deep tendon reflex (DTR) is elicited when a brisk tap from a reflex hammer is applied to a tendon. The tap stretches both the tendon and its muscles, which stimulates the spindles (stretch-sensitive receptors located within each skeletal muscle) to send a signal. This signal travels via a sensory tract to the posterior horn of the spinal cord, where there is a synapse with an interneuron, which crosses the signal over to the anterior horn of the spinal cord, where there is a synapse with a motor tract, which then sends the signal back to the muscle. The muscle then contracts, finishing the reflex arc (Fig. 1-23). In essence, reflex arcs are functional within themselves and are independent of the upper motor neuron tracts. However, they are components of the whole motor system and as such are affected by the upper motor neuron tracts (pyramidal, extrapyramidal) as well as by the cerebellar system.

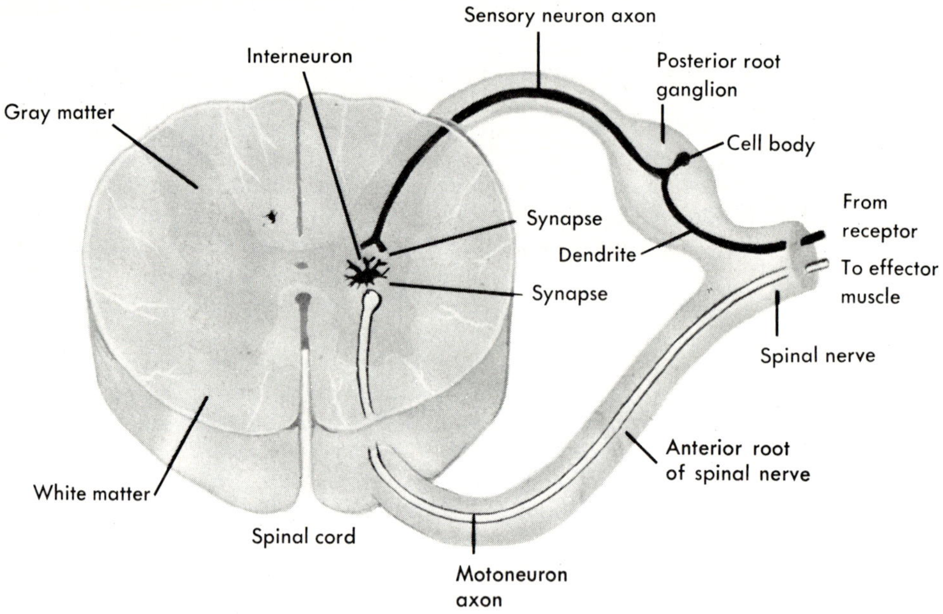

Fig. 1-23 Ipsilateral reflex arc. (From Anthony, C.P., and Kolthoff, N.J.: Textbook of anatomy and physiology, ed. 9, St. Louis, 1979, The C.V. Mosby Co.)

Grading the strength of each reflex is done on a 0 to 4+ scale. Extremities are compared.

4+	Hyperactive
3+	Stronger than normal
2+	Normal
1+	Weaker than normal
0	No response

Reinforcement is used when the reflexes are symmetrically weak or absent. This involves using isometric contractions of muscle groups other than those being tested to improve reflex activity in the tested muscles. For example, have the patient make a fist with his right hand or clench his teeth to increase reflex activity in his left hand. If reinforcement is used, this needs to be documented.

Possible causes of hyperreflexia include: (1) upper motor neuron tract disorders (see Motor system) and (2) strychnine poisoning, tetanus, and hypocalcemia.

Possible causes of hyporeflexia include (1) lower motor neuron tract disorders (see Motor system) and (2) conditions such as neurosyphilis, hypothyroidism, lead poisoning, coma, increased intracranial pressure, deep sedation, anesthesia, diabetes, and hypokalemia.

Testing procedures

These general principles should be remembered when doing a reflex test:

1. The area being tested must be totally relaxed.
2. The muscle being tested should be slightly stretched.
3. Use a sudden, brisk tap of the reflex hammer.
4. Use the same intensity of tap on corresponding sides.

Deep tendon reflexes. Table 1-6 describes the deep tendon reflexes, testing procedures, normal responses, and the involved spinal cord segments for all groups. However, note that the motor neuron tracts of the infant are not fully mature. Therefore results of reflex testing will be variable. Also, although the testing procedures are the same for the infant as they are for the other age groups, the triceps and Achilles reflexes require special comments regarding their use with infants:

1. Triceps: This reflex is not present until 6 months of age.
2. Achilles: Commonly there are multiple rapid and rhythmic plantar flexions. If the flexions are continuous, it may be indicative of central nervous system disease.

It is also impotant to note that in the older adult the nurse will find a reduced amplitude and speed of reaction to the stimulus, particularily in distal areas. This may be the result of aging changes in the extrapyramidal system, vertebral column, and intervertebral discs and of fibrotic changes in tendons and muscles.

Superficial reflexes. A superficial reflex occurs when there is stimulation of the sensory receptors in the skin resulting in a reflex arc. There is also some involvement of higher

Table 1-6 **Deep tendon reflexes**

Reflex	Procedure	Normal response	Involved segments of spinal cord
Biceps	1. Hold patient's arm in your own. 2. Slightly flex patient's arm at the elbow. 3. Place your thumb firmly on the biceps tendon. 4. Briskly tap your thumb with reflex hammer (Fig. 1-24).	Flexion of elbow; biceps contraction should be felt	C5, C6
Triceps	1. Flex patient's arm at elbow with forearm held across abdomen. 2. Briskly tap triceps tendon 2 inches above the elbow.	Extension of arm at elbow	C6, C7, C8
Brachioradialis	1. Hold patient's hand below the wrist. 2. Semipronate the hand. 3. Briskly tap the radius of the tendon 1 to 2 inches above wrist.	Flexion and supination of forearm	C5, C6
Patellar	1. Have patient sit with legs hanging freely over edge of bed or table. 2. Briskly tap patellar tendon just below the patella.	Extension of lower leg at knee	L2, L3, L4
Achilles	1. Flex patient's leg at the knee. 2. Support the foot and dorsiflex the ankle. 3. Briskly tap the Achilles tendon (Fig. 1-25).	Plantar flexion of foot; note speed of relaxation	S1, S2

neural tracts. The superficial reflexes in an infant are tested as they are in the adult (Table 1-7). However, the abdominal and cremasteric reflexes do not appear until 6 months of age. The plantar reflex does not appear until 12 to 18 months of age. Before this time, the infant will have a positive Babinski sign. In the older adult there is an increased difficulty in eliciting the abdominal reflexes. This is a result of the increased frequency with which the musculature has been overstretched, usually because of adiposity or childbearing.

Pathological reflexes. A pathological reflex is an abnormal response to sensory stimulation as a result of upper motor neuron disease (Table 1-8).

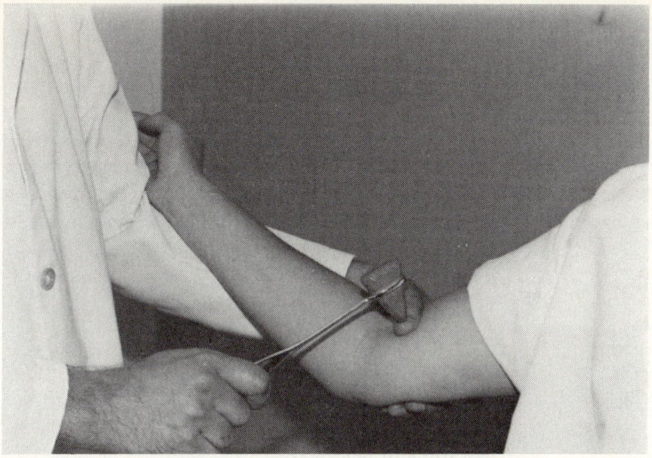

Fig. 1-24 Testing biceps reflex.

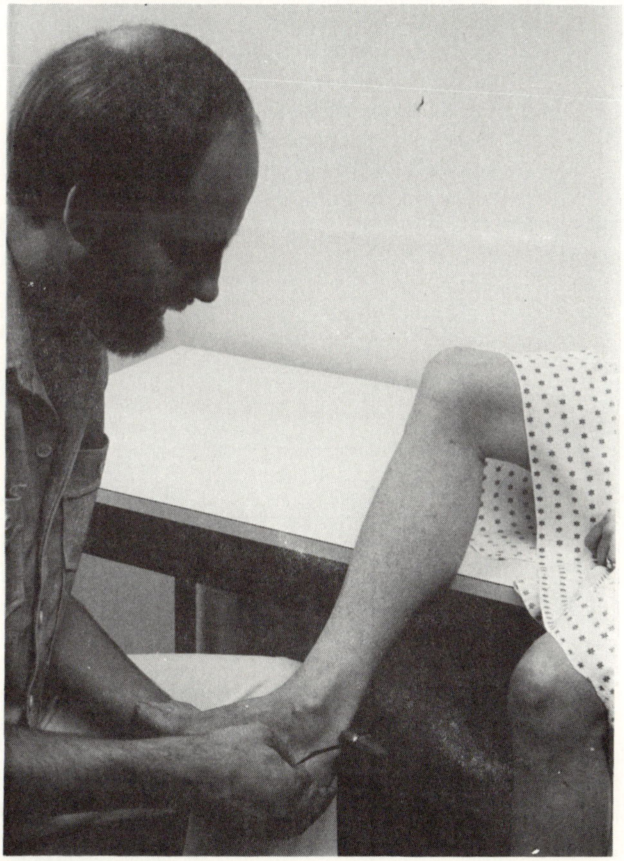

Fig. 1-25 Testing Achilles tendon reflex.

Table 1-7 **Superficial reflexes**

Reflex	Procedure	Normal response	Involved segments of spinal cord
Upper abdominal	1. Have the patient lying supine. 2. Stroke right upper quadrant of abdomen with an applicator stick 3. Stroke left upper quadrant with an applicator stick.	Movement of umbilicus toward side being tested	T8, T9, T10
Lower abdominal	1. Have the patient lying supine. 2. Stroke right lower quadrant of abdomen with an applicator stick. 3. Stroke left lower quadrant with an applicator stick.	Movement of umbilicus toward side being tested	T10, T11, T12
Cremasteric	1. Have the male patient lying supine. 2. Stroke inner aspect of the upper thigh. 3. Stroke inner aspect of the other thigh.	Testicle elevation on side tested	L1, L2
Plantar	1. Lightly stroke the lateral aspect of the sole, starting at the heel upward to the ball of the foot and across the ball (Fig. 1-26).	Flexion of toes	S1, S2

Table 1-8 **Pathological reflexes**

Reflex	Procedure	Response	Upper motor neuron disease
Babinski	Same as plantar reflex. If too much pressure is applied, one may cause a withdrawal response that may be mistaken to be a positive Babinski sign. Observe the response carefully. Babinski sign is positive in the normal infant up to approximately 12 months of age (Fig. 1-27).	Dorsiflexion and fanning out of toes	Pyramidal tract
Gordon	Firmly squeeze the calf muscles.	Same response	Same
Chaddock	Stroke lateral aspect of foot.	Same response	Same

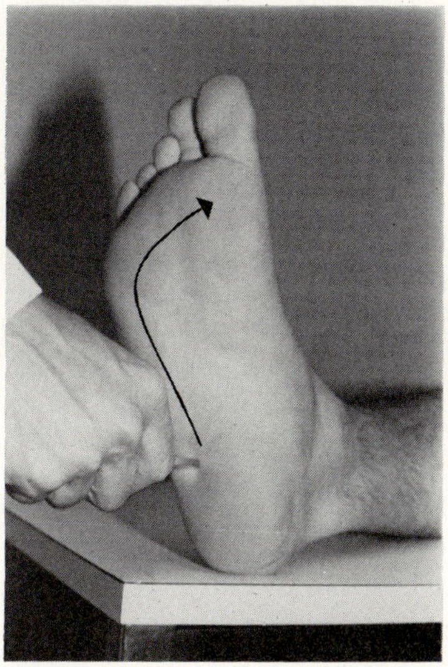

Fig. 1-26 Testing plantar reflex.

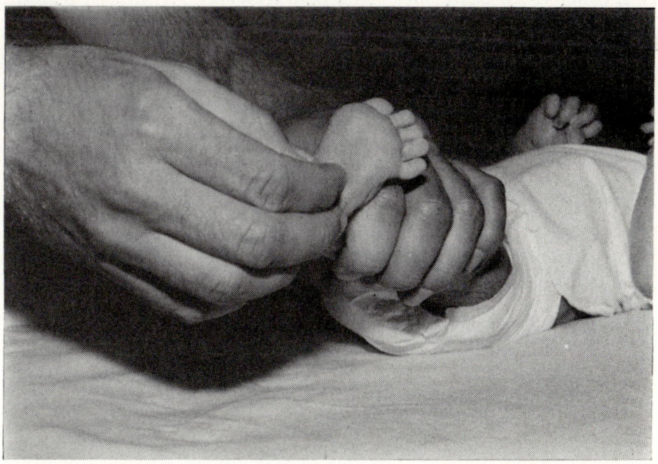

Fig. 1-27 Babinski reflex.

MENINGEAL SIGNS

Meningeal signs are elicited when there is an inflammatory process involving the meninges, which are the membranes covering the brain and spinal cord. Common causes of this inflammatory process are infectious diseases and intracranial hemorrhages.

Observe the infant for the following signs:

1. Nuchal rigidity (a very stiff neck)
2. Severe retraction of the head
3. Arm and leg extension
4. A high-pitched, shrill cry

For all other age groups assess for the following signs:

1. Nuchal rigidity (a very stiff neck)
2. Kernig's sign
   a. Have the patient lie supine.
   b. Flex one leg at the hip.
   c. Straighten the leg. A positive Kernig sign is when the patient cannot completely extend the leg. The patient may also have pain or resistance during the procedure.
3. Brudzinski's sign
   a. Have the patient lie supine.
   b. Raise the patient's head to flex the neck with your hand. Note resistance. The patient may complain of pain. Observe for flexion of the knees and hips while flexing the head. A positive Brudzinski sign involves neck flexion resistance and possibly pain and flexion of knees and hips.

VITAL SIGNS

The vital signs are a very important component of a neurological assessment. A slowly falling pulse and respiratory rate with an associated rise in blood pressure may be indicative of increasing intracranial pressure. The patient's temperature may fluctuate very rapidly from being hyperthermic to hypothermic. The frequency of recording the vital signs may need to be every 4 hours to every 15 minutes. Refer to individual disorders for a description of the specific changes that may occur in vital signs.

Suggested readings

Alexander, M., and Brown, M.N.: Pediatric history taking and physical diagnosis for nurses, New York, 1979, McGraw-Hill Book Co.

Anthony, C.P., and Thibodeau, G.A.: Textbook of anatomy and physiology, ed. 10, St. Louis, 1979, The C.V. Mosby Co.

Bates, G.: A guide to physical examination, ed. 2, Philadelphia, 1979, J.B. Lippincott Co.

Block, G.J., Nolan, J.W., and Dempsey, M.K.: Health assessment for professional nursing: a developmental approach, New York, 1981, Appleton-Century-Crofts.

Carotenuto, R., and Bullock, J.: Physical assessment of the gerontologic client, Philadelphia, 1981, F.A. Davis Co.

Chaplin, J.P., and Demers, A.: Primer of neurology and neurophysicology, New York, 1978, John Wiley and Sons, Inc.

DeJong, R.N., and others: Essentials of the neurological examination, ed. 6, Philadelphia, 1979, Smith-Kline Corp.

Hillman, R.S., and others: Clinical skills: interviewing, history taking and diagnosis for nurses, New York, 1979, McGraw-Hill Book Co.

Kart, C.S., and others: Aging and health: biologic and social perspectives, Menlo Park, Calif., 1978, Addison-Wesley Publishing Co.

Malasanos, L., and others: Health assessment, ed. 2, St. Louis, 1981, The C.V. Mosby Co.

Rudy, E.B., and Gray, V.R.: Handbook of health assessment, Bowie, Md., 1981, Robert J. Brady Co.

Taylor, J.W., and Ballenger, S.: Neurological dysfunctions and nursing intervention, New York, 1980, McGraw-Hill Book Co.

Wong, D.L., and Shaley, L.F.: Clinical handbook of pediatric nursing, St. Louis, 1981, The C.V. Mosby Co.

CHAPTER 2

Diagnostic tests

To substantiate or differentiate the diagnosis of neurological dysfunction occurring concomitantly or as a result of nonneurological disease, a battery of general diagnostic tests is ordered. These tests commonly include:

Blood glucose and pH level.

Serum electrolytes and enzymes.

Serological tests.

Arterial blood gases.

Liver function tests.

Creatinine clearance.

Endocrine function tests.

In addition to these general tests and the neurological assessment of the patient, neurodiagnostic tests are performed to pinpoint the diagnosis. While undergoing diagnostic testing, the patient can be under great stress. Stress levels can be minimized or alleviated if the patient and family are provided with a general description of the procedure including:

Who will perform it.

Where and when it will be done.

What it is intended to reveal.

Specific preparation measures and their rationale.

The patient's part in the test and the anticipated degree of discomfort.

Specific posttest measures including rationale.

In general, nursing responsibilities during diagnostic testing include:

1. Patient and family teaching regarding the procedure to be done.
2. Physical preparation of the patient.
3. Obtaining/witnessing written consent for invasive diagnostic procedures.
4. Assembling equipment for and assisting with tests done on the unit, such as lumbar punctures and caloric testing.
5. Maintaining accurate records of patient preparation, tests completed, posttest measures, and patient responses.
6. Accompanying patients requiring special care during testing to other departments, such as those patients with cervical traction, oxygen therapy, positioning limitations.
7. Transporting necessary patient-care equipment such as oxygen and suction if it is not available in other locations.

8. Initiating prescribed posttest measures and independent nursing measures to prevent sequelae and promote patient comfort.

In this chaper the following diagnostic tests will be discussed: radiographs, scans, angiography, cerebral blood flow studies, lumbar puncture and cerebrospinal fluid (CSF) examinations, myelography, pneumoencephalography, echoencephalography, B-mode ultrasound scanning, electroencephalography, electromyography, nerve conduction time studies, computerized evoked response potentials, caloric stimulation tests, electonystagmography, edrophonium testing, and intracranial pressure monitoring. The format for the discussion of these tests will include the purpose, patient preparation (teaching, physical, consent), procedure, and posttest measures.

RADIOGRAPHS

Skull radiographs

The skull x-ray film is the most common of the neurological diagnostic tests.

Purpose. Skull radiographs are obtained to diagnose:

1. Skull fractures. Four views may be taken: anteroposterior (Fig. 2-1, *A*), lateral (Fig. 2-1, *B*), Water's view (Fig. 2-1, *C*), and Towne's view (Fig. 2-1, *D*). Water's view allows for the examination of frontal and maxillary sinuses, facial bones, and the eye orbits. Towne's view permits visualization of the occipital bone.
2. Space-occupying lesions that cause a shift in the calcified pineal gland (Fig. 2-2).
3. Calcium-encased tumors of the brain.
4. Abnormal vasculature.
5. Skull or sella turcica erosion caused by pressure exerted by space-occupying lesions.

Patient preparation

Teaching. Inform the patient that he will be transported to the x-ray department by cart or wheelchair. The x-ray film will be taken by radiology personnel. There is no pain associated with the procedure in which at least two x-ray films will be taken: anteroposterior and lateral views. When sinus infection, facial fractures, or eye orbit injuries are suspected, Water's view is obtained. When occipital bone fracture is suspected, Towne's view is taken.

Physical. No specific physical preparation.

Consent. Not required in most agencies.

Procedure. Patient is positioned flat on the x-ray table and is asked to lie still.

Posttest measures. No specific measures.

Spinal x-ray films

Purpose. Spinal x-ray films are taken when the patient has experienced vertebral trauma, is complaining of back pain, or has motor or sensory deficits in the extremities.

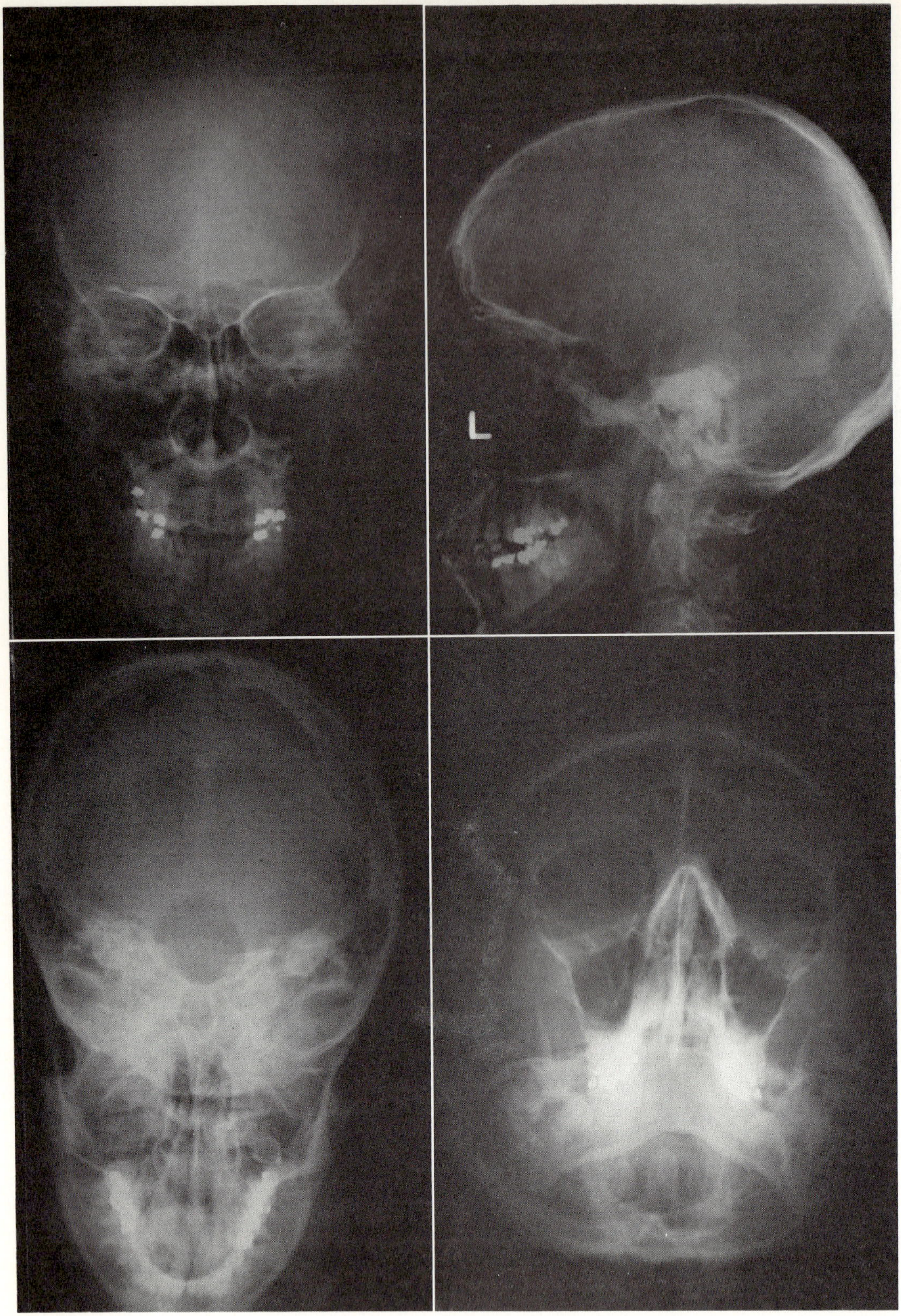

A B

C D

Fig. 2-1 For legend see opposite page.

Fig. 2-1 Skull x-ray films. **A,** Normal anteroposterior view. **B,** Normal lateral view. **C,** Normal Water's view. **D,** Normal Towne's view. (Courtesy Dr. P.D. Mahoney, Radiology Department, St. Joseph Hospital, Omaha, Nebraska.)

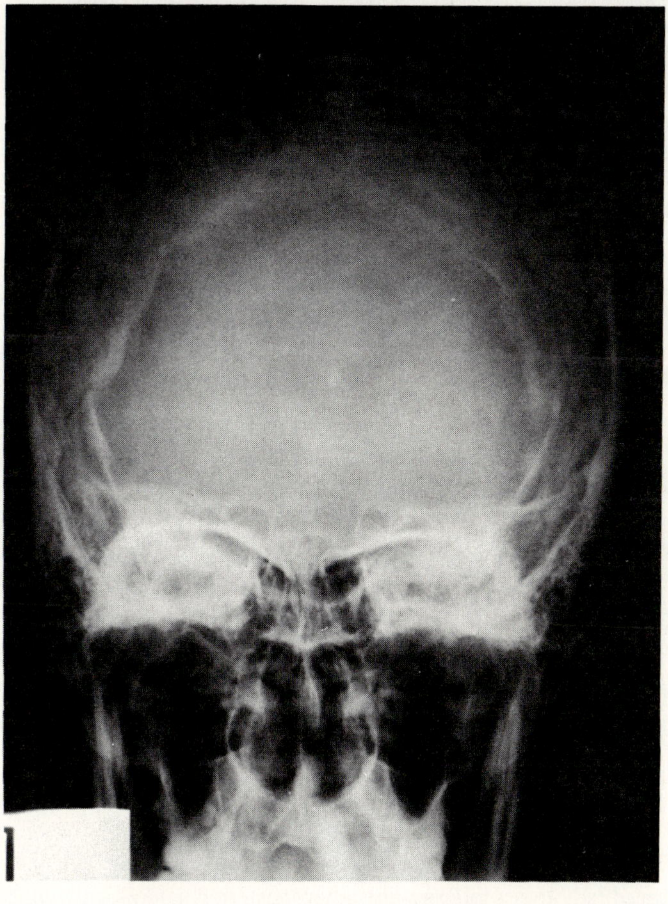

Fig. 2-2 Skull x-ray film showing 3 mm to left pineal shift. (Courtesy Dr. P.D. Mahoney, Radiology Department, St. Joseph Hospital, Omaha, Nebraska.)

A

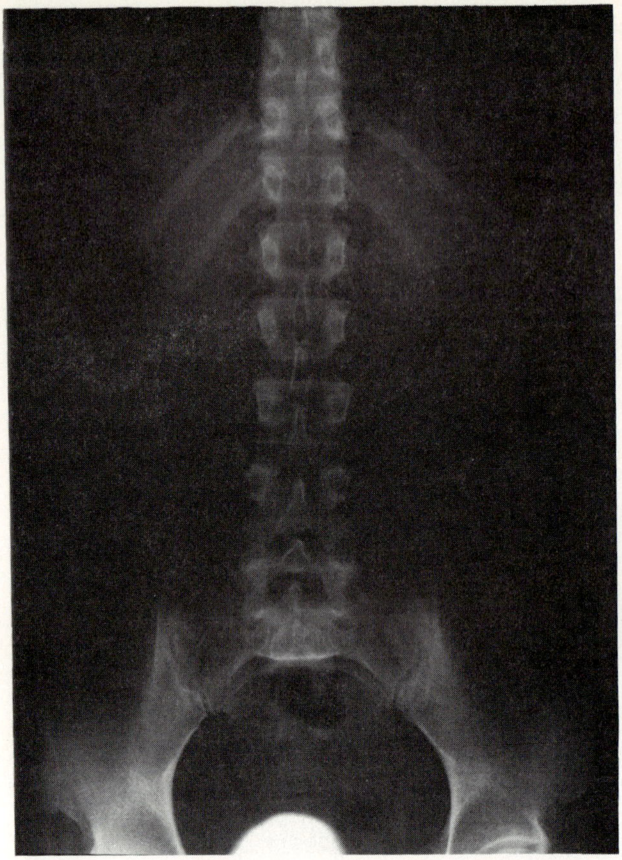

Fig. 2-3 Spine x-ray film. Normal lumbar spine. **A**, Anteroposterior view.

Complete vertebral x-ray films include cervical, thoracic, lumbar, and sacral segments. Fig. 2-3, *A* and *B*, illustrate a normal lumbar spine. Spinal x-ray films can reveal:

1. Vertebral fractures or dislocations.
2. Narrowing of the vertebral canal caused by a herniated intervertebral disk (Fig. 2-4) or neoplasms.
3. Vertebral irregularities such as spondylosis, abnormal curvatures, spurs.
4. Calcium-encased inflammations or tumors.

Because vertebral fractures can be easily missed, some agencies require that an experienced radiologist interpret the anteroposterior, lateral, and sometimes oblique vertebral films.

B

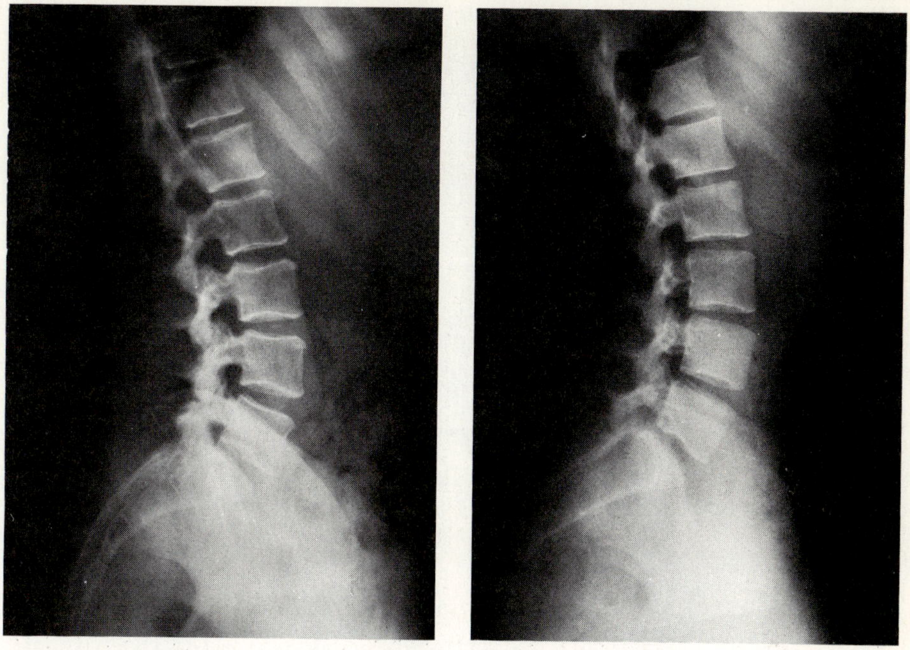

Fig. 2-3 cont'd

Spine x-ray film. **B**, Lateral view. (**B** From Ballinger, P.W.: Merrill's atlas of radiographic positions and radiologic procedures, ed. 5, St. Louis, 1982, The C.V. Mosby Co.)

Patient preparation

Teaching. Inform the patient that he will be transported to the radiology department by cart and positioned flat on the x-ray table. Several films will be taken by radiology personnel. NOTE: If skeletal cervical traction is in place, either portable x-ray machine should be used or the patient should be transported in his bed and be accompanied by the nurse. Care must be taken to maintain traction and to prevent traumatic jerking or twisting motions during transport and the x-ray procedure.

Physical. No specific preparation.

Consent. Generally not required.

Procedure. Patient lies flat and still on the x-ray table while films are taken.

Posttest measures. No specific measures.

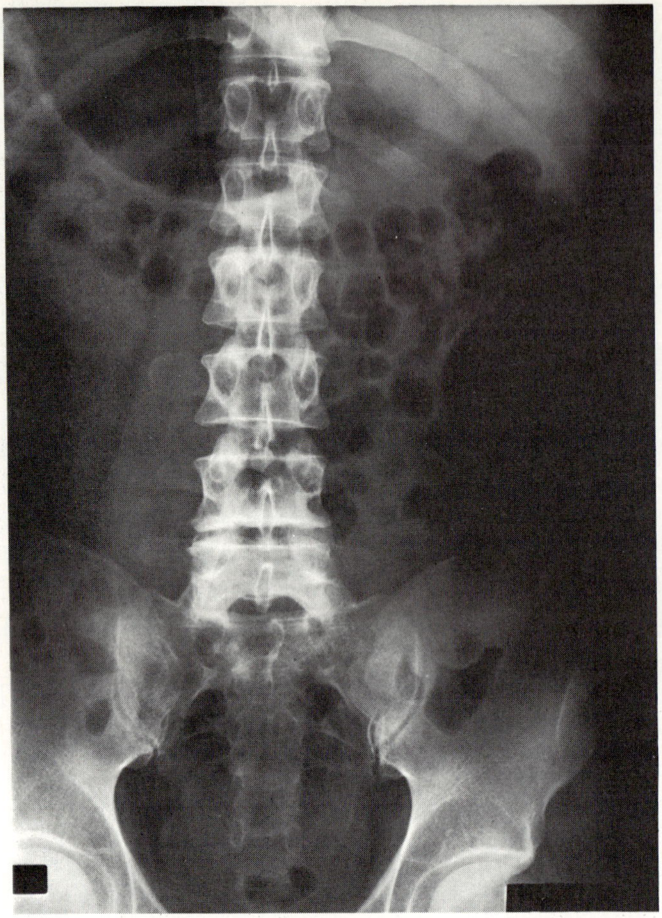

Fig. 2-4 Spine x-ray films. Herniated disc with narrowing of L4-5 interspace. (Courtesy Dr. P.D. Mahoney, Radiology Department, St. Joseph Hospital, Omaha, Nebraska.)

SCANS

Computerized axial tomography

The development and refinement of the computerized axial tomography (CAT) scanner during the 1970s has significantly improved the accuracy in diagnosis of brain dysfunction. CAT scanning is a low-risk procedure in which serial images of thin cross sections of the brain and skull are made from a variety of angles. The various densities of tissue are photographed (Fig. 2-5), recorded, and stored in a computer. This diagnostic tool can be used to visualize other body organs as well as the brain and skull. Because of the specificity of information obtained and the atraumatic nature of the procedure, the CAT has largely replaced other diagnostic methods, especially pneumoencephalography and brain scans. However, the cost for a CAT scan of the brain is

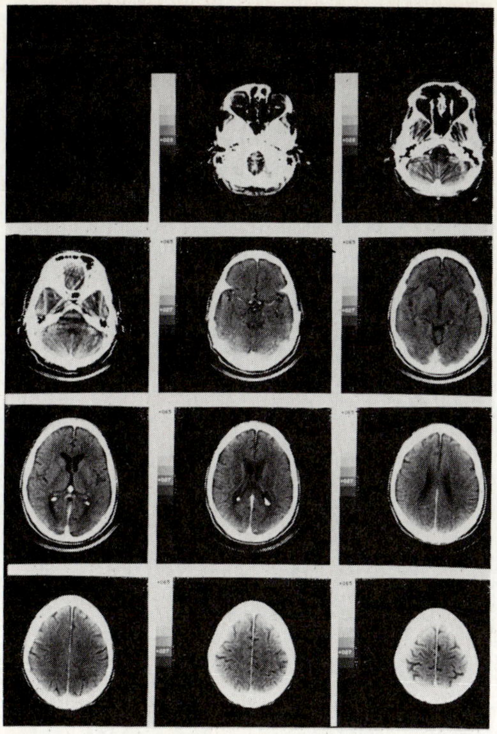

Fig. 2-5 Normal CAT scan. (Courtesy Dr. P.D. Mahoney, Radiology Department, St. Joseph Hospital, Omaha, Nebraska.)

currently higher than that for a brain scan. There are also several patient limitations for use of the CAT scanner including:

1. Weight. Patients should weigh under 290 pounds because a person over this weight may not fit through the circular opening in less recent scan machines. More recent CAT scanners have a larger opening making the weight requirement obsolete. Check with your scan department.
2. Ability to lie flat and still on the table for 20 to 40 minutes: Patients with severe headache, increased intracranial pressure, altered levels of consciousness, and infants or young children may require pretest analgesia.
3. Allergies: In cases in which visualization of the vasculature of the brain is necessary, an iodine-based contrast material (300 ml of Reno M30) is injected intravenously. Question the patient about allergies to iodine.
4. Adequate kidney function: The contrast material is eliminated through the kidneys within 24 hours.

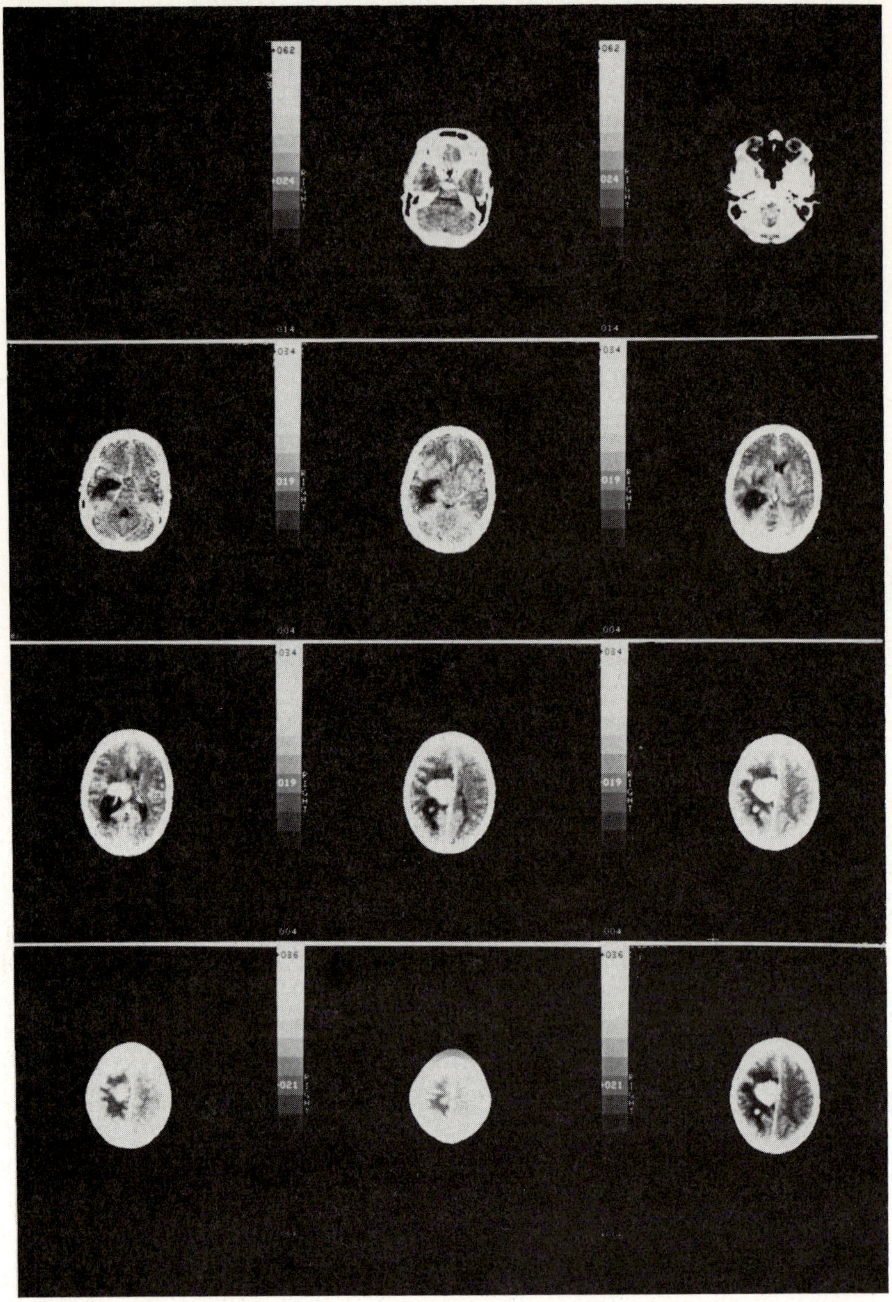

Fig. 2-6 CAT scan. Right hemisphere tumor metastatic from a right breast adenocarcinoma in a 37-year-old female. (Courtesy Dr. P.D. Mahoney, Radiology Department, St. Joseph Hospital, Omaha, Nebraska.)

Purpose. CAT scanning can reveal accurate information regarding:

1. Space-occupying lesions: tumors (Fig. 2-6), hematomas, abcesses.
2. Vascular changes: malformations, increases or decreases in vascularity, infarctions.
3. Brain contusions.
4. Brain atrophy.
5. Hydrocephalus.
6. Inflammations/infection.

Patient preparation

Teaching. Inform the patient that he will be transported to the scan department by cart or wheelchair and positioned on the CAT scan table. Show a picture of the scan machine (Fig. 2-7) or a videocassette of the procedure, if available. Scan department personnel will perform the test. Patient participation includes:

1. Lying still and flat on the table.
2. Holding breath when requested.
3. Following directions to facilitate the intravenous injection by the physician or technician of the contrast material when it is used.

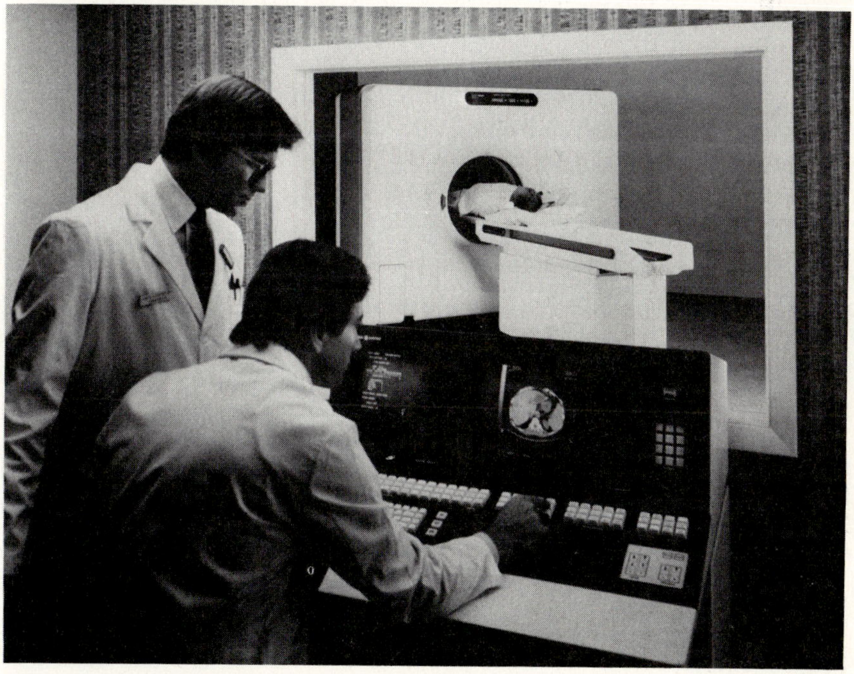

Fig. 2-7 CAT scan equipment. (Courtesy General Electric Company, Medical Systems Operations, Milwaukee, Wisconsin.)

The procedure is painless except for the contrast material injection. Warn the patient that a flushed, warm face and a metallic taste during injection of the contrast material are normal. There are no specific posttest measures. Because the contrast material is eliminated in the urine within 24 hours, there is no retention of radioactive substances.

Physical. Obtain an allergy history, focusing on iodine allergy. Ask about allergic responses to (1) ingestion of iodized salt, (2) shellfish, (3) previous diagnostic intravenous pyelogram or gallbladder x-ray films. Administer prescribed analgesics for body pain or headaches; minor tranquilizers may be prescribed for excessive anxiety. Make sure that the hair is clean and that hair fasteners and wigs are removed. Do not braid hair. If the patient requires suctioning or electronic monitoring during the procedure, the nurse should accompany the patient.

Consent. When intravenous injection of the contrast material is anticipated, many agencies require written consent.

Procedure. The patient is positioned on his back on the scan table, occasionally with a leg restraint applied. The table electronically moves through the rotating circular structure that houses the scan equipment. There are several types of machines available: CAT, EMI, delta, and ACTA. Use of the EMI scanner requires application of a head bag filled with water. The patient must lie absolutely still for the duration of the scanning procedure, which takes from 20 to 45 minutes depending on the machine. Health care personnel in the room wear protective lead aprons.

Posttest measures. Observe for allergic responses to the contrast material: rash, urticaria, pruritus. Administer prescribed diphenhydramine (Benadryl), 50 mg, for allergic responses. Provide back rubs for persons experiencing back pain as a result of the immobility on the hard table. Encourage fluid intake and monitor intake and output to ensure elimination of the contrast material.

Brain scan

Purpose. Brain scans are prescribed when a space-occupying lesion or cerebrovascular dysfunction is suspected. Presence of lateralizing signs, persistent headaches, or altered mental functioning are common reasons for a brain scan to be prescribed. The scan requires the intravenous injection of a small amount of a radioactive isotope (technetium 99m), a waiting period of 15 minutes to 2 hours, followed by the scanning procedure itself. The uptake of radioactive isotopes in normal brain tissue is minimal. A concentration of radioactive isotopes in the brain indicates the *size* and *location* of cerebral lesions (Fig. 2-8). However, the type of lesion (whether tumor, abcess, cyst, or hematoma) cannot be determined by a brain scan.

Patient preparation

Teaching. Inform the patient that brain scans are done in the nuclear division of the radiology department by nuclear medicine personnel. The scan requires the intravenous injection of a minute amount of radioactive material followed by a 15-minute to

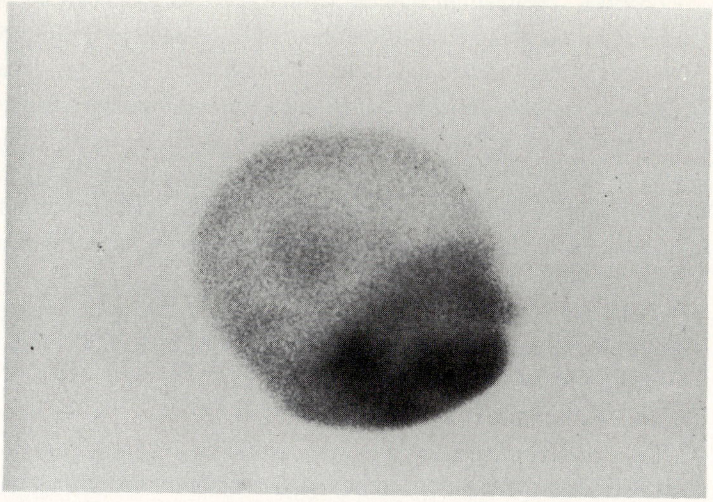

Fig. 2-8 Brain scan showing tumor metastatic from lung. (Courtesy Dr. P.D. Mahoney, Radiology Department, St. Joseph Hospital, Omaha, Nebraska.)

2-hour period to allow for absorption in the brain. After the waiting period the patient is transported to the nuclear division by cart and positioned on an x-ray table that has an overhead isotope detector that makes a ticking noise. Show pictures of the machine, room, and procedure if available. The machine moves back and forth over the head and records the uptake of the injected material on a scan sheet. The procedure takes from 30 to 60 minutes. In some instances additional scans are done 24 and 48 hours after the injection.

NOTE: The patient's hands must be kept at his sides because technetium 99m is readily absorbed by saliva and tears. Therefore if the patient coughs or rubs his eyes and then his head, the scan is inaccurate. With some machines four positions are required (supine, prone, and the right and left sides) to obtain the necessary anterior, posterior, and lateral projections.

The amount of radioactive material injected is minimal. It is excreted within 24 hours in the urine. Therefore infertility or sterility is not a sequela. However, brain scans are contraindicated during pregnancy to protect the fetus.

Physical. In some agencies certain medications (such as vasodilators, vasoconstricting agents, antihypertensive medications) are withheld for 24 hours before the scan. These medications, which affect the vasculature of the brain, are withheld to increase accuracy of test results.

Consent. Because of the injection of radioactive material, most agencies require written consent. Check your agency's consent policy.

Procedure. Technetium 99m is administered intravenously by nuclear medicine personnel in the patient's room. Following a waiting period of 15 to 120 minutes, the patient is transported to the nuclear division of the radiology department by cart for the test. The Geiger-Müller sensor passes back and forth over the patient's head for 20 to 30 minutes, recording radioisotope uptake in the brain tissue on scan sheets. In some agencies color instant photographs are taken. Because of the increased vascularity of a tumor, there is an increased isotope uptake that increases the density, causing a red appearance of the lesion in the photograph. Some refer to this as a "hot spot."

Posttest measures. All previous activities can be resumed. Provide fluid intake to produce sufficient urinary output permitting elimination of isotopes. No urinary or patient radiation precautions are necessary.

Nuclear magnetic resonance

Nuclear magnetic resonance (NMR), presently in clinical trial, is a new diagnostic tool used to determine the location and size of brain neoplasms and abnormalities. It is anticipated that NMR, which uses sound imagery, will replace CAT scans within several years. Major advantages of NMR are that it is noninvasive and requires no patient preparation other than explanation of the procedure. It can be used to diagnose:

1. Hydrocephalus.
2. Localized abnormalities such as aneurysms, tumors, and hematomas.
3. Cystic lesions.
4. Hemorrhages.

Because of the sophistication of this technique, interpretation of the findings requires the interdisciplinary collaboration between a spectroscopist and the physician or biochemist. Fig. 2-9 illustrates the configuration obtained from the NMR procedure.

Positron emission (transaxial) tomography

The positron emission tomography (PET or PETT) test is currently in clinical trial at research centers in the United States. The procedure is similar to a CAT scan using contrast media. The difference is that PET is a colorimetric test. Photons resulting from the chemical collision of positrons and electrons incorporated in the intravenous injection of glucose and radioactive flourine are detected and processed by a computer. The resulting colored images are displayed on a screen. The color shades and the patterns indicate the level of glucose metabolism. At present, this test is very expensive because of the specialized equipment and personnel required. (Conway-Rutkowski, 1982).

Purpose. PET can be used to:

1. Identify areas of abnormal brain metabolism causing mental illness and/or neurological dysfunction.
2. Determine the effectiveness of pharmacotherapeutic agents and neurosurgery.

Patient preparation and posttest measures. Patient preparation and posttest measures are the same as for a CAT scan using contrast media (see p. 56). NOTE: Another

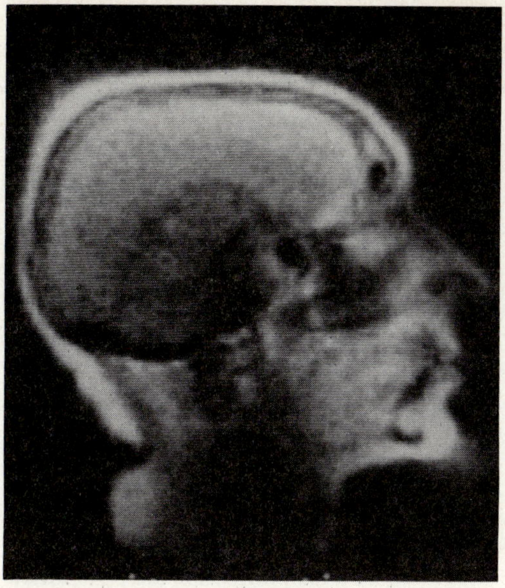

Fig. 2-9 NMR imagery. (From Hawkes, R., et al.: J. Comput. Assist. Tomogr. **4**(5):77, 1980.)

diagnostic test in current clinical trial that uses the same principles as PET is xenon enhancement tomography (XET). The primary disadvantage of XET is that it requires intubation and anesthesia of the patient.

Doppler scan

The Doppler scan is a noninvasive technique used to assess blood flow through arteries proximate to the surface. The primary use in neurology is to assess the blood flow in the carotid artery. By amplifying the ultrasounds of blood flow, Doppler imagery constructs an outline or map of moving blood.

Purpose. The Doppler scan is used to assess blood flow through the carotid arteries.

Patient preparation

Teaching. Inform the patient that the Doppler scan is not an invasive test. After being transported to the radiology department, the patient will be positioned on a table and asked to lie very still. A surface probe will be moved horizontally across the side of the patient's neck. This test is done either by the physician or by scan department personnel. Signals from the probe are displayed on a screen.

Physical. No restrictions of food, fluids, or activity. However, the patient should void before the test.

Consent. Not usually required. Check your agency's consent policy.

Procedure. After positioning the patient in a recumbant position, the physician or scan personnel move the transducer laterally across the common carotid to above the bifurcation towards the mandible. The signals are displayed on a screen and processed, stored, and printed out in graphics by the computer.

Posttest measures. None. Patient may resume previous activities.

NOTE: Directional Doppler ultrasonography is used to detect the direction of blood flow in an artery. When an occlusion of a major artery such as the internal carotid occurs, the blood flow in a more distant branch is altered. For example, when the internal carotid is occluded, the blood flow in the ophthalmic artery is reversed. Blood flow in the ophthalmic artery is normally outward or distally toward the facial skin. With a significant occlusion of the internal carotid artery, the blood flows inward toward the brainstem.

ANGIOGRAPHY

Purpose

To visualize the vascular system in the brain and spinal cord, a radiopaque iodine-based contrast material is injected directly into the carotid or vertebral arteries or indirectly into them through the brachial, subclavian, or femoral arteries. Fluoroscopy and timed-interval radiographic films are taken after the injection. This test is used to diagnose:

1. Cerebral or vertebral vascular malformations, such as congenital anomalies or those resulting from tumor formations.
2. Displacement of blood vessels caused by herniation or edema of the central nervous system parenchyma or by space-occupying lesions, such as hematomas, abscesses, tumors.
3. Occlusion, stenosis, or aneurysms of central nervous system blood vessels (Fig. 2-10).

Patient preparation

Teaching. Explain the procedure to the patient. Angiography is done in the radiology department by a neurologist or neurosurgeon. The patient is positioned on his back: In the case of children or uncooperative patients, the arms and legs are lightly restrained. Local and/or general anesthesia is used, depending on the patient's status. For local anesthesia, a local anesthetic agent such as procaine hydrochloride (Novocain) is injected into the area surrounding the artery to be injected. For systemic anesthesia phenobarbital, 100 mg, and atropine, 0.4 mg, are administered intramuscularly 30 minutes before the test.

Inform the patient of the pain and discomfort to be experienced during the dye injection: (1) There may be a burning sensation for 6 to 10 seconds behind the eyes, and in the tongue, cheeks, lips, and teeth. (2) When the carotid artery site is used, some people experience a feeling of difficulty in breathing because the intracatheter injection site is adjacent to the trachea.

Patient participation. Emphasize the need for the patient to lie very still and caution against talking and coughing. The patient should follow the directions of the

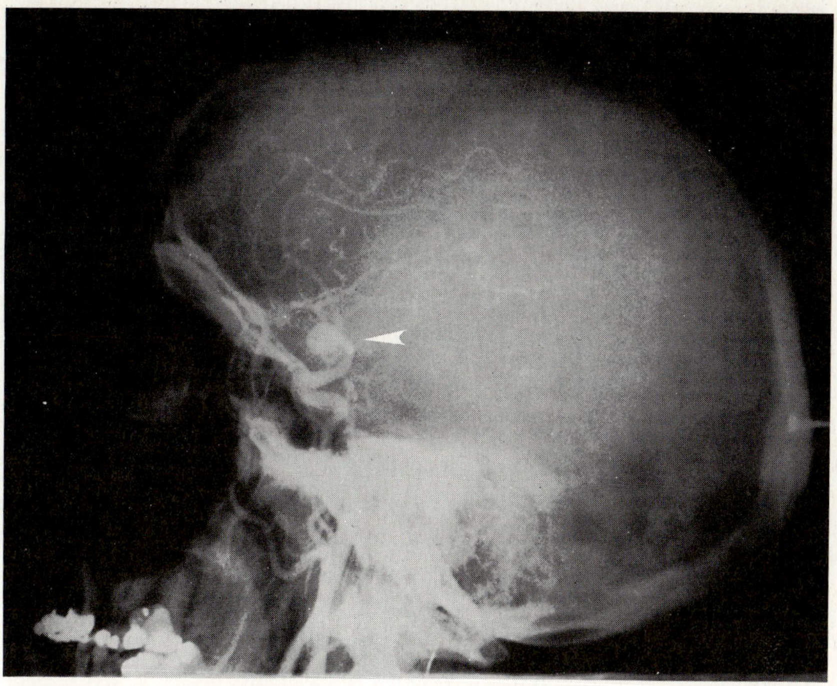

Fig. 2-10 Cerebral angiogram, lateral view. Arrow pinpoints aneurysm. (From Conway-Rutkowski, B.L.: Carini and Owens' neurological and neurosurgical nursing, ed. 8, St. Louis, 1982, The C.V. Mosby Co.)

neurologist to take a deep breath and hold it during catheter insertion. Inform the patient that a tight dressing will be applied over the catheter insertion site. Posttest measures are explained below.

Physical

1. Ask the patient about allegies to procaine and iodine.
2. Encourage fluids 2 days before the test to ensure adequate hydration. The patient should take nothing by mouth for 6 to 12 hours before testing.
3. Perform and record results of sensitivity tests to iodine and procaine 24 hours before testing when allergies are suspected.
4. Skin preparation: Shave 2 to 3 inches around the injection site in the neck, femoral, clavicular, or brachial areas. This is sometimes done in the radiology department just before testing.
5. Dentures, glasses, and hair fasteners are removed.
6. Obtain and record baseline neurological assessment data.
7. Administer and record prescribed pretest medications.

Consent. Because angiography is an invasive procedure that involves a degree of risk, written consent is required. The neurologist explains the procedure and risks involved including (1) allergic reactions to the dye, (2) stroke (1%), (3) hematoma formation and rarely (4) pulmonary or cardiac emboli. Written consent from the patient and/or the family must be obtained before pretest sedation.

Procedure

The sedated patient is placed in a supine position on the x-ray table. Arms and legs may be restrained. Following administration of the anesthetic, the skin site preparation, and arterial puncture, the contrast material is injected. The cerebral vasculature is visualized on the fluoroscope and rapid time-interval films are taken. The procedure generally takes from 30 to 45 minutes. Because of the danger of anaphylactic shock, resuscitation equipment must be readily available. After the injection needle is removed, direct pressure is applied to the insertion site for 5 to 10 minutes to prevent hematoma formation. Neurological assessment data are obtained and recorded, and a pressure dressing is applied to the puncture site before returning the patient to his room. When the brachial or femoral artery has been used, the arm or leg is immobilized. Distal pulses, color, and temperature are assessed and recorded hourly.

Posttest measures

1. Assess and record neurological assessment data on a flow sheet every 15 to 30 minutes until the vital signs are stable.
2. Bed rest with the head elevated 15 to 30 degrees for 24 hours is prescribed when the subclavian, brachial, or carotid artery is used. Flat bed position is indicated when the femoral artery is used.
3. Check puncture site dressings hourly. Report bloody drainage exceeding 1 cm to the neurologist.
4. Immobilize puncture site for 6 to 8 hours.
   a. Use an ice collar for carotid or vertebral punctures.
   b. Use lateral trochanter rolls with the arm or leg in straight alignment for femoral or brachial punctures.
5. Assess and record distal pulses, color, and temperature for femoral or brachial punctures.
6. Observe for signs and symptoms of complications including:
   a. Allergic responses: pruritis, skin rash, hypotension, tachycardia, fever.
   b. Puncture site edema or hematoma:
      (1) For carotid punctures: dysphagia, dysphasia.
      (2) For femoral punctures: decrease or absence of pedal pulse, pallor, and coldness of feet and toes with parethesias.
   c. Vascular complications:
      (1) Stroke: hemiparesis/hemiplegia, dysphasia, decrease in level of orientation, visual disturbances.
      (2) Cardiac or pulmonary emboli: chest pain, dysnpea, dysrrhythmias.

Digital subtraction angiography

Digital subtraction angiography (DSA) is a computerized radiological procedure. It requires an intravenous rather than arterial catheterization and uses a contrast medium injection to allow examination of selected arterial circulation. By using computer technology, DSA provides an alternative to cerebral angiography for high-risk patients.

Purpose. The DSA procedure is prescribed in order to:

1. Assess for cerebral arterial disease.
2. Screen patients for potential aneurysms, emboli, or stenosis.
3. Determine the effectiveness of neurosurgery.

Patient preparation

Teaching. Inform the patient that he will be transported to the radiology department and will be positioned on his back. Warn the patient that he will be requested to lie very still and hold his breath upon request. An intravenous line will be started in one arm near the elbow after the area has been anesthetized with procaine or lidocaine. Tell the patient that a "pinching" will be felt when the catheter is inserted in the vein and that an intravenous solution will be hung. After the contrast material is injected, images will be seen on the screen. The test takes 20 to 40 minutes.

Physical

1. Ask the patient about allergies to lidocaine or iodine. Inform the physician if the patient is allergic to these substances.
2. There are no fluid nor activity restrictions.
3. The patient should have no food for 2 hours before testing.

Consent. Because of the intravenous insertion, many agencies require written consent. Check your agency's consent policy.

Procedure

1. The brachial or cephalic area is prepped with an antiseptic and draped to enlarge the sterile field. NOTE: The brachial vein is preferred because of its direct route to the superior vena cava.
2. Lidocaine is injected subcutaneously in the tissue surrounding the vein. A wait of 5 to 8 minutes ensures that the area is anesthetized.
3. The physician nicks the skin over the vein and inserts a 16-gauge angiocatheter, threading it up the vein with adjunct fluoroscopy to guide correct placement of the catheter.
4. A 7 Fr. 65 cm pigtail catheter is threaded over the guidewire and positioned at the junction of the superior vena cava and the right atrium. A 500 to 1000 ml bag of dextrose in water is attached to the catheter.
5. The initial reference film is taken.
6. Then 30 to 45 ml of iodine-based contrast material is injected at sequential intervals.

Between injections the intravenous solution is infused to maintain the patency of the catheter.

7. Images of the cerebral vasculature are shown on the screen. These same images are transmitted to the computer, which processes the sequential information by subtracting later contrast-medium-enhanced images from the initial reference image. This process yields a contrast-enhanced picture of the cerebral arteries.
8. Following the procedure the angiocatheter is removed and pressure is applied to the insertion site for 3 to 5 minutes.

Posttest measures

1. Observe the intravenous insertion site for oozing or inflammation.
2. Assess and document pulses and capillary refill times distal to the infusion site hourly for 4 hours. NOTE: Check your agency's policies for the time schedule. Increase the patient's fluid intake (to at least 2000 to 3000 ml) for 24 hours to enhance excretion of the contrast material.
3. Observe for allergic responses to iodine such as nausea, vomiting, and dizziness.

CEREBRAL BLOOD FLOW STUDIES

Purpose

Cerebral blood flow studies (CBFS) are used to measure blood flow through the vasculature of the brain, thus estimating cerebral perfusion (Fig. 2-11). CBFS are used to:

1. Assess regional and total cerebrovascular profusion.
2. Determine the effect of stenosed arteries on brain perfusion.
3. Determine the presence and/or degree of collateralization of vasculature after the stenosis or occlusion.
4. Compare profusion in the two hemispheres and differentiate between white and gray matter profusion.
5. Identify focal seizure-producing sites when correlated with electroencephalogram (EEG) data.
6. Evaluate effectiveness of therapeutic measures including surgery and medications.
7. Differentiate between communicating and noncommunicating hydrocephalus.
8. Identify brain death.

Patient preparation

Teaching. Inform the patient that the test is done in a radiological diagnostic laboratory, by a neurologist or a trained technician. Explain that accurate results are dependent on the patient's lying still on the table with muscles and mind relaxed. Inform the patient that the head of table can be raised if difficulty in breathing is experienced. Thoroughly explain the procedure to allay fears and promote relaxation. Explain that a minute amount of a radioactive substance will be injected or inhaled by the patient and that this material will be excreted by the lungs or kidneys within hours. Emphasize that this is a painless procedure except for the injection. NOTE: Mental and physical relaxation by the patient is imperative because anxiety increases cerebral blood flow, resulting in erroneously high readings.

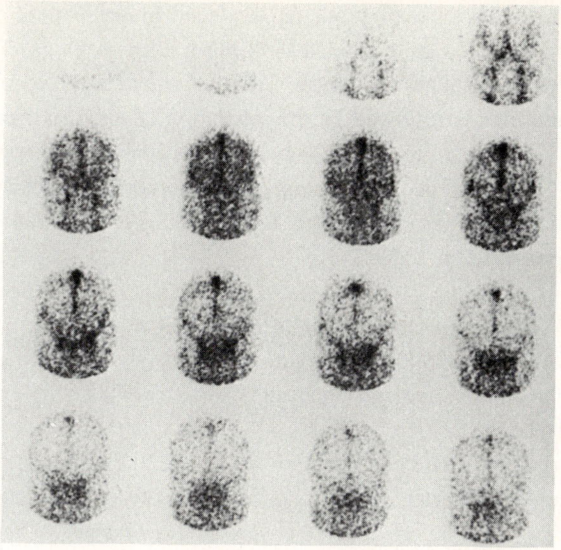

Fig. 2-11 Normal cerebral blood flow studies using injectable radioactive isotope.

Physical. No food or fluid restrictions. Central nervous system stimulant and depressant medications are withheld for 24 hours before testing in some agencies. Obtain and record an accurate health history focusing on (1) obstructive respiratory diseases such as emphysema and asthma; (2) cardiovascular diseases, including hypertension and congestive heart failure; and (3) seizure activity/epilepsy. Record recent hemogloblin and hematocrit. No pretest medication is required. Wash patient's hair and remove hair fasteners. Record pretest vital signs.

Consent. Written consent is required by most agencies.

Procedure

1. Patient is positioned in a supine or semi-Fowler's position on a padded table.
2. Usually 16 probes are placed on specified areas of the scalp and they are affixed in place with a pastelike substance. Some machines require 16 to 32 detectors that do not need paste and these are placed directly on the scalp. The probes are attached to the computer.
3. Injection method: Xenon 133, technetium 99, or krypton 85 is injected into one or both carotid arteries. Radiosensitive probes pick up and record the isotope flow. The rate of clearance is calculated. Normal is 50 ml/min/gm. Following the procedure, a pressure dressing is applied to the injection site.

4. Inhalation method: A mouthpiece is placed in the patient's mouth or a mask is applied. The nares are occluded with nasal clips or plugs. The patient is asked to breath deeply through the mouth. The gaseous form of xenon 133 is inhaled for 1 minute and this is followed by the inhalation of air for 10 minutes. Xenon readily diffuses across the cell membranes in the brain. The normal rate is 56 to 91 ml/min/100 gm. Probe monitoring and the computerized calculation are identical to those used with injection method. CBFS results are correlated with specific neurological problems in Table 2-1.

Posttest measures

1. Monitor and record vital signs and neurological status.
2. Following the injection:
   a. Check the injection site dressings.
   b. Apply an ice collar.
   c. Bed rest with the head elevated for 4 to 12 hours is prescribed.
   d. Provide fluids after assuring the presence of the gag reflex.

LUMBAR PUNCTURE

Purpose

Lumbar puncture involves the aseptic insertion of a hollow 18-gauge needle with a stylet into the subarachnoid space between the third and fourth or fourth and fifth lumbar spaces. A lumbar puncture can be done for diagnostic or therapeutic reasons. Diagnostically, the lumbar puncture is done to:

1. Measure cerebrospinal fluid (CSF) pressure.
2. Obtain CSF for examination in order to diagnose:
   a. Infections/inflammations such as meningitis, syphilis, ruptured abcesses, and multiple sclerosis.
   b. Hemorrhage, either subarachnoid or intracerebral.
   c. Neoplasms.
3. Determine blockage of CSF flow (Queckenstedt's test).
4. To introduce contrast materials (air or a radiopaque dye) for radiographic examination.

Therapeutically, a lumbar puncture precedes:

1. Intrathecal injections of antibiotics or antiinflammatory medications.
2. Spinal anesthesia.

Contraindications

Patients with severely increased intracranial pressure are at risk for uncal or brainstem herniation during lumbar puncture. If determining CSF pressure is the only reason for the lumbar puncture, an alternative noninvasive means of measuring intracranial pressure, the Ladd fiberoptic sensor, should be considered. The risk/benefit ratio of a lumbar puncture must be carefully weighed by the neurologist. Another contraindication to a lumbar puncture is the presence of lumbar-area skin or bone infection because during the puncture the infectious organisms can be introduced into the subarachnoid space.

Table 2-1 Use of cerebral blood flow studies in diagnosis of neurological problems*

Problem	Comments
Stroke Ischemia (TIA)	Carotid → ↑ in middle cerebral artery flow Vertebral basilar → ↓ occipital and ↓ posterior temporal areas
Infarction	Critical value for F, on nrCBF 40 ml/100 brain/min.
Occlusion of cerebral and carotid arteries (including endarterectomies)	Initially diffuse ↓ in nrCBF. After 1-3 weeks mean nrCBF ↑ and zone of infarction ↓
Subarachnoid hemorrhage (aneurysm and arteriovenous fistula)	Topographic ↓ in rCBF correlated with angiographically demonstrated vasospasm or intracerebral hematoma
Headache Migraine, cluster	nrCBF often documents changes in cephalic blood flow. Prodrome nrCBR ↓ in clinically appropriate region → ↑ lactate → hyperemia
Seizures Epilepsy	CBF and metabolism ↑ four times during generalized seizures. nrCBF may show ↑ rCBF over epileptogenic focus
Increased intracranial pressure	As cerebral edema ↑ CBF ↓ when intracranial pressure equals arterial blood pressure CBF = 0
Trauma Concussion, contusion	Concussion ↑ CBF (temporary loss of autoregulation of blood flow) Contusion with damage to microcirculation → ↓ CBF
Degenerative diseases Dementia, hydrocephalus	nrCBF ↓ in most organic dementias. nrCBF ↓ in normal pressure hydrocephalus (white matter and grey matter weight in ant. cerebral artery area)
Schizophrenia and other mental problems	No change in mean CBF. Distribution of CBF ↓ in frontal areas.
Metabolic disorders Diabetic coma Hypoglycemic coma Hepatic, uremic encephalopathy Hyperthermia	↓ in nrCBF in coma from diabetes, renal or liver dysfunction. ↑ in temp (39°) → ↑ rCBF. Above temp 42° C, EEG slows, and CBF abruptly ↓.
Hypertension	Normal CBF with autoregulation but have ↑ in cerebral vascular resistance. Do not tolerate rapid ↓ in blood pressure.

*Reprinted with permission of Marilyn Lyons, RN, MA, and J. Neurosurg Nurs. **13:**289, 1981.

Patient preparation

Teaching. Inform the patient that the lumbar puncture will be done by the neurologist in the patient's room or in the unit examination room. Show a diagram of the spinal cord and vertebrae depicting the location of the end of the cord and the site of needle insertion and demonstrate this on the patient's back. This alleviates patient's fears of the puncturing of the spinal cord itself. Demonstrate the fetal position in which the patient will be placed. Explain posttest measures and their rationale (see below). Answer questions regarding possible sequelae, such as headache and leg pains, and explain preventative measures that will be used.

Physical

1. Ascertain medications currently being taken. NOTE: Patients on anticoagulants are at risk for posttest hemorrhage.
2. Obtain a sterile lumbar puncture tray, two syringes, local anesthetic agents, and gloves for the physician.
3. Aseptically set up equipment on the bedside or on a Mayo stand.
4. Have the patient void.
5. Position the patient in a latereal recumbant fetal position near the edge of the bed to ensure maximum separation of spinous processes. In some instances, the patient requires assistance to maintain the fetal position.
6. Thoroughly cleanse the lumbar skin area with antiseptic. Warn the patient about the cold liquids before application.
7. Assist with the procedure (see below) and record gross appearance and manometer readings.

Consent. Written consent must be obtained before this invasive test.

Procedure

Lumbar punctures are done by a physician. Following skin preparation, local anesthesia, and aseptic draping, an 18-gauge spinal needle with a removable stylet is introduced into the subarachnoid space at L3-4 or L4-5. At this point the patient should be requested to relax his position slightly. Tenseness of back and leg muscles yields a falsely elevated pressure reading. The stylet is removed and the manometer is attached to obtain pressure readings (normal is 60 to 80 mm water). The nurse records two readings: opening and closing pressures. Three to five CSF samples (3 to 5 ml each) are obtained in sterile test tubes. The nurse numerically labels the tubes. Gross CSF appearance data are recoded, that is, blood and color. When the CSF is bloody, differentiation between a central nervous system hemorrhage and a traumatic tap is necessary (see Table 2-2). After the CSF samples are obtained, the needle is removed. Slight pressure and a bandage on the puncture site area applied.

Laboratory request forms are completed. For the most accurate results the CSF samples should be taken to the laboratory for immediate examination. Changes in CSF can occur in as little as 20 minutes. Normal CSF values and reasons for common abnormal findings are summarized in Table 2-3. Procedure and patient responses are documented.

Table 2-2 Differentiating CNS hemorrhage from traumatic lumbar puncture

Characteristics	Normal	CNS hemorrhage	Traumatic puncture
Color of CSF	Clear	All samples bloody Xanthochromia	Initial sample bloody, then clear
Microscopic appearance of RBCs	None	Scalloped edges (crenated)	Normal shape
Aggregation of RBCs	None	None	Collect in bottom of test tube

Table 2-3 Normal CSF values, abnormal findings, and possible causes*

Constituent	Normal	Abnormal	Causes
Protein	15-45 mg/100 ml	Elevated	CNS infection, hemorrhage, tumor
Glucose†	45-75 mg/100 ml	Decreased Normal	Bacterial meningitis Viral meningitis
Cells	0-8 cells/μl	Elevated	CNS bacterial infections
Chloride	Adult: 118-132 mEq/L Child: 120-128 mEq/L	Decreased	Tubercular meningitis
Colloidal Gold curve‡	0001111000‡	First or mid zone increase	Neurosyphilis
Fluorescent Antibody	Negative	Positive	Neurosyphilis
Cytology	No cell growth	Positive	Neoplasm
Xanthochromia	Negative	Positive	Previous CNS hemorrhage

*Adapted from Tilkian, A., Conover, M., and Tilkian, S.: Clinical implications of laboratory tests, ed. 3, St. Louis, 1983, The C.V. Mosby Co.

†Blood glucose levels should be obtained to determine significance. Normally CSF glucose is two-thirds the blood glucose level.

‡Not as reliable as fluorescent antibody.

Posttest measures

1. The patient lies flat in bed for 6 to 24 hours depending on the persistence or presence of headache. The head is elevated 15 degrees for meals. Upright positioning can cause or aggrevate headaches.
2. Neurological assessment data are obtained and recorded every hour until stable. Then patient activity can be resumed.
3. Provide and encourage intake of fluids preferred by the patient for 48 hours. Intake should exceed 3000 ml daily to facilitate CSF production.
4. Administer prescribed oral analgesics for headaches.
5. Maintain accurate intake/output records for 24 hours.

6. Assess bladder distention. Occasionally patients have difficulty in voiding for 24 hours after a lumbar puncture.
7. Encourage range of motion and leg exercises to reduce muscle spasms.
8. Observe for meningeal signs resulting from a septic puncture such as nuchal rigidity, fever, photophobia.

MYELOGRAPHY

Purpose

Myelography is done to detect abnormalities of cord or vertebrae or to find the location of an obstruction in the flow of CSF in the vertebral subarachnoid space. The most common cause of obstruction is a herniated intervertebral disk (Fig. 2-12). Other causes of obstruction may be a ruptured or degenerated disk, a neoplasm, or an abscess.

Patient preparation

Teaching. Myelography is done in the radiology department generally by a neurologist or orthopedic surgeon. Medications (phenobarbital or meperidine and atropine) are administered by injection 1 hour before the test to promote relaxation and cause drowsiness. Food and fluids are withheld for 4 hours before the test. The patient is transported to the radiology department by cart and placed in a fetal position on an

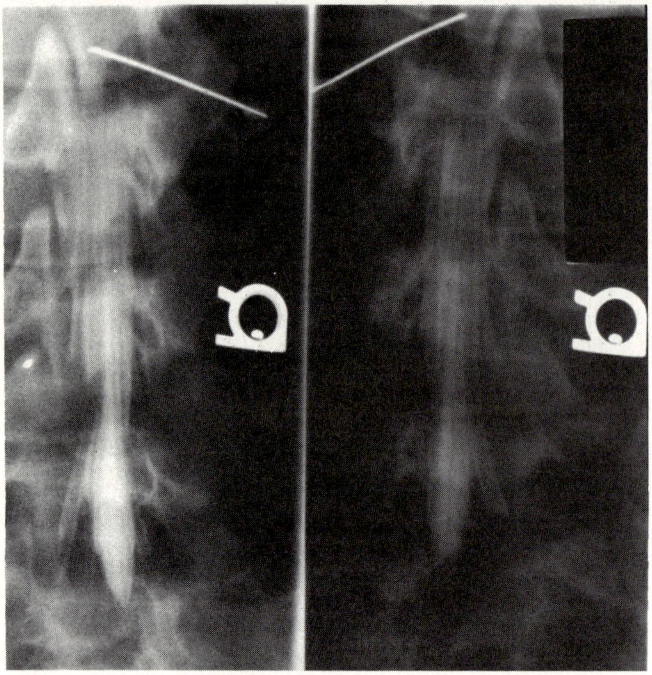

Fig. 2-12 Myelogram using metrizamide. Herniated lumbar disc. (Courtesy Dr. P.D. Mahoney, Radiology Department, St. Joseph Hospital, Omaha, Nebraska.)

x-ray tilt table. The pretest lumbar puncture (see above) and the myelography, including the table-tilting procedure, should be explained to the patient. Explain posttest measures and their rationale.

Physical

1. Depending on the contrast material to be used, obtain an allergy/health history. With metrizamide (Amipaque) ask about any history of epilepsy, chronic alcoholism, or respiratory disease. With iodophenylundecylic acid (Pantopaque) ask about allergies to iodine.
2. Withhold foods and fluids for 4 to 6 hours before the myelogram.
3. Have the patient void. Administer prescribed premyelogram medications. Raise the side rails following medication administration.
4. If the patient is taking phenothiazines, record this fact on the request form and on the patient's record. There is an increased incidence of seizures when metrizamide is used.

Consent. Written consent is required following the physician's explanation of the test and of the common sequela (headache).

Procedure

Following a lumbar (occasionally cervical) puncture and removal of 10 to 15 ml of CSF, one of two available contrast materials is injected into the vertebral subarachnoid space. Table 2-4 differentiates between the two available contrast materials regarding their composition, mechanism, test procedures, and potential adverse effects. The contrast material mixes with CSF, outlining the vertebral canal, thus making obstructions visible on the fluoroscope. Time-sequenced films are taken. Tilting of the table is necessary when iodophenylundecylic acid is used. Also when this medium is used, the contrast material is removed before removal of the spinal needle. Following myelography, the puncture site is covered with a sterile bandage.

Posttest measures

1. Obtain and record neurological assessment data every 2 to 4 hours for 24 hours.
2. When iodophenylundecylic acid has been used, the patient remains flat for 6 to 24 hours to prevent or minimize postmylogram headache. When metrizamide has been used, a semi-Fowler's position (15 to 30 degrees) for 8 hours is recommended. NOTE: When metrizamide has been used, flat positioning can precipitate seizures.
3. Administer prescribed analgesics for headache: acetaminophen or aspirin for mild headache, propoxyphene (Darvon) or codeine for more severe ones.
4. When allowed, assist males to stand for voiding.
5. Provide and encourage fluid intake of the patient's preference. Over 2500 ml intake is recommended.
6. Maintain accurate intake/output records for 24 to 48 hours.
7. Assess for distended bladder. The potential for urinary retention is enhanced by immobility.

Table 2-4 Differentiation between contrast materials used in myelography

	Metrizamide (Amipaque)	Iodophenylundecylic acid (Pantopaque)
Composition	Water base	Oil base, iodine
Mechanisms	Upward diffusion superior to injection site	Not diffused
Test procedure	Limited tilting of table	Requires considerable table tilting
Excretion	Urinary, within 72 hours	Removed following myelogram
Nursing observation	Seizure activity if contrast material ascends to cranium*; to prevent cranial ascension: (1) inject slowly, (2) increase hydration before testing	Signs of meningeal irritation: Fever; Headache; Nuchal rigidity
Adverse effects	Mental abberations: disorientation, hallucinations, depression (rare); Visual disturbances; Dysphasia; Chest pain; Dysrhythmias	Neck/back/leg pain that is accentuated by movement; Photophobia

*There is an increased incidence of seizure activity for patients taking phenothiazines.

8. Assess for the adverse effects listed in Table 2-4. Notify the physician if or when they are observed.
9. Provide a restful environment.

PNEUMOENCEPHALOGRAPHY

Pneumoencephalography involves the injection of air into the subarachnoid space. This procedure has largely been replaced by more effective testing procedures. For adults it has been replaced by scanning procedures; in infants by direct ventriculography. This procedure is contraindicated when intracranial pressure is increased.

Purpose

Pneumoencephalography is used to diagnose:

1. Hydrocephalus (Fig. 2-13).
2. Ventricular hypertrophy or neoplasms.
3. Congenital anomalies.
4. Pituitary or posterior fossa tumors.

Patient preparation

Teaching. Inform the patient about the pretest sedation. Food and fluids are withheld for 6 to 8 hours before the procedure. Explain the procedure including the fact that multiple positions (seated, supine, prone, and head-down) with be used. Discuss the common feeling of "bubbling in the brain" that follows the injection of air after a lumbar or cisternal puncture. Inform the patient/family of the common sequela of

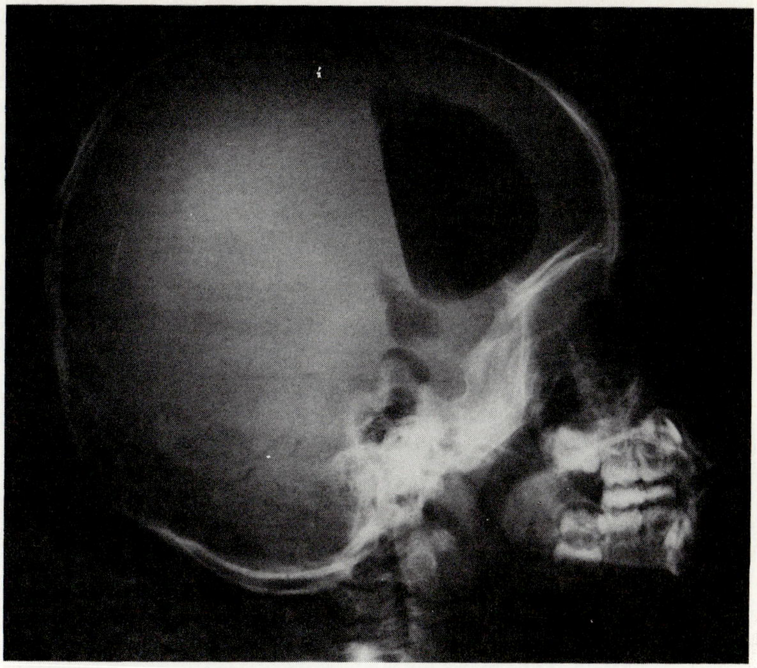

Fig. 2-13 Pneumoencephalogram. Hydrocephalus. (Courtesy Dr. P.D. Mahoney, Radiology Department, St. Joseph Hospital, Omaha, Nebraska.)

headache and about the methods used to prevent or minimize it. Discuss posttest measures.

Physical

1. Withhold food and fluids for 6 to 8 hours before the test to prevent vomiting.
2. Obtain and record baseline neurological assessment data.
3. Remove dentures and hair fasteners.
4. Provide a hospital gown with an open back.
5. Administer prescribed sedatives/hypnotics such as phenobarbital, 100 mg, and atropine, 0.4 mg

Consent. Written consent is obtained after the neurologist thoroughly explains the procedure and the common posttest sequelae.

Procedure

Pneumoencephalography is done in the radiology department by a neurologist. The patient is secured in a chair adjacent to the x-ray machine. Warning: Some elderly

A

B

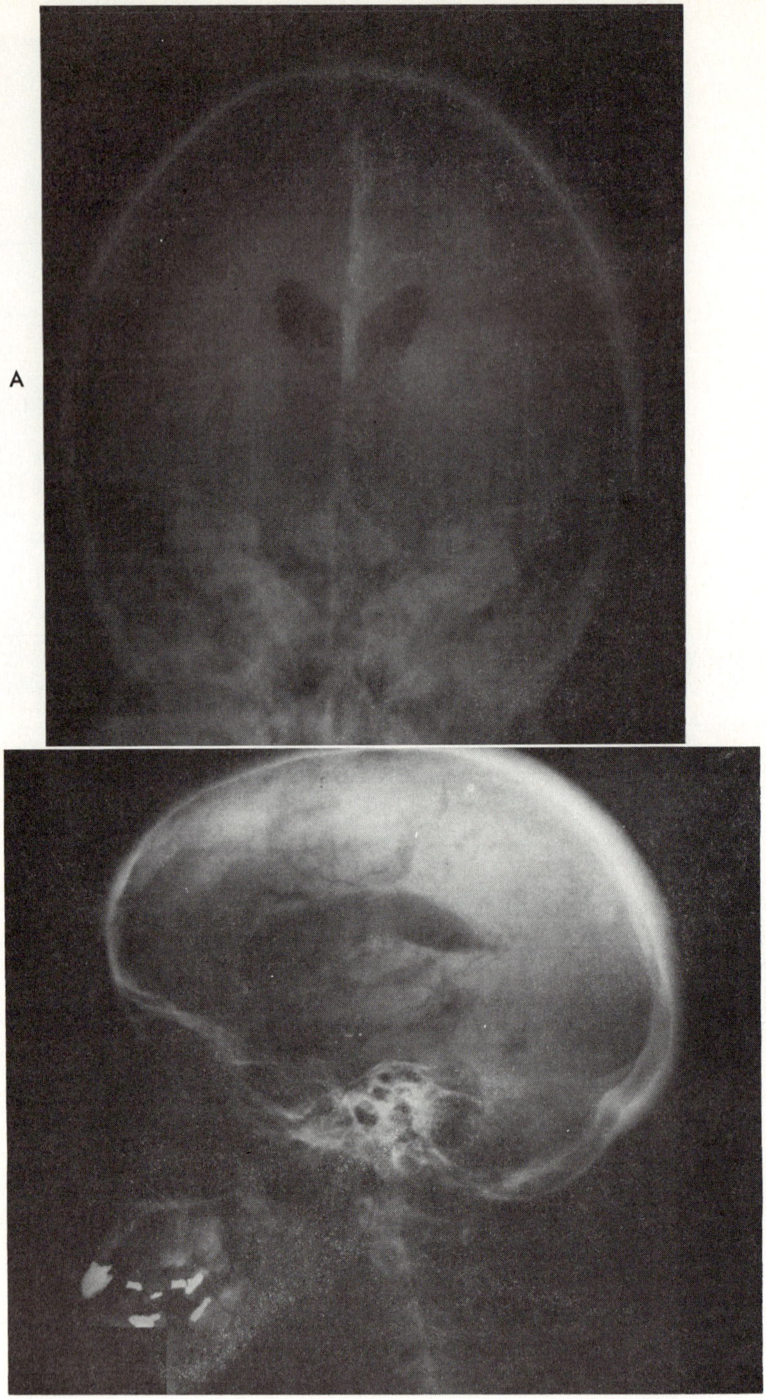

Fig. 2-14 Pneumoencephalogram. **A,** Normal anteroposterior view. **B,** Normal lateral view. (Courtesy Dr. P.D. Mahoney, Radiology Department, St. Joseph Hospital, Omaha, Nebraska.)

patients experience hypotensive syncope during the procedure. With the patient in the seated position, a lumbar or cisternal puncture is done and 5 ml of CSF is removed and replaced by 5 cc of air until 25 ml of CSF has been removed and replaced by 25 cc of air. The spinal needle is then removed and a sterile bandage is applied to the puncture site. Fluoroscopy and x-ray films are taken in the various positions (Fig. 2-14). Following completion of the procedure, which takes 45 to 60 minutes, the patient is returned to his room by cart.

Posttest measures

1. Position the patient flat in bed for 24 to 48 hours.
2. Monitor and record neurological status hourly. Fevers of 101° F are not uncommon for 24 to 48 hours after the test.
3. Administer prescribed analgesics for headache.
4. Provide and encourage fluid intake of 3000 ml every 24 hours for 2 days. NOTE: Citrus juices increase the potential for stomach upset. If oral intake is not possible, intravenous fluids are prescribed and infused.
5. Maintain accurate intake/output records.
6. Administer prescribed antiemetics for nausea/vomiting.
7. Apply an ice cap, as prescribed, to minimize headache.
8. Minimize environmental stimuli (light and noise).
9. Maintain side rails in an up position because of the increased potential for seizures.
10. Observe for and report immediately potential sequelae such as seizure activity or air emboli.

ECHOENCEPHALOGRAPHY

Purpose

Echoencephalography is used to determine:

1. The presence and location of midline (third-ventricle) shift caused by space-occupying lesions.
2. Brain atrophy.

Echoencephalography is a nonspecific diagnostic test. However, because is requires a small amount of time (1 to 5 minutes) and patient participation is not necessary, echoencephalograms are a useful diagnostic method for agitated or comatose patients. Correlation of the echogram with the results of other diagnostic tests is necessary for a definitive diagnosis. CAUTION: Bilateral pathology, which prevents a midline structure shift, yields a normal echoencephalogram.

Patient preparation

Teaching. Inform the patient that the test will be done either in a diagnostic laboratory or in the patient's room. It is done by an echo technician. Explain that a small crystal probe will be secured with a strap to the temporal areas of the head. Show a picture of the placement and the oscilloscope, if available. Inform the patient that he will lie in a supine position on a cart or bed with arms at his sides. The test is painless and takes approximately 5 minutes.

Physical. Remove all hair fasteners. No food or fluid restrictions. No pretest medications.

Consent. Written consent is not required in most agencies because of the noninvasive nature of the test.

Procedure

A crystal probe containing a transducer is secured to the temporal skull bones with a head strap. The probe emits a high frequency sound wave that travels at varying speeds depending on tissue density. The sound waves, which are reflected by the skull bone and the third ventricle, are recorded on an oscilloscope tracing. Time-sequenced instant photographs of the waves on the oscilloscope are obtained to measure deviations from normal. In an adult, a ventricular M-spike shift of 5 mm or more is considered abnormal. With unilateral space-occupying lesions, the M spike shifts away from the lesion (Fig. 2-15).

A

B

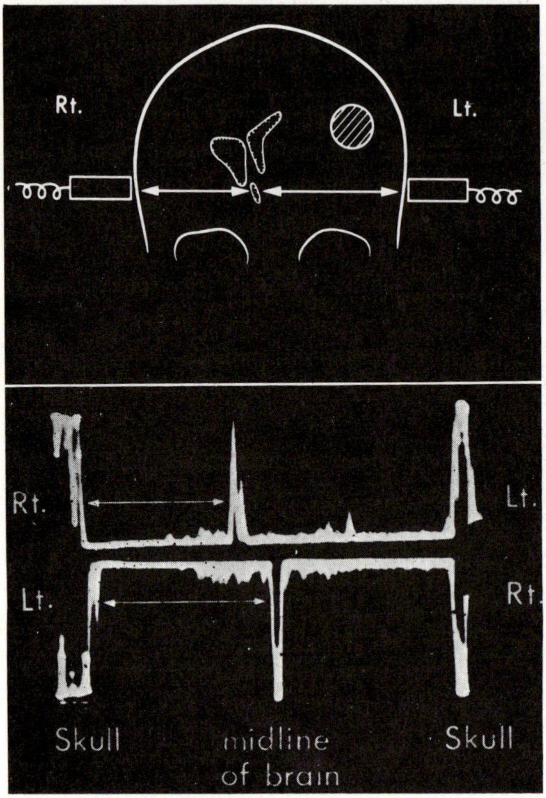

Fig. 2-15 Echoencephalography. **A,** Probe is applied in turn to temporal scalp on back side in case of left-sided mass, causing shift to right. **B,** Polaroid print of oscilloscope tracing, indicating midline closer to right side of skull. (From Jennett, W.B.: In Wells, C., and Kyle, J.: Scientific foundations of surgery, William Heineman Medical Books, Ltd.)

Posttest measures No specific posttest measures.

B-MODE ULTRASOUND SCANNING B-mode ultrasound scanning registers amplified echoes through a surface probe with a transducer, which is placed over the temporal lobe and directed toward the third ventricle. The sound images are converted into electrical impulses and concurrently recorded on an oscilloscope and graph paper. This procedure is most effectively used with infants because of the thinness of their skull bones.

Purpose B-mode ultrasound scanning is used to:

1. Detect shifts of the lateral ventricles associated with expanding lesions.
2. Evaluate the width of the lateral ventricles. If the ventricles are enlarged, either hydrocephalus or diffuse brain atrophy is suspected.

Patient preparation **Teaching.** Inform the patient that this is a noninvasive, painless test. Explain that after being transported to the ultrasound lab, the patient will be positioned on a table and a surface probe will be placed on the skull bone just above and behind the ear. Tell the patient that the probe will be connected to a recording device and that the sound images will be displayed on an oscilloscope and recorded on graph paper. The test takes 30 to 45 minutes.

Physical. No restrictions or special preparations.

Consent. Usually none is required. Check your agency's consent policy.

Procedure A surface probe is either placed on or moved back and forth over the temporal skull area. The probe is connected to a recording device. The ultrasonic waves are converted into electrical impulses and these impulses are seen on the oscilloscope and recorded on graph paper.

Posttest measures None. The patient may resume previous activities.

ELECTROENCEPHALOGRAPHY
Purpose Electroencephalography (EEG) is the graphic recording of electrical activity (brain waves) in specified bilateral cortical areas of the brain. Because of the significant amount of patient participation required, patient cooperation is necessary for accurate results. An EEG is done to:

1. Diagnose epilepsy.
2. Differentiate organic from functional brain dysfunction.
3. Identify the location of vascular infarctions or space-occupying lesions, (tumors, hematomas, abcesses).
4. Diagnose mental retardation or drug overdose.
5. Determine brain death. In many states, three flat EEGs are required before disconnecting patients from life-sustaining equipment.

Patient preparation

Teaching. Inform the patient that EEGs are done in a quiet room in the diagnostic laboratory by an EEG technician. No hair cutting or shaving is required, simply clean hair. Explain that 16 to 24 small electrodes are affixed to the scalp with a pastelike substance. The electrodes are connected to the EEG machine. Show a picture of a patient having an EEG if available. Assure the patient that the 45 to 60 minute procedure is painless and that there is no danger of electrical shock. Correlating EEG testing with the more familiar electrocardiogram procedure can decrease anxiety. The electrical activity only comes *from* the patient. None goes *toward* the patient. Encourage the verbalization of fears or anxieties regarding the EEG to promote the relaxation necessary for accurate results. Explain the patient's part in the procedure including:

1. Sitting or lying in a relaxed, motionless manner in a recliner chair or bed.
2. Following the instructions of the technician:
   a. To hyperventilate for 3 to 5 minutes.
   b. To keep the eyes closed when a flickering light is focused on the patient (photic stimulation).
   c. To sleep. If the patient is unable to sleep, a hypnotic sedative is administered.

Inform the patient that the physician will explain the EEG findings, usually the following day.

Physical

1. Medications such as central nervous system depressants (including alcohol and tranquilizers) or stimulants are withheld for 24 hours before testing because they alter the electrical activity of the brain. If the danger of precipitating seizures is minimal, some physicians withhold anticonvulsant medications 24 to 48 hours before testing.
2. Fluid containing caffeine, such as coffee, colas, and tea, are withheld for 24 hours before EEGs.
3. Hair must be clean and free of sprays, oils, lotions, and hair fasteners.
4. Usually, the patient has breakfast before testing. This is because hypoglycemia causes abnormalities in electrical potentials.
5. Advise the patient to go to sleep later than normal the night previous to the test. Sleeping immediately before the EEG test should be discouraged.

Consent. Written consent is not required in most agencies unless the less common scalp electrode implant method is used. This does not negate the need for a thorough explanation of the procedure.

Procedure

The patient is transported by wheelchair or cart to the EEG diagnostic room. He is positioned in a recliner chair or on a bed and made comfortable. The EEG technician affixes 16 to 24 electrodes in specific locations on the scalp and connects them to the

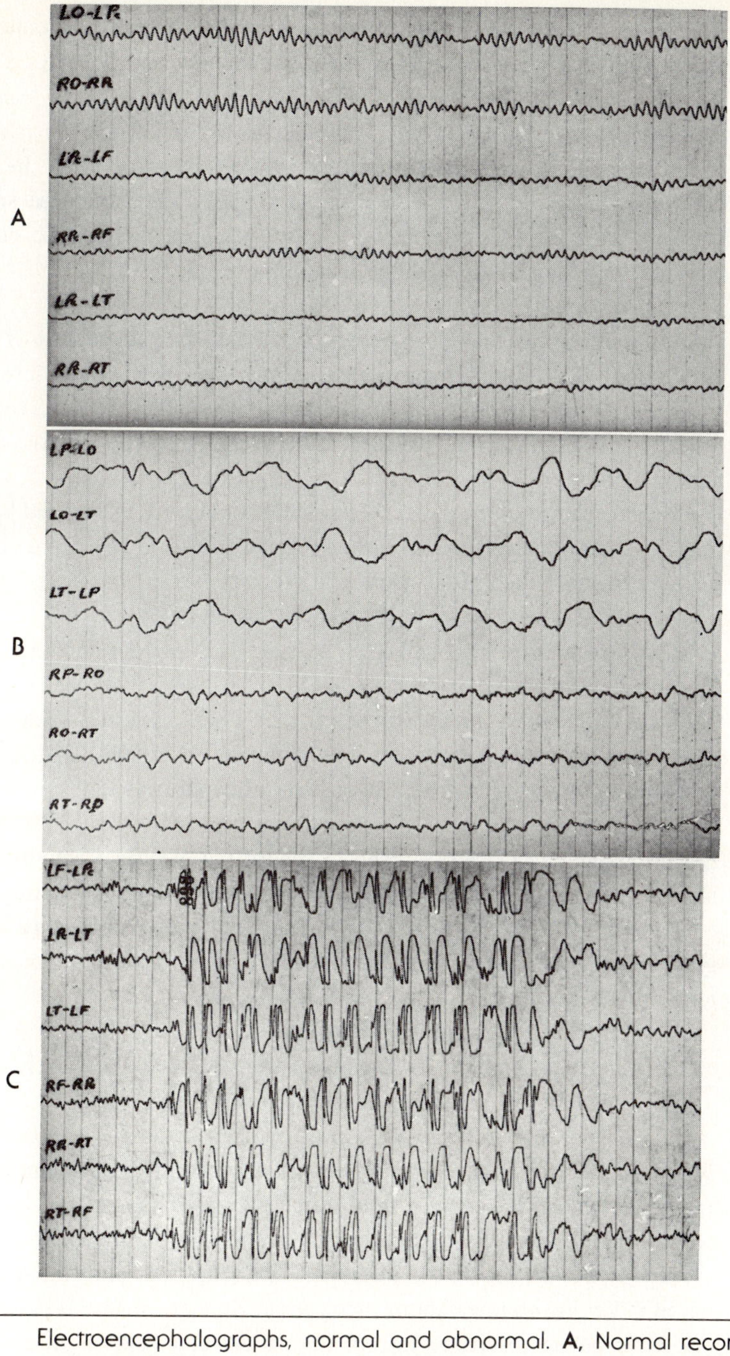

Fig. 2-16 Electroencephalographs, normal and abnormal. **A,** Normal record with regular, 10-per-second alpha waves dominant throughout. **B,** Irregular high-amplitude delta waves (1 to 2 per second) prominent over the left side. This client had intracranial tumor. **C,** Three-per-second, synchronous "spike and dome" waves present in all areas, as seen in minor epilepsy. (From Conway-Rutkowski, B.L.: Carini and Owens' neurological and neurosurgical nursing, ed. 8, St. Louis, 1982, The C.V. Mosby Co.)

lead wires attached to the machine. A baseline printout is obtained. Three testing phases follow: Hyperventilation, photic stimulation, and sleep.

Hyperventilation. The patient is requested to hyperventilate (to take 30 to 40 deep breaths through the mouth per minute) for 3 to 5 minutes. NOTE: Increased serum pH (approximately 7.8) increases neuron excitability and can cause seizure activity in epileptic patients. Electrical activity is recorded on the graphic printout. The time required for return to the baseline reading is noted.

Photic stimulation. A flickering light is focused on the patient, who is asked to keep his eyes closed. This stimulus may cause seizure activity in seizure-prone patients.

Sleep. The patient is asked to sleep. If he is unable to do so, a fast-acting hypnotic is administered.

The recordings of the patient's electrical activity are interpreted by the neurologist. Specific patterns correlate with certain diagnoses (Fig. 2-16). Following the procedure, the patient is returned to his room.

Posttest measures

1. Remove the paste from and wash the hair. Nail polish remover dissolves the paste.
2. Provide a restful environment.
3. Place side rails in the up position if a hypnotic agent has been administered.
4. Administer prescribed medications withheld before the EEG.
5. Observe for seizure activity in seizure-prone patients.

ELECTROMYOGRAPHY

Purpose

Electromyography (EMG) is used to record the electrical activity of the peripheral nerves. Muscles are tested at rest and with minimal and maximal voluntary muscle contractions. The electrical activity is recorded on an oscilloscope and on a print-out graph. The nerves and muscles tested depend on the patient's clinical signs and symptoms. Electromyography is used to diagnose:

1. Muscular dystrophy or other degenerative myopathies.
2. Muscle denervation as a result of specific nerve pathology.
3. Reinnervation and the potential for rehabilitation.

Patient preparation

Teaching. Inform the patient that electromyography is done in a neurodiagnostic laboratory, to which the patient is transported by wheelchair or cart. Explain that discomfort, varying from mild to considerable, is felt during the insertion of sterile needle electrodes into the muscles to be tested. The sensation is much like the feeling experienced in getting an injection of medication. Skin at the injection site is cleansed with antiseptic before insertion. Inform the patient that both slight and maximal muscle contraction and relaxation will be requested by the EMG technician. The length of the test is dependent on the number of neuromuscular testing sites. The usual time required is 30 to 45 minutes.

Table 2-5 **EMG action potentials**

Muscle activity	Normal	Abnormal	Reason
At rest	None	2-10 sec with fasciculations	Lower motor neuron disease
Minimal voluntary contraction	5-10 sec	1-5 sec with fibrillations	Lower motor neuron disease
		Large, polyphasic waves	Irregular nerve regeneration
Maximal voluntary contraction	Numerous	Decreased amplitude and duration of contractions	Muscle disease

Physical. No food or fluid restrictions. No pretest medication except when the patient is apprehensive, in which case a minor tranquilizer is prescribed. The patient should shower before testing. Lotion should not be applied to the skin in test site areas.

Consent. In many agencies written consent is required because of the invasive nature of the test.

Procedure

The skin at needle electrode injection sites is cleansed with an antiseptic agent, such as chlorhexidine gluconate (Hibiclens) or alcohol. The needle electrode is inserted into the muscles to be tested and connected to a recording device. Normal and abnormal action potentials and the type of dysfunction indicated are summarized in Table 2-5. Following completion of the test, the needle electrodes are removed and bandages are applied to insertion sites if necessary. The patient is returned to his room. NOTE: Technicians should be notified if the patient is on anticoagulant therapy so they can anticipate bleeding from needle insertion sites.

Posttest measures

No specific interventions. Check needle electrode insertion sites for signs of inflammation/infection.

NERVE CONDUCTION TIME STUDIES

In some agencies nerve conduction time studies are part of the EMG.

Purpose

Nerve conduction studies are used to measure and compare the excitability and conduction velocity of both the motor and the sensory components of peripheral nerves in the limbs. These studies are useful in determining:

1. Presence or extent of regeneration following peripheral nerve trauma or compression. This is done by comparing the traumatized limb with the uninjured extremity.

2. Extent of peripheral neuropathy caused by metabolic dysfunction, particularly diabetes, nutritional deficiencies, or hepatic disease.
3. Improved nerve conduction following Guillain-Barré syndrome.

Patient preparation

Teaching. Inform the patient that nerve conduction time studies are done in the neurodiagnostic laboratory, usually by a technician or physical therapist. Explain the procedure (see below). Assure the patient that the procedure is painless because electrodes are placed on not under the skin. There is no danger of electrical shock. Results of the test will be explained by the physician following the necessary calculations, which are usually completed within 1 day.

Physical. No food or fluid restrictions. No pretest medication. Skin in the areas to be tested must be clean and free of lotion.

Consent. None required in most agencies.

Procedure

For motor testing two electrodes, one for stimulation and one for recording, are moved and positioned in different areas along the nerve path of both extremities to permit comparison studies. The recording electrode measures the number of seconds it takes for the impulse to travel a specific number of meters. Because of the differing lengths and thicknesses of nerves, motor conduction times vary. Normal conduction times are (1) ulnar and median nerve, 50 to 60 m/second; (2) popliteal nerve, 45 to 55 m/second. Conduction times below 40 m/second correlate with neuropathy.

For sensory testing, the following procedure is used: With sensory electrodes in place, sensory stimulation is applied to an area distal to the point of injury or dysfunction. Sensory action potentials are then measured proximal to the stimuli.

Posttest measures

No specific posttest interventions. Continue monitoring and recording of motor and sensory functions.

COMPUTERIZED EVOKED RESPONSE POTENTIALS

Computerized evoked response potentials (ER or CER) are sensitive neurodiagnostic tests involving the measured stimulation of specific cranial or peripheral nerves with a computerized summation and averaging of the tested nerve's response. Currently the acoustic, optic, and median nerves are being tested. (Adams and Victor, 1981).

Purpose

The purpose of visual evoked response (VER) testing is to:

1. Assess retinal and optic nerve integrity.
2. Determine the location of lesions causing half-field visual losses; that is, to relate a half-field visual loss to a lesion in the anatomical areas of the optic chiasm, visual cortex, or optic nerve radiations.

The auditory evoked response (AER) is used to evaluate acoustic nerve dysfunction. NOTE: Some refer to this test as brainstem auditory evoked response (BAER). The somatosensory evoked response (SSER) differentiates peripheral median nerve dysfunction from cervical cord or brainstem lesions.

Patient preparation

Teaching. Inform the patient that evoked response testing is similar to an EEG and is done in the EEG lab. However, fewer electrodes are used and these are positioned according to the nerve being tested. Tell the patient that he will be positioned on a table or in a recliner chair and that sensory stimulation involving flashing lights (like a strobe light), or clicking sounds, or low-voltage electrical stimuli will be administered. Testing takes 30 to 45 minutes.

Physical. No food, fluid, or activity restrictions. Hair must be clean and free of metal fasteners.

Consent. Usually none is required. Check your agency's consent policy.

Procedure

1. Lead electrodes are affixed to the areas being tested and are attached to the computer.
   a. For AER testing the electrode is placed near the ear.
   b. For VER testing the electrodes are placed near the eyes and on the back of the skull.
   c. For SSEP testing the electrodes are placed on the area below the elbow and high on the back of the neck.
2. The measured stimulation is administered. NOTE: Patients prone to seizure activity should be monitored carefully. For some the photic stimulation precipitates seizure activity.
3. The results are processed by the computer and recorded on graph paper. The averages of the responses are recorded in numerical terms.
4. Following testing the patient is returned to his room.

Posttest measures

None. Patient may resume previous activities.

CALORIC STIMULATION TEST

Purpose

Caloric stimulation testing is done to:

1. Test vestibular function of the acoustic (VIII) nerve.
2. Differentiate cerebellar from brainstem dysfunction.
3. Corroborate the diagnosis of Meniere's syndrome or acoustic neuromas.

Patient preparation

Teaching. Inform the patient that caloric testing is done in the examining room on the unit by the physician. Explain the procedure. Inform the patient that:

1. The physician will use both cold and warm water to irrigate in both ears.
2. Observations for eye movements will be made.
3. The physician will request finger-to-nose and occasionally heel-to-toe testing (Romberg) following the irrigation.
4. Some patients become nauseated, and when that occurs testing is stopped.

Physical

1. Examine both ear drums for intact tympanic membranes. Perforation of the tympanic membrane is a contraindication for this test.
2. Food and fluids are withheld for 8 hours before testing to decrease the potential of vomiting.
3. Assemble necessary equipment in the treatment room:
   Otoscope
   Water thermometer
   Containers with hot (112° F or 44° C) and cold (86° F or 30° C) water
   Irrigation set-up, IV stand, and large bore irrigation tip
   Ear syringe
   Emesis basin
   Stopwatch
   Two chairs
   Caloric testing flow sheet
   Cotton for drying ear
   Towels and rubber apron or sheeting
4. Have the patient void and then transport him to the examining room by wheelchair.
5. Assist the patient to a seated position with the head tilted forward 30 degrees for vertical canal testing and drape him with protective covering.
6. Assist in changing the head position (to 60 degrees backward) for horizontal canal testing.

Consent. Written consent is not usually necessary. Check your agency's policy.

Procedure

The ear on the affected side is tested first to ensure accurate data.

Vertical testing

1. Position the patient with the head tilted forward 30 degrees. Ask the patient to fix his gaze forward on a specific object.
2. Cold fluid is directed into the auditory canal on the affected side initially. Normally within 30 seconds nystagmus and complaints of nausea and dizziness occur.
3. The direction of nystagmus is recorded. Normal with cold water is downward and away. With warm water it is upward and toward the irrigated ear. No nystagmus is an abnormal finding. The diagnostic significance of caloric testing is summarized in Table 2-6.

Horizontal testing. Reposition the patient with the head tilted backward 60 degrees. Patient must fix his gaze forward before the irrigation. Direct 250 ml of irrigation fluid (cold followed by warm) into the auditory canal for 30 seconds or until symptoms of nystagmus, nausea, or dizziness appear. Maximum irrigation time is 3 minutes. With warm water the gaze is *toward* the irrigated ear. With cold water the gaze is *away from*

Table 2-6 Caloric testing responses

Water temperature	Irrigated ear	Time before nystagmus appears	Direction of nystagmus	Type of nystagmus	Diagnosis
30° C	Left	2 min	To right	Rapid	Normal response
	Right	2 min	To left	Rapid	
44° C	Left	1 min	To left	Slow	
	Right	30 sec	To right	Slow	
30° C	Left	2 min	To right	Rapid	
	Right	15 sec	To left	Rapid	Acoustic neuroma
44° C	Left	1 min	To left	Slow	
	Right	45 sec	To right	Slow	
30° C	Left	45 sec	To right	Rapid	
	Right	2 min 15 sec	To left	Rapid	
44° C	Left	2 min	To left	Slow	Temporal lobe neoplasm
	Right	45 sec	To right	Slow	
30° C	Left	3 min		None; slow	
	Right	3 min		None; slow	Meniere's syndrome
44° C	Left	3 min		None; slow	
	Right	3 min		None; slow	

the irrigated ear. A 5-minute wait between irrigation of the ears is recommended. Times, symptoms (nystagmus, dizziness, nausea, vomiting), and patient responses to requests for finger to nose and heel to toe (Romberg) are recorded. Following the procedure the patient's ears are dried, the protective draping is removed, and the patient is returned to his room by wheelchair.

Posttest measures

1. Bed rest with the head elevated for 1 to 3 hours is prescribed.
2. Provide a quiet environment, tissues, and an emesis basin.
3. Observe for nausea, vomiting, dizziness.
4. Initial safety measures: Put the side rails up and provide assistance with mobility for patients experiencing dizziness.
5. Resume pretest diet and activity after 2 to 3 hours or when symptoms disappear.

Alternative methods

The Hallpike method of caloric testing requires a shorter time and an increased force of water flow. In Nelson's method a small amount (0.2 ml) of ice water is used.

ELECTRONYSTAGMOGRAPHY
Purpose

Electronystagmography is an electronic test used as an alternative to or to substantiate findings of caloric testing. It decreases subjectivity in determining the presence and type of nystagmus.

Patient preparation

Teaching. Inform the patient that the test is done in the diagnostic laboratory by a technician with the patient lying on a couch. Small electrodes are affixed to the skin near the eyes and attached to a recording machine. Eye movements are recorded on graph paper. Inform the patient that positional changes will be requested during testing. In some agencies cold- and warm-water ear irrigation (0.2 ml) is used as a stimulus.

Physical. No food, fluid, or activity restrictions before testing.

Consent. Written consent is usually not required. Check your agency's policy.

Procedure

Patient is in a supine position. Electrodes are affixed with a pastelike substance to the skin near the eyes and attached to the recording machine. Eyes must remain closed. Either positional changes or caloric testing or both provide the stimulus. Eye movements are recorded on graph paper as either fast or slow nystagmus.

Posttest measures

No specific interventions. Pretest activities may be resumed.

EDROPHONIUM TESTING

Purpose

Edrophonium (Tensilon) testing is done to:

1. Diagnose acetylcholine deficiency at the myoneural junction (myasthenia gravis).
2. Differentiate between myasthenia gravis and Bell's palsy, muscular dystrophy, or hypotonia caused by carcinoma or myositis.

Patient preparation

Teaching. Testing is done in the patient's room. An intravenous injection of edrophonium is administered by the physician. Within 1 minute the limb, eye, and facial muscles of myasthenia gravis patients will respond to volition, and an improvement in muscle tone will be observed. Because of the short duration of its action, edrophonium is used solely for diagnostic and not for therapeutic reasons. In the myasthenic patient pretest hypotonia reoccurs within 5 minutes.

Physical. No food, fluid, or activity restrictions.

Consent. Because of the possibility of cholinergic crisis, most agencies require written informed consent.

Procedure

Before initiating this test, have atropine, 0.6 mg, drawn up in a syringe. Edrophonium chloride, total dosage of 10 mg, is injected intravenously using the following schedule:

1. Initially inject 2 mg within 30 seconds.
2. Test muscle strength. Wait 1 minute.
3. Inject 3 mg over the next 30 seconds.
4. Test muscle strength. Wait 1 minute.

5. Inject 5 mg.
6. Test muscle strength.

Within 1 minute of injection, voluntary muscle activity is improved and facial and eye muscle tone is increased dramatically. This dramatic improvement lasts less than 5 minutes. CAUTION: During edrophonium testing, patients taking anticholinesterase medication (neostigmine, pyridostigmine, ambenonium) should be observed for signs and symptoms of cholinergic crisis. If such signs and symptoms occur, the atropine is administered.

Alternative procedure. The neostigmine test is used as an alternative procedure. Neostigmine, 1.5 mg, and atropine, 0.6 mg, are given intramuscularly. A dramatic improvement in muscle tone and motor ability is observed within 10 to 45 minutes, particularly in the limbs. The positive neuromuscular effects last for 4 to 5 hours.

Posttest measures

Observe for the return of decreased volitional muscle power and muscle tone. Resume pretest food, fluid, and activities. For patients with myasthenia gravis, provide encouragement and emotional support when signs and symptoms return.

INTRACRANIAL PRESSURE MONITORING

Currently, intracranial pressure (ICP) can be monitored with three types of devices: (1) intraventricular catheters or cannulas; (2) subarachnoid screws; (3) epidural fiberoptic sensors. Although these methods are primarily employed to objectify clinical patient assessment, the intraventricular catheter and subarachnoid screw also have therapeutic uses. They can be used to (1) drain excessive CSF; (2) obtain serial CSF samples for laboratory examination; and (3) administer medications such as diuretics, steroids, barbiturates, or antibiotics.

Purpose

These devices are used to monitor changes in ICP. The sensor, catheter, cannula, or screw is attached to a transducer through which pressure changes are recorded on an oscilloscope and/or on graph paper. Intracranial monitoring is employed when:

1. Suspicion of cerebral edema, hematoma, or hemorrhage exists.
2. Clinical signs and symptoms of increasing ICP or an expanding lesion are observed.
3. Obstruction of CSF flow, as with hydrocephalus, is suspected.
4. Uncal or brainstem herniation is suspected.
5. The effectiveness of clinical management (as with barocoma, osmotic diuretics) needs to be assessed.

Patient preparation

Teaching

1. Inform the patient and family that the physician will explain the procedure, which is generally done in surgery.
2. Show a picture of a monitored patient or the equipment to be used. Correlate this procedure with the more familiar cardiac monitoring.

3. Demonstrate the position that is essential to accurate monitoring; that is, a semi-Fowler's position with a head elevation of 15 to 30 degrees. NOTE: Hip flexion of over 80 degrees can result in inaccurate readings. Neck flexion is prohibited and this necessitates immobilization of the head. The prone position is also contraindicated. All of these positions cause an increase in ICP.
4. Explain the need to avoid certain activities and the means used to prevent or minimize their possible occurrence:
   a. Valsalva maneuver: Stool softeners not enemas are used.
   b. Holding breath during position changes: Exhale slowly when changing position.
   c. Neck flexion: Trochanter rolls or small sandbags are placed on both sides of the neck.
   d. Extertion causing muscle contraction: Assistance in position changes and passive range of motion exercises will be provided.
   e. Pooling and hardening of secretions in the throat: Fluids are provided at regular intervals and oral/pharangeal suctioning is provided as necessary.
   f. Vomiting: Medications to reduce nausea (antiemetics) are prescribed. In some instances a nasogastric tube is inserted and connected to low-grade suction.
5. Explain that normal activities, such as breathing and REM sleep, cause expected fluctuations in pressure.
6. Reinforce that the usual length of time for intracranial monitoring is 2 days to 3 weeks. The average length is 7 days. No posttest disfigurement occurs.

Physical

1. Wash hair if dirty. Cut hair in 3 to 5 cm area at the insertion site.
2. Prepare the insertion site: Shave area and scrub for 3 to 5 minutes with antiseptic.
3. Complete the preoperative care consistent with agency policies.

Consent. Because of the invasive nature of intracranial monitoring, informed written consent is required following a thorough explanation by the physician.

Procedure

The procedure varies slightly depending on the device being used.

Intraventricular catheter or cannula. Following a surgical scrub of the insertion site, a burr hole is made on the lateral aspect of the cranium in the nondominant hemisphere (Fig. 2-17). A catheter or cannula is inserted into the lateral ventricle. The catheter or cannula is connected via a stopcock to pressure tubing with a transducer. This is attached to monitoring equipment and provides for direct measurement of CSF pressure within the lateral ventricle. A sterile dressing is placed around the catheter or cannula. The disadvantages of using intraventricular catheters or cannulas are (1) difficulty in placement when a ventricular shift has occurred, (2) infection, and (3) difficulty in maintaining patency. In infants the burr hole is not necessary. The catheter or cannula is passed through an incision made over the fontanel.

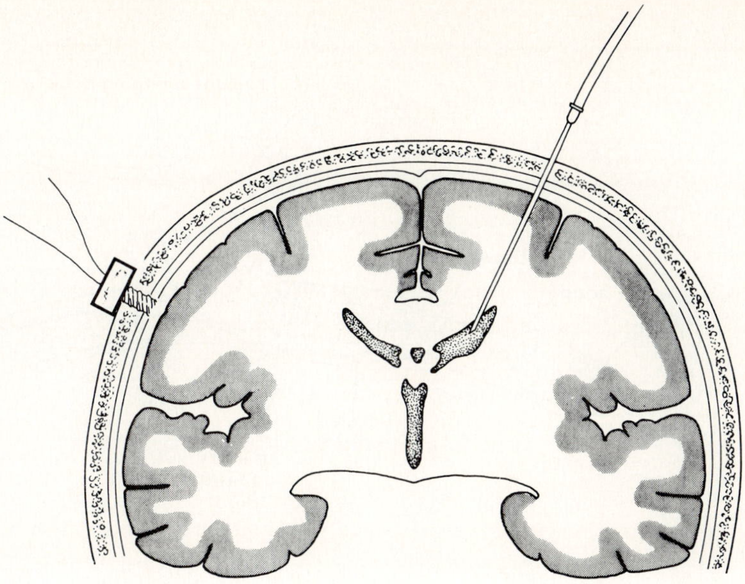

Fig. 2-17 Subarachnoid screw monitoring (left) and intraventricular (right) devices for measuring intracranial pressure. Both require attachment to transducer using a stopcock and/or pressure tubing. (From Budassi, S.A., and Barber, J.M.: Emergency nursing: principles and practice, St. Louis, 1981, The C.V. Mosby Co.)

Subarachnoid screw. Following a surgical scrub, a ⅜-inch drill burr hole is made in the superior frontal cranium over the dural sinuses. A screw device (Viries) is twisted into the hole. A sterile three-way stopcock, which is connected to pressure tubing and a transducer, is attached to the screw and connected to the monitoring equipment (Fig. 2-17). A sterile dressing or collodion is placed around the insertion site. The disadvantages of the subarachnoid screw are (1) its infection potential; (2) when occluded it requires flushing with intravenous saline by experienced personnel; and (3) it cannot be used for children under 5 years of age because of skull bone instability.

Epidural sensor. The major advantage of epidural monitoring is that it does not require invasion below the protective dura. A pressure- and light-sensitive membrane sensor is implanted between the skull and dura through a burr hole (Fig. 2-18). The sensor is then connected to a transducer and recording device.

Posttest measures

1. Following return from the surgery department, attach tubing to the monitoring/recording devices.

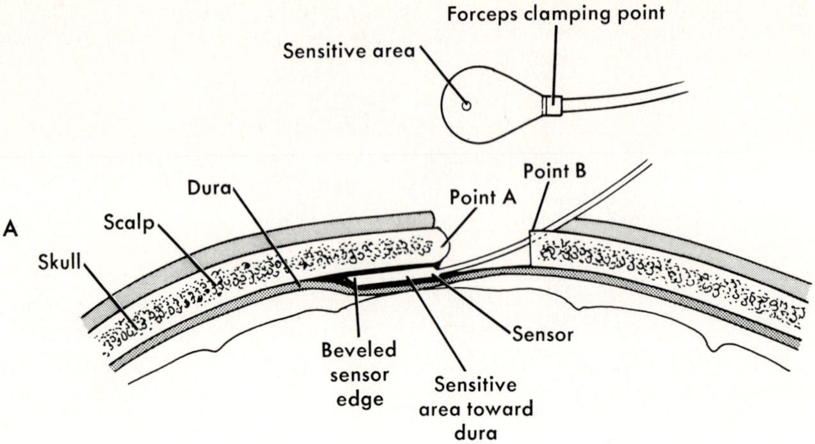

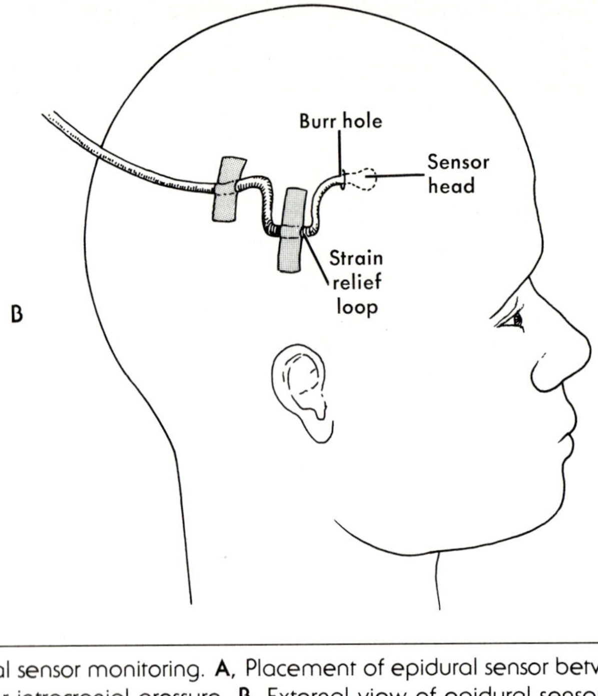

Fig. 2-18 Epidural sensor monitoring. **A,** Placement of epidural sensor between skull and dura to monitor intracranial pressure. **B,** External view of epidural sensor. (From Budassi, S.A., and Barber, J.M.: Emergency nursing: principles and practice, St. Louis, 1981, The C.V. Mosby Co.)

Table 2-7 Flushing procedure for subarachnoid screw

Indications:	Flat waves; rounded peaks; straight lines; tubing leaks
Procedure:	1. From flush intravenous saline solution, withdraw 0.1 ml into the syringe. 2. Attach syringe to stopcock. 3. Open stopcock to syringe. 4. Infuse 0.1 ml saline very slowly. 5. Reposition stopcock to open between screw and monitor. 6. Check waves on monitor.
Precautions:	1. Use strict aseptic technique. 2. Use of more than 0.1 ml saline should be done by the physician. 3. If single flushing does not yield results, consult physician. 4. Always return stopcock to original recording position.

2. Calibrate the subarachnoid or ventricular transducer according to the manaufacturer's directions.
3. Position the patient with the head elevated 15 to 30 degrees. Position the patient to ensure that there is no hip or neck flexion.
4. Follow your agency procedures for flushing the cannula or subarachnoid screw. Table 2-7 details the indications, procedures, and precautions for the flushing process.
5. Assess and record clinical neurological data hourly.
6. Check the insertion site four times daily for signs of infection.
7. Aseptically change dressings surrounding insertion site following cleansing with hydrogen peroxide or prescribed antiseptic.
8. Interpret readings and notify physician of abnormalities (Fig. 2-19).
9. Recognize patient conditions and activities, such as the following, which cause transient alterations in ICP:
   a. Causes of increased ICP
      (1) Defecation
      (2) Coughing
      (3) Airway obstruction
      (4) Abdominal breathing
      (5) Vomiting
      (6) Suctioning
      (7) REM sleep
      (8) Position changes and the supine position
      (9) Muscle exertion or tensing
      (10) Active range of motion exercises
   b. Causes of decreased ICP
      (1) Inspiration

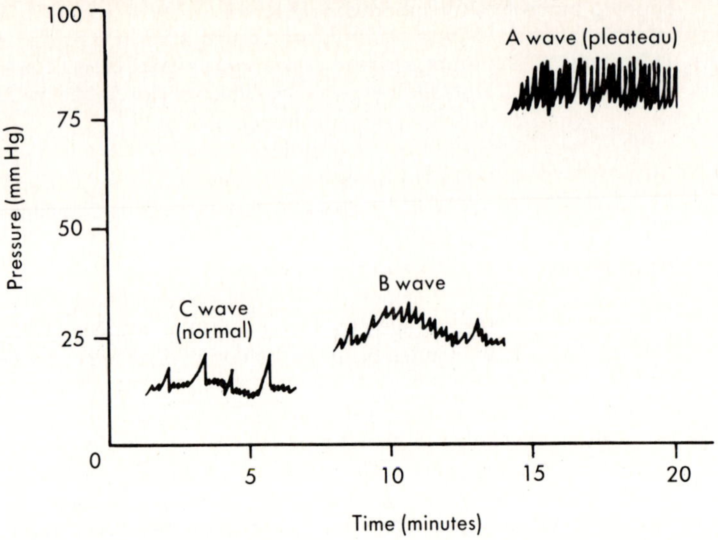

Fig. 2-19 ICP monitoring parameters.

(2) Central nervous system depressant medications, including analgesics and tranquilizers.

10. Schedule activities causing increases in ICP, such as suctioning or position changes, at intervals.
11. Change flushing tubing and saline solution every 24 hours.
12. Encourage deep-breathing by patient every 2 hours.
13. Administer prescribed medications including steroids and prophylactic antibiotics.
14. Provide adequate nutrition: soft, easily masticated and digested foods for oriented patients; gavage with nutritionally balanced solutions for nonoriented, comatose patients.
15. Observe for leakage in system. If leakage occurs:
    a. Clamp tubing with hemostat as close to the screw or catheter insertion site as possible.
    b. Notify the physician immediately.
    c. Close the stopcock and cover leaking area with sterile dressings.
16. Maintain normal body functions in order to prevent common dysfunctions such as:
    a. Loss of skin integrity.
    b. Joint deformity.
    c. Malnutrition.
    d. Underhydration or overhydration.
    e. Elimination dysfunction.

17. Provide a calm environment:
    a. Limit stimuli such as light or noise.
    b. Explain all procedures before their initiation.
    c. Use an emphathetic approach with the patient and family.
    d. Remind the patient and family of the purpose of the monitoring and the usual time frame.
    e. Reinforce the fact that there is no change in physical appearance following removal of monitoring devices.

Suggested readings

Adams, R., and Victor, M.: Principles of neurology, New York, 1981, McGraw-Hill Book Co.

Alterman, P., editor: An overview of NMR in medicine, NCHCT Monograph Series, Washington, D.C., 1981, U.S. Department of Health and Human Services.

Bickerstaff, E.: Neurological examination in clinical practice, ed. 4, Oxford, 1980, Blackwell Scientific Publications, Ltd.

Conway-Rutkowski, B.: Carini and Owens' Neurological and neurosurgical nursing, ed. 8, St. Louis, 1982, The C.V. Mosby Company.

Criss, E.: Digital subtraction angiography (DSA), Am. J. Nurs. **82:**1706-1707, 1982.

Haughey, C.: What to say and do when your patient asks about C.T. scans, Nursing81 **11:**72-77, Dec., 1981.

Hickey, J.: The clinical practice of neurological and neurological nursing, 1981, Phildelphia, J.B. Lippincott Co.

Lyons, M., and Wilson, D.: Regional cerebral blood flow—a newer non-invasive neurodiagnostic test, J. Neurosurg. Nurs. **13:**286-293, 1981.

O'Reilly, B.: Preparing the patient for computerized tomograpy, J. Neurosurg. Nurs. **11:**41, 1979.

Tilkian, S., Conover, M., and Tilkian, A.: Clinical implications of laboratory tests, ed. 2, St. Louis, 1979, The C.V. Mosby Company.

CHAPTER 3

Alterations in comfort: pain

Pain is a common manifestation of many disease conditions. Pain is the response to a stimulus that occurs either from within the organism or from an external environmental source. The organism perceives this stimulus as a feeling of discomfort that may be a threat to the total integrity of that person. Pain is an individualized, unpleasant experience that can only be shared with others as a subjective event. The individual experiencing pain is the only one who can fully know the sensation of his pain.

Pain is a common patient-care problem that is associated with a large number of organic disorders. The management of pain is a challenge to the practitioner, and the nurse learns to assess, interpret responses to pain, and utilize the nursing process to apply interventions to provide relief of pain.

PATHOPHYSIOLOGY

Pain perception

The nurse must understand the anatomical and physiological bases for pain in order to understand pain and its effect on the individual, since the experience of pain is expressed in a person's behavior. Simply described, pain is a feeling, sensation, or warning. It is initiated at the cellular level and is communicated to the brain via the spinal cord through afferent fibers. The end result is the behavior of the person in response to pain.

Perception variables

The integrity of the nervous system influences pain perception. Perception is the point at which the individual perceives the pain experienced. Pain is a means of calling attention to the individual as well as alerting the individual to other internal problems related to disease processes or other disorders. If the individual is fatigued, angry, lonely, or bored, pain perception is increased. There are numerous other variable factors that influence pain perception. These variables include:

1. Altered consciousness that is associated with analgesics, anesthesia, or cerebral disturbances resulting from hypoxia or trauma.
2. Threshold level, which is the perception of the intensity of pain. Sociocultural factors can influence pain tolerance level for individuals. Pain is present when stimuli to the pain receptors reach a predetermined threshold level.
3. Age. In children the nervous system is immature and pain perception is different from in adults. Likewise, deterioration of the nervous system in elderly individuals affects pain perception.
4. Pain tolerance, which is variable among individuals because of the self-concept and body image conceptualized by those individuals.

5. Absence of pain, which occurs in individuals who have experienced a physiological trauma or a chemical or surgical transection of a part of the nervous system that makes transmission of pain impulses to the brain impossible. These persons, having lost the ability to perceive pain, have a high risk of injury.
6. Sociocultural factors, which include an individual's religious, cultural, and philosophical background.
7. Personality and the ability to cope with pain and life stresses.
8. Previous pain experience.
9. Pain trajectory or the expected painful experiences as perceived by the individual.
10. Pain control, which is dependent on the individual's ability to cope.
11. Anxiety, which is a major influence on pain perception. Anxiety may be an outward expression of pain, or persons with high anxiety levels may tolerate pain more poorly and be more vulnerable to painful experiences. Persons with chronic pain undergo mental and physical deterioration and increase their anxiety level. Reduction of anxiety is a prime focus of nursing intervention.
12. Females and males usually react differently to pain. Cultures allow women to express pain more fully through emotional outlets. However, the question of which gender is more tolerant of pain is not resolved.
13. Environmental factors that influence pain perception including the time of day and activity. Persons perceive pain more intensely at night and in darkness because of fear. When individuals are more active, they seem to have a better self-image and feel better about themselves, and pain experiences are lessened. Weather conditions affect pain perception, especially cold and damp environments.
14. Birth order. Some theories indicate that the firstborn may be less tolerant of pain because of inexperienced parents who overemphasized concern with minor painful incidents (Jones, Dunbar, and Jirovec, 1978).

Theories

The nature of pain has been controversial for years. There are three common theories of pain perception: (1) specificity theory; (2) pattern theory; and (3) gate control system. The gate theory will be defined here because it is the basis for current pain management techniques. The gate theory was developed by Melzack and Wall. According to this theory, there is a special gating mechanism that is made up of large and small fibers, of substantia gelatinosa cells, and of transmission or T cells. Pain travels from the periphery to the central nervous system via T cells located in the spinal cord. Peripheral afferent nerve fibers are either large or small in diameter. These cells either facilitate or inhibit the transmission of afferent impulses to the T cells. The substantia gelatinosa cells extend the length of the spinal cord. Large-fiber impulses stimulate the substantia gelatinosa activity and inhibit T-cell activity (closed gate). Small-fiber impulses inhibit substantia gelatinosa activity and facilitate T-cell transmission (open

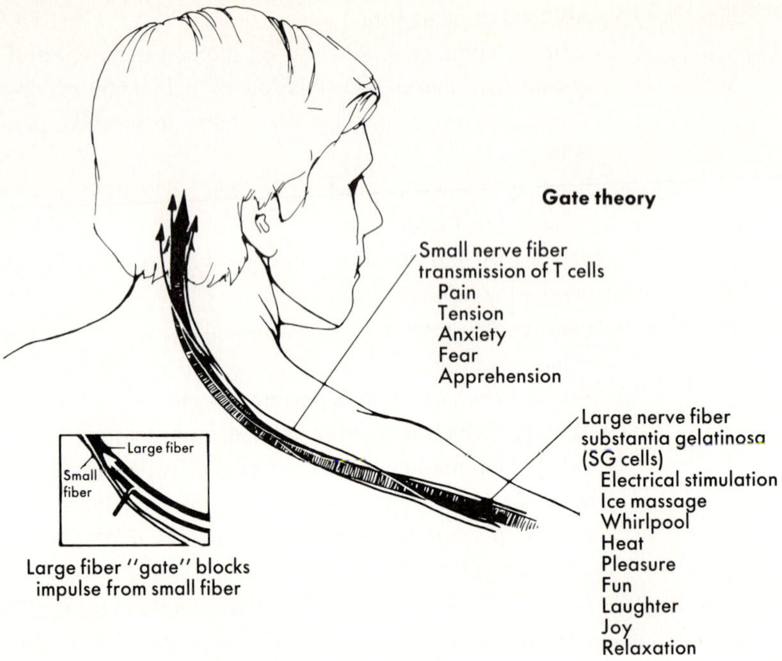

Fig. 3-1 Schematic illustration to demonstrate what stimuli facilitate or inhibit the transmission of afferent impulses to the brain. This is based on the gate theory of pain management. The small fibers allow stimuli to reach the brain and the large fibers "close" the gate and inhibit transmission of stimuli.

gate). The gate theory then is based on the fact that large fibers close the gate and small fibers open the gate. Through this mechanism the psychological and physiological aspects of pain are balanced (Fig. 3-1).

A new key to understanding pain is the endorphins. Endorphins are chemical compounds located in various body parts, and particularly where the neural transmission of pain is mediated. Endorphins possess an opiatelike property and inhibit the transmission of painful stimuli at various points along the central nervous system. Chemically, the endorphins are peptides. The parent molecule of the endorphins is beta-lipotropin, which is 1 of the 91 amino acids that make up the opiatelike compounds identified as endorphins and enkephalins (Wilson and Elmassian, 1981).

Endorphins as natural pain relievers were first identified in 1970 in animal brain receptors (Wilson and Elmassian, 1981). More research needs to be done to link the functions of the brain and the central nervous system in the perception and response to pain. One group of researchers discovered that patients with high tolerance and pain thresholds had above average levels of endorphins in their cerebrospinal fluid (Wilson and Elmassian, 1981). If endorphins could be synthetically manufactured, a possibly nonaddicting analgesic could be available for pain control, which would be a monumental breakthrough in pain management.

ETIOLOGY

Sources of pain may be physiological or psychic in nature and are dependent upon the variables that affect the perception of pain:

Sources of pain

Physical

1. External environment (such as heat and cold)
2. Physical trauma
   a. Cuts
   b. Inflammation or infection
   c. Force to body
   d. Hemorrhage
   e. Pressure

Internal environment

1. Organic disorders
2. Childbirth
3. Pathological processes
4. Muscle spasms
5. Cellular obstruction or ischemia
6. Calculi
7. Distention in ducts or canals
8. Fluid accumulation and fluid loss (such as a spinal-tap-caused headache).
9. Cramps
   a. Menstrual
   b. Constipation
   c. Labor contractions
10. Chemical irritation

Psychological

1. Tension
2. Stressful situations
3. Emotional response or coping mechanism
4. Phantom pain (a pain that persists after destruction of the neural pathways, such as following amputation of a limb)
5. Psychic pain resulting from overwhelming sorrow and grief

Environmental

1. Noise
2. Drafts and wind

CLASSIFICATIONS

Acute pain

Pain is described as acute or chronic. Acute pain is of a severe nature and occurs unexpectedly. Acute pain is associated with anxiety, such as in anticipation of scheduled therapies, diagnostic tests, surgical procedures, or childbirth, as well as the anxiety provoked by fear or a threat to body integrity. The anxiety accompanying acute pain affects the coping mechanisms of the individual experiencing pain. Acute pain is managed by eliminating the source of pain, comfort measures, decreasing anxiety, reducing the stimulus, altering the perception of the painful stimuli, and increasing pain tolerance.

Chronic pain

Chronic pain is prolonged over a period of time, usually greater than 6 months. It is (1) pain associated with terminal illnesses that are pain producing; (2) pain that is caused by organic conditions that do not respond to therapy; and (3) pain that is primarily psychogenic in origin and that has become an adaptive behavior for the individual. The managment of chronic pain is more involved than the management of acute pain because it deals with a multiplicity of health care problems.

Pain clinics. In the past decade pain management programs have been developed for the management of chronic pain. The focus of these programs is on the long-term physical and emotional disability produced by chronic pain. Persons seeking treatment in these pain clinics are physically incapacitated and suffer emotional turmoil and degeneration of the total holistic integrity of the body. Many also suffer from drug abuse problems as a result of their pain. These individuals have suffered pain for such a long period that their activities are greatly reduced, and they are no longer productive members of society.

The success of the pain management program is dependent upon the desire of the individual to gain independence and improve his self-concept. Motivation is the key to effecting the change necessary for the individual to alter his life style. Encouragement and support from family will facilitate the achievement of independence and wellness sought by the individual desiring to change.

The focus of the pain management program is on the whole individual. The patient is not sick, but disabled. The program is designed to replace the symptoms displayed by chronic pain and bring about the change in life-style. Independence and assertiveness are stressed in the program. The patient enters the program to help himself. A rigid schedule of activities including swimming, walking laps, exercises, and self-control are emphasized. Through a structured program involving both the patient and his family, the patient can overcome the disabilities caused by pain.

The primary goals of the pain management program are the readjustment of the physical state of the patient by use of physical conditioning, release from drug dependence, and recognition and release of the emotional stress that prolonged suffering can place on the individual and his relationships. Pain management in structured pain clinics is a new field of nursing practice. The nurse in this setting meets a challenging reward when interventions help patients conquer chronic pain.

The holistic person is considered in planning interventions to utilize in a pain management program. The emotional, physical, social, and sexual factors are all considered in the establishment of realistic individual goals for the patient in achieving a new life-style. Therapeutic measures such as relaxation, stimulators, biofeedback, contracting, ventilation about pain (''pain talk''), placebos, and heat and cold therapies are all instituted in assisting the patient to overcome his disability. A strong involvement with the family structure and its members must be included. Pain management programs use a multidisciplinary approach involving the physician, nurse, physical therapist, and psychologist. All of this can lead to a successful program in creating the emergence of a happy, independent individual who has a positive self-concept.

Headache

Headache is a common type of pain. This is a surprising phenomenon since most of the cranial structures are not sensitive to pain. Areas that are insensitive to pain include the skull, parenchyma of the brain, a large portion of the dura and pia mater, the ependymal lining of the ventricles, and the choroid plexus. Cranial areas sensitive to pain include:

- Intracranial structures
  - Afferent veins
  - Cranial sinuses
  - Arteries of the dura mater
  - Arteries and major branches at the base of the brain
  - Portions of the dura mater near large vessels
- Extracranial structures
  - Mucosa
  - Arteries
  - Muscles
  - Fascia
  - Scalp
  - Skin
- Nerves
  - Second and third cervical nerves
  - Trigeminal, facial, glossopharyngeal, and vagal cranial nerves

Pathways of headaches arise in structural areas from either above or below the tentorium (see Fig. 3-2). Pain in areas above the tentorium is transmitted through the trigeminal nerve and experienced in the parietal, temporal, or frontal aspects of the brain. Pain that originates from the area below the tentorium is transmitted through the upper cervical spinal roots and the glossopharyngeal and vagal nerves. This pain is expressed in the occipital portion of the brain.

Three broad categories of headaches are related to the underlying mechanisms that cause them. These include:

1. Intracranial problems
   a. Meningeal processes (encephalitis meningitis).

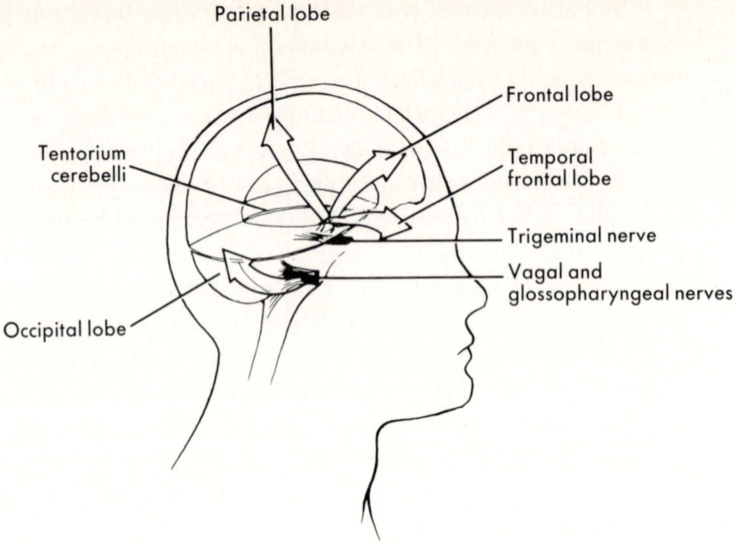

Fig. 3-2 Schematic drawing of the transmission of headache pain to specific lobes of the brain, showing the cranial nerves that transmit the stimuli to the brain lobes where pain is expressed.

b. Decreases in intracranial pressure (ICP) that occur after a spinal tap or pneumoencephalogram.

c. Hematomas, tumors, abscesses, aneurysms, hemorrhage, increased ICP.

2. Extracranial problems. The pain is a result of direct stimulation to the pain sensitive structures, of vascular and muscle contractions, or of referred pain from spasms in another area. These types of pain occur in the eye, nasal sinuses, teeth, mouth, ears, cervical spine, and neck and head muscles, and from inflammation of the cranial arteries.
3. Generalized conditions. Arterial hypertension resulting from the dilation of the entry and exit cranial arteries with the addition of edema. These headaches are produced by pyrexia, anoxia, intoxication, and vasodilators such as alcohol, nitrates, and histamines.

For simplicity in understanding the types of headaches and successful nursing intervention for each group, Table 3-1 defines the three major groups of headaches. These groups are vascular, psychogenic, and traction-inflammatory. Alternate methods of classifying headaches include muscle contraction and tension, which correlate with vascular and psychogenic. The table also discusses the causes and therapy for facial pain.

Table 3-1 Headaches: classifications, causes, and therapy

Classification	Cause	Therapy
Vascular headaches		
1. *Migraine* a. Familial "sick headache": These occur more in women with onset at puberty and with termination at menopause; however, they may occur in childhood and continue throughout a life span. Symptoms: visual hallucinations, transitional impaired vision; severe, unilateral throbbing pain; vomiting; strange odors; tingling in the arm; sudden euphoric feeling. b. Common migraine: Aura is nondescript or absent. c. Cluster headaches: These involve severe unilateral pain that occurs at approximately the same time each day and may last for weeks up to months, then disappear for years. They occur most often in males age 20-40. Pain affects the eye of the affected side and is accompanied with tearing, runny nose, perspiration, drooping eyelids, or constricted pupils. These headaches are seasonal and are believed to be related to an allergic reaction.	Caused by intracranial vasoconstriction followed by extracranial vasodilation of the cerebral arteries. Familial history of headaches. Attack is precipitated by emotional disturbances, fatigue, tension, noise, bright lights, and crowds. The following factors precipitate all types of migraine headaches: 1. Sudden drop in high estrogen levels that occurs just before the onset of the menstrual period. 2. Barometric conditions, changes in temperature, especially falling temperatures. 3. Food: Nitrates and nitrites. Preservatives contained in canned meats are vasodilating agents. Monosodium glutamate (MSG), caffeine, coffee, tea, cola beverages, chocolate. Amines: cheese (except cottage and cream cheese); alcohol, especially red wine, beer, liquors; citrus fruits; chicken livers; smoked or pickled fish; yogurt. 4. Stress 5. Sun's glare or flickering lights. 6. Fasting 7. Fever	Prevention of the occurrence of the headaches is the primary therapy. Patient education is important. The patient must be instructed on medications, removal of precipitating factors, coping mechanisms, and what organ problems are manifested by headache or a symptom. *Drugs:* 1. Ergotamine tartrate (Ergomar, Gynergen) 2. Dihydroergotamine mesylate (D.H.E. 45) 3. Propranolol (Inderal) 4. Methysergide (Sansert) 5. Cyproheptadine (Periactin) 6. Prednisone (Detasone, Orasone) 7. Tricyclic antidepressants (Elavil, Tofranil) 8. Isometheptene (Midrin) 9. Ergotamine/caffeine (Cafergot) 10. Ergotamine/caffeine/belladonna (Wigraine) 11. Codeine-narcotic analgesic for severe pain. 12. Aspirin and other analgesics for mild pain. (Refer to pharmacology books for descriptions of what these do and how they work.) Remove precipitating factors: Eliminate foods high in tiramine or MSG. Avoid excessive carbohydrates. Eat regular meals. Avoid hypoglycemia and fasting. Eat a high protein diet. Decrease sugar intake. Slow down and provide rest and nonstressful situations.

Continued.

Table 3-1 Headaches: classifications, causes, and therapy—cont'd

Classification	Cause	Therapy
Vascular headaches—cont'd		
2. Hemiplegic headaches are manifested by head pain and neurological deficits: paresthesia of the hand, face, leg, or, if more severe, weakness; speech disturbances; impaired consciousness; or visual disturbances.	Family history is usually reported by these patients.	
3. Hypertension headaches are an emergency and are of a severe nature.	Occur when diastolic blood pressure is above 120.	Lower blood pressure immediately, usually with medications.
4. Temporal arteritis occurs in persons over 60 years of age. It is a throbbing, unilateral pain that produces visual loss, psychiatric symptoms such as confusion or disorientation, and occasional fevers.	Swollen, tender temporal arteries.	Corticosteroids
Psychogenic headaches (tension or muscle contraction)		
Tension, muscle contraction, depression, anxiety. Pain occurring in these types is bilateral in nature and lacks the throbbing that migraines produce. The pain originates in the occipital area of the brain and radiates to the frontal area.	Persons with these types of headaches are depressed or anxious. Continuous muscle contractions of the neck, poor posture, chronic tension and stress in combination with fatigue and psychic conflicts predispose a person to these headaches.	1. Assess the level of anxiety or depression. 2. Drugs such as aspirin or analgesics and antidepressants or tranquilizers (diazepam [Valium], chlordiazepoxide [Librium]) may be used. 3. Other treatment methods: relaxation, massage, counseling to relieve emotional stress or alter coping mechanisms. Change life situations. Use biofeedback, hypnosis, meditation, and warm baths.

Involve brain, sinuses, teeth, eyes, nose, blood vessels, meninges.	Head pain caused by increased ICP or pressure caused by space-occupying processes in the cranium. Extracranial lesions. Brain tumor, subarachnoid hemorrhage. Patient will have symptoms that increase in severity and produce neurological deficits. Diseases of facial structures, throat, and ears. Infection (meningitis, encephalitis). Occlusive vascular disorder. Phlebitis. Arteritis. Postconcussion syndrome (occurs after head trauma and produces no neurological deficits). Acute glaucoma (dizziness, blurred vision). Sinusitis (facial pain near frontal and maxillary sinuses). Malocclusion of teeth (shift in jaw strains the facial muscles). Persons who grind their teeth when under stress will have headaches.	Treat the cause.

Table 3-1 Headaches: classifications, causes, and therapy—cont'd

Classification	Cause	Therapy
Facial pain		
1. Trigeminal neuralgia (tic douloureux). A painful condition involving the fifth cranial nerve (trigeminal). If affects the second and third divisions of the fifth nerve, maxillary and mandibular, respectively. The trigeminal nerve conveys impulses of heat, cold, pain, and touch from the scalp, face, and mucous membranes of the head (see Fig. 3-3). The condition occurs most frequently in persons over 40 years of age. The pain occurs in paroxyms and may last only a few seconds or occur repetatively for minutes to hours. The pain may subside completely and then recur several weeks later. Persons are fearful of the pain and remain inside, avoid eating and become malnourished, avoid laughing, crying, talking, and personal hygiene, since movement or touching the face will often provoke the intense pain.	Symptoms involve attacks that occur suddenly and are stimulated or triggered with tooth brushing, chewing, drafts of air, washing face, shaving, talking, heat, and cold. Recent studies have proven that trigeminal neuralgia is caused by compression of the trigeminal nerve adjacent to the brainstem. This is most often related to an enlarged vascular loop.	Nursing management: Comfort measures to treat any type of pain may be instituted. Patient education is important so that the patient learns precipitating factors that cause the pain and will be able to avoid that stimuli. Emphasize daily hygiene. Encourage activity. Discourage isolation. If surgical methods are instituted to manage the pain, routine postoperative nursing care measures are necessary. Medical management: Carbamazepine (Tegretol) is used to treat trigeminal neuralgia with good results. Phenytoin (Dilantin) has proven effective in pain relief for some patients but the mechanism of its action is not known. Alcohol injections into the gasserian ganglion have also provided relief, and propanolol (Inderal) is also being used.

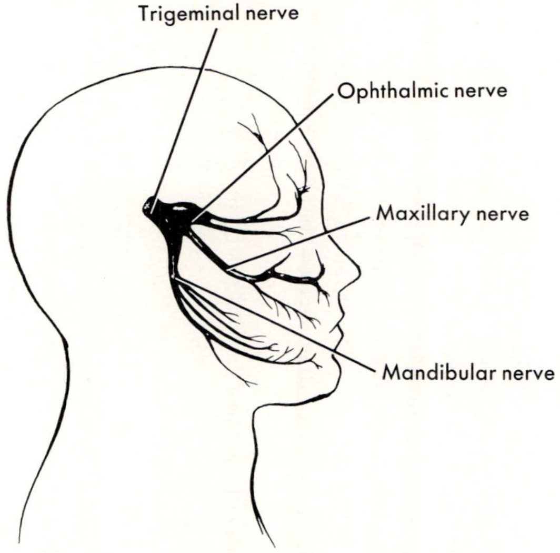

Fig. 3-3 The trigeminal nerve and its three divisions.

Surgical procedures:

1. Sheldon procedure. Electrocoagulation of the gasserian ganglion. Radio frequency electrodes are implanted into the nerve fibers and cause destruction of the pain-related fibers while the tactile fibers are spared.
2. Microsurgery. The Jannetta procedure is a new technique that is utilized in the relief of pain caused by trigeminal neuralgia. The procedure is done via an occipital craniectomy and a microscope is used to locate the nerve fibers. The trigeminal nerve fibers are cut and sensations of pain and temperature are eliminated with the preservation of touch and the corneal reflex. Microsurgical techniques have been perfected and are being performed successfully with minimal serious complications.

Peripheral nerve and muscle disorders causing pain

Carpal tunnel syndrome (CTS) results from compression of the median nerve against the transverse carpal ligament, which is the fourth wall that composes the carpal canal in the hand. The canal is a four-sided tunnel composed of nine tendons and the median nerve. A variety of conditions may crowd this space and cause the median nerve to be pinched, which is manifested by pain, paresthesia, and atrophy of the thenar (thumb) muscle after prolonged damage. Conditions that cause CTS include trauma such as a Colles' fracture of the wrist, rheumatoid arthritis, benign growths like lipomas or ganglion cysts, gout, edema, occupations (such as typist, butcher, hairdresser, truck driver), and hobbies (such as knitting). CTS occurs more frequently in females and involves the 30 to 60 age group. It is diagnosed following a physical examination of the hand that reveals decreased sensation in the palm and fingers, a positive Tinel sign, and a positive Phalen test.

Tinel's sign is elicited by lightly percussing the median nerve at the wrist. The patient with CTS will feel a tingling sensation radiating into the affected hand.

Phalen's test is a wrist flexion test in which the patient is instructed to sit at a table or desk and place the elbows on the edge and then to let the wrists drop into a flexion for 30 to 60 seconds. The test is positive if the patient experiences paresthesia and numbness. A variation of Phalen's test is the forced wrist-flexion test. This test is performed in the same manner as Phalen's test with the exception that after the elbows are propped on the table edge, one wrist is held in flexion first, and then the other wrist is held in flexion. A positive test will present symptoms immediately.

Electroneuromyography may be performed to test for CTS. This test measures the velocity of the median nerve or the speed at which the nerve transmits impulses to the muscle fiber. If the velocity is decreased 5 or more milliseconds below normal, the test is positive. Velocity of the median nerve may measure a normal value even when nerve compression is present in CTS; therefore both hands must be examined utilizing more than one diagnostic test. The dominant hand is most often affected, but both can be involved in CTS.

Patients with CTS usually relate a history of "a pain that awakens them at night" (a paresthesia) and numbness of the fingers that is relieved with exercise to "wake up" the hand. The middle finger, index finger, and thumb are the primary fingers involved.

Therapy for CTS is usually surgery to relieve the median nerve compression. Drug therapy may be instituted initially in an attempt to relieve the symptoms with use of anti-inflammatory preparations such as phenylbutazone (Azolid, Butazolidin). Hydrocortisone injection into the carpal tunnel is sometimes done to relieve the compression. The use of a canvas or plastic splint is encouraged to avoid activity that produces prolonged wrist activity. In the presence of other disease processes as the cause, these conditions are treated as a measure to abolish the CTS symptoms.

Nursing care involves patient education and assessment measures in determining that symptoms of CTS are present. Following surgical repair of the CTS, postoperative nursing interventions are utilized to manage the patient's recovery. Nursing care measures included postoperatively are elevation of the operative hand to reduce swelling, frequent neurovascular checks of the fingers, encouraging the patient to move the fingers at frequent intervals, and educating the patient as to how to check the nailbeds for circulation and the fingers for neurosensation. Activities of daily living such as eating, dressing, and bathing will be inhibited with the use of only one hand. The nurse will teach the patient how to perform these activities with one hand and will make life easier for the patient. Nursing interventions to achieve this are cutting meat, buttering bread, opening containers, and pouring beverages at meal time; providing a sling for the operative arm to help elevate it; providing a gown with snaps on the sleeves to facilitate dressing; providing a bar of soap with a string attached to hang around the patient's neck during showers, and slipping a plastic bag over the cast or dressing, also for showers.

Isometric and passive postoperative exercises should be instituted soon after surgery to preserve mobility and facilitate healing by increasing the circulation. The isometric exercises are done by making a fist and then relaxing the fingers. Passive exercises are performed by exercising the affected fingers using the opposite hand. Active exercises to encourage mobility are encouraged as soon as possible. Other activities include instructing the patient to avoid lifting heavy objects, to wear the splint or sling when involved in play or work activities, to carry a shoulder bag instead of a hand bag, and to carry small objects in the arms rather than in the hands. Recovery following surgical repair of CTS may take up to 1 year, but the patient eventually has full return of sensation and is painfree and able to perform previous activities.

NURSING CARE AND TREATMENT

The nurse must be sure to listen to what the patient in pain is telling him or her because the subjective data is the primary assessment tool. As stated earlier, pain is a personal experience. It is difficult to assess a person's pain. Persons in pain have attitudes about how it should be evaluated and treated based on social, cultural, and personal values. The individual assessing the pain has also developed attitudes about how pain should be expressed and tolerated. The variance in the assessment of the intensity of the pain between the one experiencing pain and the assessor will create problems for both.

Nursing assessment of pain is composed of objective and subjective data. Objective data includes increased pulse, blood pressure, respirations, perspiration, cool moist skin, pallor, facial grimaces, posture, gait, clutching of the painful site, and verbal expressions such as moans or cries. Subjective data is the patient's description as he relates the pain experience to the assessor. Data collection is based on the following:

1. Review of past history
2. Clinical description
   a. Subjective evaluation
   b. Coping mechanisms
3. Description of the location of pain
4. Onset
5. Evolution of pain
6. Quality and characteristics of the pain; e.g., dull, sharp, aches, radiating,

pressure, burning, itching, localized. Neurological pain is generally described as cold, burning, crawling, itching, "pins and needles," numbness, grabbing

7. Duration, intensity, and severity of pain
8. Any changes that occur after the onset of the pain
9. Precipitating factors
10. Relief measures
11. Any symptoms associated with the pain
12. What the pain experience means to the individual
13. Clinical observation and validation of data collected
14. Analysis of pain behavior (setting in which it occurs, frequency, what the individual will gain or lose from the experience, who provides the attention or support the person in pain seeks)

Dependent and independent interventions in pain management

The goals of pain management are centered on prevention, patient education, and promotion of wellness utilizing the holistic approach. Patient education is the key to success of pain management. The nurse teaches the patient how to identify precipitating causes of pain and cope with the pain experience. The support of family members or significant others is essential to the control of pain by the individual. Comfort measures can be provided to enhance the effects of other pain management measures. Simple comfort measures include rest, a quiet environment, bathing, backrub or massage of painful body parts, positioning, presence of a supportive individual, taping well the tubes and other equipment utilized in treatment for the hospitalized patient.

In the succeeding paragraphs, specific dependent and independent interventions will be discussed.

Pharmacological control

1. Analgesics
   a. Antipyretics relieve pain by a peripheral mechanism. They cause few central nervous system side effects. Common antipyretics are:
      Aspirin
      Acetaminophen (Tylenol)
      Indomethacin (Indocin)
      Phenylbutazone (Butazolidin)
      Oxyphenbutazone (Tandearil)
   b. Narcotics relieve pain by means of an unknown central action in the nervous system. Pain is relieved through an altered consciousness and obtundation of other sensory stimuli. Narcotics act as a blunting mechanism in relieving pain. Narcotic drugs include:
      Morphine
      Hydromorphone (Dilaudid)
      Meperidine (Demerol)
      Codeine

Levorphanol (Levo-Dromoran)
Methadone (Dolophine)
Pentazocine (Talwin)
Propoxyphene (Darvon)

2. Psychotropic drugs are most effective in intractible pain. A common combination is phenothiazine tranquilizers and a tricyclic antidepressant.
3. Carbamazepine (Tegretol) and phenytoin (Dilantin) are useful in alleviating brief neurotic pain associated with conditions such as trigeminal neuralgia, multiple sclerosis, tabes dorsalis, and some pains that follow spinal cord injury.
4. Baclofen (Lioresal) is useful in controlling painful flexor and extensor spasms of spinal cord diseases (multiple sclerosis, spinal cord trauma or compression).
5. Placebos. The use of placebos in pain management is based on the strong psychological aspect of pain. Placebos may be used in diagnostic measures for pain since they are used in carefully observed clinical settings.

Noninvasive techniques

Distraction. By directing the attention of the person experiencing pain to something else, the perception of pain is altered.

1. An example of how to use distraction: Concentration on a simple task makes distraction more effective. Therefore have the patient tell the nurse about an exciting ball game, interesting movie, stimulating book or joyful personal experience.
2. Encourage active listening to music and emphasize the rhythmic pattern of music. Tell the patient to stare at an object, close the eyes, and concentrate as on a pretty picture, or peaceful mountain lake as he listens to the music and concentrates on the rhythm.
3. Teach the patient to concentrate on rhythmic breathing. During deep breathing teach the patient to look at an object and breathe in and out slowly, counting 1-2-3-4—as he does so. As he becomes more relaxed, he counts silently. The patient should inhale through the nose; exhale through the mouth.
4. Stroking or massaging a body part during rhythmic breathing may facilitate the distraction.

Relaxation techniques. Relaxation techniques require more concentration and knowledge than distraction and also previous use of relaxation techniques. Meditation is one popular technique of relaxation. Relaxation is based on the control of mind over body. Relaxation is effective in relieving ongoing pain and produces both mental and physical relief from stress and discomfort. Dr. Herbert Benson implemented the use of relaxation techniques for stress and pain control in the early 1970s (Benson, 1975).

1. Type of relaxation techniques:
   a. Rhythmic breathing
   b. Relaxation to music

2. Effects:
   a. Reduce anxiety
   b. Ease muscle tension
   c. Decrease fatigue
   d. Provide a rest period that is as beneficial as actually sleeping
   e. Enable the patient to fall asleep
   f. Increase the effectiveness of other pain relievers
   g. Help the patient to remove himself from the painful experience

Stimulators. The purpose is to close the pain pathway "gate" and to block the conduction of the pain.

ACUPUNCTURE. Acupuncture techniques were developed in China and have become used worldwide to treat neuralgia, phantom limb pain, and pain related to surgical procedures. The Chinese theory for acupuncture is based on two universal forces being expressed at the human level. These levels are the spirit (yin) and the blood (yang). The theory is based on the belief that yin and yang are in disharmony. With insertion of acupuncture needles at certain sites along the meridians of the transmission avenues of yin and yang, harmony is allowed to return to yin and yang.

Acupuncture is performed by insertion of stainless steel needles along sites. The needles are stimulated by use of electrical impulses, heat, or herbal essence. The best explanation for the effects of acupuncture is based on the gate theory. The acupuncture needles stimulate the large fibers and close the gate. Needles are placed along neuronal input sites and control pain transmitted from body organs to the brain by creating an inhibitory effect on the brain and gate control mechanism.

ELECTRICAL STIMULATION. Transcutaneous stimulation (TENS) is used for relief of intractable pain and surgical procedure pain. Its function is based on the gate control theory, and it uses electrical stimulation to the large fibers, which decreases transmission activity of the small fibers.

Patients are instructed how to control the radio frequency of the electrical impulses transmitted through a pocket-sized transmitter. Electrodes are placed over the painful area or nerve pathway and the transmitter is attached to these electrodes. When the patient desires to supersede the painful sensation, the transmitter is adjusted until the sensation is relieved. Patients feel a tingling sensation at the site of the electrodes when this is achieved.

SPINAL CORD STIMULATION. The spinal cord stimulation (SCS) system is used to manage chronic intractable pain. The patient can apply electrical stimulation to various spinal cord tracts that influence chronic pains. SCS is indicated to control pain of trunk and limbs, especially in low back pain and phantom limb pain. The technique involves surgical implantation of tiny electrodes into the epidural space and then connecting them to the leads of a small battery-operated stimulator. Stimulation to relieve pain is assessed for 24 hours postoperatively, and then another operation is performed to internalize the system. Internalization is done by implanting a radio receiver under the skin below the rib cage and reconnecting the electrode lead wires to this radio receiver via an extension wire. The patient is taught to care for the antenna and the wireless transmitter system.

COLD PACKS. Cold packs slow the conduction of impulses to the brain and motor impulses to the muscles. Frequently used cold applications are ice bags, cool damp towels, and gel packs. Cold also decreases swelling and bleeding after surgery or trauma and provides quick relief for sprains, strains, headaches, sore throats, joint pain, muscle spasms, or back pain associated with childbirth.

MENTHOL OINTMENTS. The mechanism of menthol ointments is not known for sure. Menthyl salicylate is the substance in the majority of these ointments and it relieves pain through its analgesic effect. The ointment provides warmth to the site and is thought to function by way of gate control. Ointments have a strong odor and the patient should be asked if he objects to this odor before the use of ointments.

TOUCH. The use of touch provides both psychological and physical relief of pain. Touch indicates a feeling of caring for the individual who is suffering pain. Application of massage or pressure to the pain site relieves pain using the gate control theory. (Do not rub a painful calf as this may dislodge a thrombus or clot.)

Mind-control

HYPNOSIS. Hypnosis techniques work by decreasing levels of pain by reducing anxiety and creating a positive aspect of pain by the use of distraction, the power of suggestion for analgesia to decrease pain, and the use of creative imaginative and thought processes to decrease pain. The motivation of the individual and the ability to be open to suggestion are important powers for hypnosis to be effective. Psychological preparation alters the awareness of pain and enables the patient to cope with the experience.

BIOFEEDBACK. Biofeedback is based on operant conditioning principles, whereby the stimulus of pain is altered and negative experiences are not recognized but rather positive behavior is recognized and rewarded. (Illness is negative. Wellness is positive). Biofeedback has been successful in treating migraine headaches as the patient learns to shunt blood from the head to the hands. This is done by squeezing the thumb tightly and concentrating on the pain at that site rather than the headache. Biofeedback is a means of distraction by forcing concentration on a feedback signal.

Surgical intervention

Nerve blocks. Nerve blocks involve the injection of local anesthetics such as lidocaine (Xylocaine) or procaine (Novocaine) close to nerve trunks to relieve discomfort. Alcohol blocks destroy the nerve fibers and are used for peripheral blocks. Alcohol blocks are used to treat trigeminal neuralgia and spasms associated with multiple sclerosis.

Neurosurgery. Neurosurgery is a last resort for the treatment of pain because it destroys nerve pathways.

1. Chordotomy is the interruption of the pain conduction pathways in the spinal cord by transection of the spinothalamic portion of the anterolateral tract. Pain

and temperature sensation are obliterated below the level severed but other sensation and motor functions are left intact. Significant nursing care measures are related to the postoperative problems of urinary retention, which is transitory, and impaired sexual functioning in males.

2. Rhizotomy is the division of the interior and posterior spinal nerve root between the ganglion and cord. Cranial and upper cervical root rhizotomies are the most successful and are useful in the treatment of conditions of the head and neck such as cancer, radiation scars, and trigeminal and glossopharyngeal neuralgias.
3. Neurectomy is the interruption of a peripheral or cranial nerve to eliminate localized pain.
4. Sympathectomy interrupts afferent pathways in the sympathetic division of the autonomic nervous system. This is also useful in the treatment of vascular disorders such as Raynaud's phenomenon, thromboangitis obliterans, and angina pectoris because it eliminates vasospasm and increases peripheral blood supply.
5. Cerebral surgery such as lobotomy, thalamotomy, and cingulotomy may alter the person's personality. Thalamotomy is being used experimentally to treat head and neck cancer, facial postherpetic neuralgia, and thalamic syndrome. This procedure involves the implantation of electrodes into the thalamic nuclei via burr holes. Tissue is destroyed by electrocoagulation of the site of pain perception.

Sphenopalatine ganglion block. The sphenopalatine ganglion block (SPAB) is a new treatment in the relief of neck, shoulder, and low back pain. Bupivacaine (Marcaine) is applied through the nasal cavity using two to four sterile applicators. The theory on which this treatment is based is that the sphenopalatine ganglion is the largest cranial ganglion and it is located in the nasal cavity. It contains nerve branches with sensory, motor, and sympathetic roots that lead to the rest of the sympathetic ganglion, which control pain to the arms, legs, body, and neck. The procedure causes no discomfort to the patient unless he has a cold, sinus congestion, or septal deviation. Rare side effects that may occur are drying of the mouth, light headedness, soreness of the tongue, nausea, or headache. The treatment works by nerve hyperstimulation, psychological factors, decreased edema, or blockage of sympathetic nerve pathways.

Implementation

The goals of nursing care are dependent on prevention of pain, provision of comfort measures, and patient education. Successful management of pain is dependent on the nursing intervention. Measures to promote relief of pain may be instituted at any point illustrated in the following diagram (Fig. 3-4).

Evaluation of the plan. Depending on what interventions have been utilized in the relief of pain, the nurse and patient will be able to determine if the patient has gained new strategies and coping mechanisms to control pain, whether pain tolerance has increased through the use of coping mechanisms, and whether behavior patterns in response to

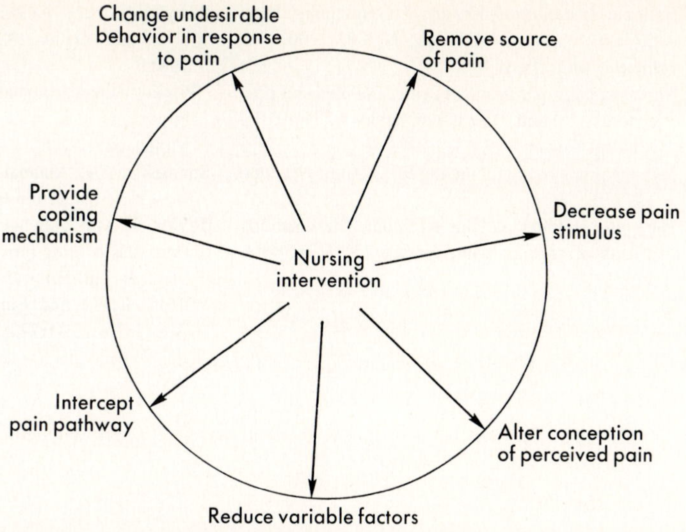

Fig. 3-4 Schematic drawing illustrating the nursing interventions to utilize in pain control.

pain have changed. Absence of physiological pain indicates that pain has been relieved or alleviated. Anxiety is lessened. The patient's overall behavior and social and family life will be improved with the reduction in pain. The patient will learn to incorporate the pain experience and management into his total life. Objectives for care will be individualized and specific for each patient because pain is an individualistic experience.

Suggested readings

Banner, A.: Publication of the Immanuel Medical Center, Omaha, **59:**4-5, Dec. 1980.

Benson, H.: The relaxation response, New York, 1975, Avm Publishers.

Berger, M.R., and Froimson, A.J.: Hands that hurt: carpal tunnel syndrome, Am. J. Nurs. **79:**264-265, 1979.

Beyerman, K.: Flawed perceptions about pain, Am. J. Nurs. **82:**302-304, 1982.

Conway-Rutkowski, B.: Getting to the cause of headaches, Am. J. Nurs. **81:**1846-1849, 1981.

Conway-Rutkowski, B.: Carini and Owens' neurological and neurosurgical nursing, ed. 8, St. Louis, 1982, The C.V. Mosby Company.

Greisner, P.B., and Meisel, S.: A guide to headaches and how to relieve their pain, Nursing81 **11:**50-57, April 1981.

Jacox, A.K.: Pain—a source book for nurses and other health professionals, Boston, 1977, Little, Brown & Co.

Jacox, A.K.: Assessing pain, Am. J. Nurs. **79:**895-900, 1979.

Jones, D., Dunbar, C.F., and Jirovec, M.M.: Medical-surgical nursing, a conceptual approach, New York, 1978, McGraw Hill Book Co.

McCaffrey, M.: Relieving pain with noninvasive techniques, Nursing80 **10**(12):55-57, Dec. 1980.

Melzack, R., and Wall, P.D.: Pain mechanisms: a new theory, Science **150:**971-978, 1965.

Miller, B.K.: Hands that hurt less, Am. J. Nurs. **79:**266-267, 1979.

Miller, B.K.: How to spot—and treat—carpal tunnel syndrome—early, Nursing80 **10**(3):50-53, March 1980.

National Institute of Health: Chronic pain, hope through research, NIH Pub. No. 82-2406, Bethesda, MD, April 1982.

Nebraska pain management center policies and procedures, Omaha, 1978, University of Nebraska Medical Center.

Nursing grand rounds, Nursing77, **7**(10):66-70, Oct. 1977.

Pace, B.: Helping patients overcome the disabling effects of chronic pain, Nursing77, **7**(7):38-43, July 1977.

Perry, S.W., and Heidrich, G.: Placebo response: myth and matter, Am. J. Nurs. **81:**720-725, 1981.

''Pisces—selectry spinal cord stimulation system, Physician and patient information booklets, Minneapolis, 1980-1981, Medtronic Inc.

Samuels, M.A.: Manual of neurologic therapeutics, Boston, 1978, Little Brown & Co.

Taylor, J., and Ballenger, S.: Neurologic dysfunctions and nursing intervention, New York, 1980, McGraw Hill Book Co.

Wilson, R.W., and Elmassian, B.J.: Endorphins, Am. J. Nurs. **81:**722-725, 1981.

CHAPTER 4

Altered states of consciousness

Altered levels of consciousness (LOC) can vary from heightened to depressed states. Heightened LOC can result from the use of abuse of central nervous system stimulants or from psychogenic causes. Depressed levels of consciousness most often are the result of trauma, cerebrovascular dysfunction, or endogenous disease. However, they can also be caused by the ingestion, inhalation, or injection of substances. Unfortunately, the use and abuse of prescribed and illicit drugs in the United States has reached epidemic proportions (Jaffe, 1980).

Accuracy in determining LOC is enhanced by describing objective patient behaviors rather than subjective impressions such as agitated, lethargic, confused. The Glascow Coma Scale (see Chapter 1) is one method of objecting data. Other methods involve the use of phrases describing patient behaviors or describing patient responses to specific stimuli. Examples of behavioral descriptions for heightened LOC include:

Talkativeness with increased rate of speech
Visual or auditory perceptual distortions
Fidgety or excessive movements of extremities and eyes
Mood swings from friendly to throwing objects, biting behaviors
Incoordination, inability to complete tasks, tremors
Numerous changes in content of conversation
Impaired intellectual functioning, decreased concentration

For depressed LOC an example of the stimulus/response method is:

Stimulus	Response
Verbal question regarding name, date, location	Oriented to person, time, place
Verbal question (as above)	Responds appropriately within 30 seconds
Verbal question and pressure/pinch	No response to verbal sound stimulus, appropriate response (flexion, withdrawal, push away) to noxious stimuli
Question/sound and pressure/pinch	No response to verbal or noxious stimuli

HEIGHTENED STATES OF CONSCIOUSNESS

As stated earlier, heightened levels of awareness can be caused by:

1. Ingestion, injection, inhalation of central nervous system (CNS) stimulants such as amphetamines, cocaine, hallucinogens.
2. Withdrawal from CNS depressants.
3. Psychoemotional imbalances such as excessive stress, manic psychosis.

Pathophysiology

The physiological effects of any of the above listed causes are those of cortical, subcortical, and sympathetic nervous system stimulation. Synaptic excitability and neural depolarization are increased. The amount and intensity of neural cellular activity is enhanced. The inhibitory function of the ascending reticular activating system is diminished. Cortical stimulation results in intensification of perceptual awareness, in increased speed in thought processes, and in a general feeling of excitement. Stimulation of the sympathetic nervous system causes tachycardia, mydriasis, hyperreflexia, tremors, and peripheral vasoconstriction. Subcortically, stimulation of the heat regulatory centers in the hypothalamus results in increased body temperature. The increased respiratory rate is caused by stimulation of the respiratory centers in the brainstem.

Classification

Drug toxicity: CNS stimulants
Drug withdrawal: CNS depressants
Psychogenic: Stress or psychosis

Assessments

Because of the diversity of potential causes of heightened LOC, the objective and subjective assessment data obtained must be both complete and accurate. Subjective data can be obtained from the patient, family, or a significant other. Explaining that accurate information is essential to specific therapeutic measures increases the potential for honest responses to questions as does the use of a nonjudgmental approach by the interviewer.

General subjective assessment data. Conduct a focused interview to determine:

1. Behavioral and physiological changes before admission:
   a. Excessive talkativeness
   b. Insomnia
   c. Visual/auditory distortions
   d. Inability to concentrate
   e. Lack of coordination: ataxia, inability to write, dress, feed self
   f. Excessive physical activity of a repetitive and stereotyped nature
   g. Increases in pulse, respiration, and blood pressure
   h. Muscle twitching/tremors
   i. Seizure activity
2. Psychoemotional changes:
   a. Acute anxiety resulting from loss of loved one, family discord, fear for life position of self or others, change in life-style or situation
   b. Withdrawal from CNS depressants
3. Type, route, and amount of ingested, inhaled, or injected CNS stimulant substances such as:
   a. Amphetamines: amphetamine, dextroamphetamine, methamphetamine
   b. Cocaine
   c. Hallucinogens: lysergic acid diethylamide (LSD), marijuana, phencyclidine (PCP)

4. Methods used to neutralize or remove the substance before admission:
   a. Induction of vomiting
   b. Administration of a counteracting substance
5. Concomitant health problems:
   a. Diabetes
   b. Hypertension
   c. Cardiovascular, liver, or kidney disease
   d. Mental imbalances
6. Medications currently used, both prescribed and over-the-counter, and known allergies

Specific assessment data. CNS stimulants such as amphetamines, cocaine, and hallucinogens are sympathomimetic agents. The exhilarating or mind-altering effects can lead to both physical and psychological dependence (Bergersen, 1979). Because of the increasing use and abuse of these drugs, familiarily with their signs and symptoms is prerequisite to the initiation of appropriate interventions to ensure maintenance of vital functions and mental, emotional, and physical homeostasis.

Amphetamines

Subjective assessment data

Feelings of euphoria and exhilaration
Improved ability to concentrate and work
Increased physical tolerance and self-confidence
Palpitations
Irritability
Dizziness
Anorexia and weight loss
Insomnia
Feelings of physical and psychological dependence
Excessive fatique and mental depression if drug is withheld or withdrawn
Formication (sensation of crawling insects under the skin)
In children the paradoxical effect of lethargy (an occasional occurrence)

Objective assessment data

Restless, fidgety behaviors
Talkative: fast with frequent content changes
Hypertension
Hyperpyrexia with flushed skin
Tachycardia
Dry mouth
Hyperactive bowel sounds
Dilated pupils
Diaphoresis

With long-term amphetamine use:

- Malnutrition
- Scratch marks and skin infections caused by scratching perceived crawling insects under the skin

Violent aggressive behaviors (occasional) directed toward self or others.

Cocaine

Subjective assessment data

Euphoria
Restlessness and apprehension
Insomnia
Anorexia and weight loss
Tactile hallucinations: formication
Delusions of persecution (intoxication)

Objective assessment data

Malnutrition with gastrointestinal upsets: hyperactive bowel sounds, vomiting
Perforated nasal septum (for chronic sniffers)
Tachycardia with dysrhythmias
Variable hypertension and hypotension
Dilated pupils
Hyperactive reflexes
Muscle twitching and spasms
Seizure activity: focal or generalized
Respiratory depression (intoxication)

Hallucinogens

LSD

SUBJECTIVE ASSESSMENT DATA

Vertigo
Perceptual alterations: intensification of sights, sounds, touch
Synthesia: transference of sensory perceptions (''see a sound,'' ''hear a color'')
Impaired value judgement: inability to distinguish between good/bad, desirable/undesirable
Flashbacks: reoccurrence of drug experiences up to a year after last dosage

OBJECTIVE ASSESSMENT DATA

Tachycardia
Dilated pupils
Hyperactive reflexes
Signs of anxiety: excessive oral behaviors such as smoking, chewing, muscle tenseness/twitching, fidgeting, decreased direct eye contact
Respiratory depression with decreased response to verbal or painful stimuli (overdose)
Clotting abnormalities: prolonged prothrombin and partial thromboplastin times

Marijuana

SUBJECTIVE ASSESSMENT DATA

Euphoria
Dizziness
Anxiety
Intestification of sensory perceptions
Chest tightness
Decreased concentration ability
Lack of goal orientation

OBJECTIVE ASSESSMENT DATA

Impaired coordination
Conjunctivitis
Tachycardia
Postural hypotension
Positive toxicology screen

Phencyclidine (PCP or angel dust)

SUBJECTIVE ASSESSMENT DATA

Alternating feelings of euphoria, agitation, apathy, and paranoia
Amnesia
Perceptual disturbances causing ataxia, falls
Physical weakness

OBJECTIVE ASSESSMENT DATA

Vertical nystagmus (differenting sign)
Blank staring into space
Miotic pupils, decreased reaction to light stimuli
Rigid, sometimes bizarre body positioning
Slurred speech
Tremors and jerky movements of extremities with muscle spasms
Hypertension, systolic and diastolic
Dysrhythmias
Fever with diaphoresis and flushed face
Excessive salivation, drooling
Vomiting
Decreased sensation capabilities
Seizure activity
Positive urine toxicology screen

Withdrawal from CNS depressants. Although CNS depressants are prescribed sparingly for patients with neurological disorders, persons with chronic pain may have been taking them for a long time. In other instances, self-medication with CNS depressants is the problem. Signs and symptoms appear within 8 hours of the last dose.

Subjective assessment data

History of taking CNS depressant
Insomnia
Restlessness
Heart palpitations
Hallucinations, visual and auditory
Nervousness/anxiety
Vision disturbances
Muscle weakness

Objective assessment data

Increased nasal and lacrimal secretions
Diaphoresis with goose flesh
Anorexia
Yawning/sneezing
Dilated pupils
Fever with alternating hot and cold flashes
Nausea
Vomiting
Diarrhea
Hypertension
Rapid, irregular respirations
Abdominal cramps/wretching
Tachycardia
Muscle twitching/tremors
Disorientation
Slurred speech
Seizures, generalized motor

Diagnostic tests. In acute overdose cases treatment necessarily precedes diagnostic testing. Screening toxicology tests, both qualitative and quantifying, are used to determine the presence of or the amount of various drugs in the urine, blood, and gastric contents. Because drugs are more easily detected in urine, *urine is the specimen of choice for toxicology screening tests* (Morgan, 1982). However, in acute overdose cases all three types of specimens should be obtained as soon as possible after admission for accurate results. Fig. 4-1 illustrates a sample report form. Time requirements, determinations, and specimens required are delineated in Table 4-1.

Toxicology screening tests (Table 4-1)

1. Urine spot tests: a qualitative colorometric examination.
2. EMIT screen: quantitative enzyme immunoassay test developed by the Ciba Company.
3. Thin layer chromatography: a multiphased examination for selected drugs in urine, blood, and gastric specimens.

Name	Date plasma obtained:
Number	Time plasma obtained:
Hospital	Dosage:
Room	Time of last dose:
Physician	

Amitriptyline	ng/ml
Desipramine	ng/ml
Doxepin	ng/ml
Imipramine	ng/ml
Nordoxepin	ng/ml
Nortriptyline	ng/ml
Total tricyclic	ng/ml

Therapeutic

	Individual variation in metabolism	Suggested starting dosage (mg/day)	Suggested trial dosage (mg/day)	Dosage range (mg/day)	Therapeutic TOTAL TRICYCLIC (ng/ml)
Amitriptyline (Elavil)	10-fold	50	150	75-300	125-250
Desipramine (Norpramine)	30-fold	50	150	75-300	150-300
Doxepin (Sinequan, Adapin)	10- to 15-fold	50	150	75-300	75-200
Imipramine (Tofranil)	30-fold	50	150	75-300	150-300
Nortriptyline (Aventyl)	10-fold	25	75	40-100	50-150

NOTE: Nortriptyline and possibly the other tricyclics are clinically less effective both above and below these therapeutic ranges.

Overdose

Biggs reported 40 patients admitted for tricyclic overdose who did not have a substantial amount of any other drug. The following are the incidence of findings in those 40 patients and the levels at which they were found.

Finding	Number	Total tricyclic level (mean ± SEM)
Unconsciousness	19	1027 ± 188
Respiratory assistance required	16	1121 ± 219
Ventricular rate over 120/min	12	1189 ± 248
QRS over 100 msec	20	1202 ± 167
Arrythmia	7	1274 ± 289
Bundle branch block	6	1287 ± 318
Cardiac arrest	3	1703 ± 151
Grand mal seizures	8	1829 ± 86
Death	2	1843 ± 97

Fig. 4-1 Sample toxicology report form.

Table 4-1 Toxicology screening tests

Test	Time	Determinations	Specimen
Urine spot test	2-4 min	Acetaminophen-phenacetin Alcohol Desipramine-imipramine Ethchlorvynol Glucose Ketones Phenothiazines Salicylate	30 ml urine.
EMIT screen	1½ hr	Amphetamines Barbiturates Benzodiazepines Cocaine Methadone Opiates Propoxyphene Phencyclidine Marijuana	50 ml urine. Specimen should be obtained as soon as possible after admission for suspected overdosage because the drug is more highly concentrated and therefore more easily detected. With incontinent patients the EMIT screen can be done with only 2 ml of urine.
Thin layer chromatography	2-3 hr	Amphetamines Antihistamines Barbiturates Benzodiazepines Cocaine Ethchlorvynol Glutethimide Meperidine Meprobamate Methadone Methaqualone Opiates Pentazocine Phencyclidine Phenothiazines Phenylpropanolamine Phenytoin Propoxyphene Tricyclic anti-depressants	Specimen collection: All three types of specimens can be analyzed by using the chromatography method. a. Venous blood: 20 ml of venous blood collected in two 10 ml test tubes (without separators) b. Urine: minimum of 20 ml, preferably 50 ml c. Gastric: initial specimen, not gastric washings NOTE: The water soluble lubricant used on nasogastric tubes interferes with test results. If used, the laboratory personnel should be informed. Laboratory personnel should also be advised about the patient's diagnosis, suspected drugs, and prescribed medications administered.
Serum spot test	After centrifuging, 2-4 min	Acetaminophen-phenacetin Alcohol Salicylate	Because thin layer chromatography is usually prescribed in addition to the spot test, collect 20 ml of venous blood in two test tubes. NOTE: The specimen for the blood alcohol screening should be collected in a fluoride tube.

4. Serum spot testing: a qualitative spot test for the presence of substances.

Arterial blood gases: These are determined if oxygenation problems are present.

Specimen: 3 ml of arterial blood collected asceptically in heparinized test tubes.

Serum electrolytes: Because of vomiting and diarrhea associated with CNS stimulant overdose, electrolyte imbalances should be suspected.

Specimen: 5 ml of venous blood.

Electrocardiogram: to determine dysrhythmias caused by hypoxia and electrolyte imbalances.

Psychogenic/psychiatric disorders. In addition to the use or abuse of drugs, LOC can be heightened by psychogenic/psychiatric disorders ranging from acute anxiety attacks to psychosis (Pisarcik, 1981).

Acute anxiety

SUBJECTIVE ASSESSMENT DATA

History: loss of loved one; inability to meet established goals; social or economic insecurity
Impaired judgment or concentration
Indecisive and dazed feelings
Choking sensation
Restlessness
Sensation of chest pressure
Feelings of helplessness or impending danger
Diarrhea and increased urinary frequency
Insomnia

OBJECTIVE ASSESSMENT DATA

Fidgety behaviors
Tremors of extremities
Dry mouth
Tachycardia
Diaphoresis
Polyuria
Increased and irregular respirations

Manic psychosis

SUBJECTIVE ASSESSMENT DATA

Variable mood elevation/depression
Intolerant of difficulties, irritable
Feelings of ''lack of control''
Vague somatic complaints
Auditory hallucinations (visual hallucinations are more common in organic psychoses)
History of taking lithium carbonate or of previous mental health problems

OBJECTIVE ASSESSMENT DATA

Talkative: humorous, loud, excessive; ask personal questions of sexual nature
Constant fidgety movements
Propulsive speech through clenched teeth
Variable pulse rate
"Pacing" behaviors

Interventions

Initial interventions are focused on maintenance of vital functions; provision of a safe, controlled environment; and establishing a one-to-one relationship to reduce the patient's anxiety level.

Safe, controlled environment

Private room with minimal furnishings: bed, desk, chair
Reduced stimuli: light, noise
Temperature: cool room with good ventilation
Remove potentially harmful objects: lamps, assessment equipment, syringes, sharp objects, light cords
Undress patient and place clothes, purse, and other personal belongings in a labeled bag for safekeeping
Nurse should position self for easy access to door.
Use cloth or soft restraints judiciously

One-to-one relationship

Stay with patient
Calm, nonjudgmental approach
Unhurried speech
Encourage verbalization of fears, anxieties
Complete mental status examination:
- General appearance: hygiene, dress, posture
- Behavior: posture and movements
- Voice and speech: vocabulary, relevance to situation
- Emotional reactions: variability; sad, happy, fearful facial expression; muscle tenseness
- Speech content: logical, relevant to situation
- Orientation level and memory abilities
- Insight: knowledge of present situation
- Decision-making ability

Reality opportunities: repeated reorientation to time, person, and place
Physical offerings: liquids (if gag reflex present), elimination opportunities, wiping perspiration, allow positioning for maximum comfort
Provide organization through use of concrete tasks such as rebreathing techniques, relaxation methods, deep breathing (Pisarcik, 1981).
Heightened states of awareness.

Nursing care plan: **HEIGHTENED STATES OF CONSCIOUSNESS**

NURSING DIAGNOSIS	EXPECTED OUTCOMES	NURSING INTERVENTIONS
Sensory overload with perceptual alterations due to effects of CNS stimulant agents or psychological imbalances	Normal sensorium	See general interventions regarding environment, safety, and patient-professional relationships. Reorient patient at frequent intervals. Administer prescribed medications: See Table 4-2 for medications prescribed for specific symptoms.
Potential for systemic poisoning due to ingested agents.	Ingested agents removed from gastrointestinal system and systemic absorption inhibited Toxiocology testing negative	For oriented patients: Induce emesis. See Table 4-3 for rationale, contraindications, procedure, and precautions. For patients who are nonresponsive (comatose, lack the gag reflex, are postictal, or have ingested acid or alkali or petroleum-based agents, initiate gastric lavage and postlavage care. See Table 4-4 for procedure and precautions.
Altered and variable cardiac output due to sympathetic nervous system stimulation	Blood pressure: 120/80 Pulse: 80 ± 10 with no arrhythmias	Monitor and document vital signs. Administer prescribed medications. See Table 4-2. Demonstrate and encourage deep breathing and relaxation techniques.
Self care deficit due to necessity of a controlled, safe environment	Physiological needs met	Provide: Privacy Blankets for warmth Toilet facilities for elimination Fluids for hydration Vomiting equipment for vomitus, i.e., basin, tissues, cool wet wash cloth, and mouth wash Explain rationale for all procedures. Because of short-term memory deficits, explanations may need to be repeated several times.
Anxiety varying from mild to severe due to unfamiliar surroundings and people and fear of personal outcome	Decreased anxiety	Reorientation at regular intervals. Introduce self and maintain open communication. Use of a nonthreatening, calm, supportive, yet controlled approach with active listening. Ensure patient's and care provider's safety through a controlled environment. Refer to specialized care provider when indicated. Encourage verbalization and provide reality testing in identification of cause of current health deficit and collaborate in defining goals to eliminate or minimize the problem.
Knowledge deficit: resources	Restates resources available Contacts referral agencies	Suggest or refer to community referral agencies: Mental health inpatient or outpatient facilities Drug abuse agencies Pastoral care Social service agencies.

Table 4-2 Medications prescribed symptomatically in heightened states of consciousness

Disorder	Medication
Hypertension	Diazoxide (Hyperstat), 300 mg IV push within 30 sec, usually followed by administration of Furosemide (Lasix)
Anxiety/tremors	Diazepam (Valium), 5-10 mg IM repeated every 2 hr or 2-10 mg oral not to exceed 40 mg/day
	Oxazepam (Serax), 10-30 mg oral not to exceed 120 mg/day
Cardiac dysrhythmias	Lidocaine, 1-5 mg/kg IV bolus, then 1-4 mg/min drip
Severe agitation, assaulting, extreme mental anguish	Haloperidol (Haldol), 0.5-5.0 mg IM; repeated at 40-50 min intervals*
Respiratory/metabolic alkalosis	Ammonium chloride, 2.75 mEq, and ascorbic acid, 2 g, added to IV solution
Seizure activity	Diazepam (Valium), 5-10 mg IV push, followed by longer acting phenytoin (Dilantin) IV drip

*Contraindicated in severe cardiac disease and pregnancy. In other cases haloperidol is preferred over phenothiazine agents, which may exaggerate psychotic reactions (Pisarcik, 1981).

Table 4-3 Procedure for inducing emesis

Rationale	Removal of ingested poisons (30%-40% optimally) to prevent systemic absorption
Contraindications	Acid, alkali, or petroleum-based agents Nonresponsive, comatose patient After seizures Absent gag reflex
Precautions	Have functioning suction equipment readily available to prevent aspiration of vomitus. Do not administer milk, milk products, sugars, or starches, which decrease utilization of charcoal (Manoguerra, 1981).
Procedure	Position patient on left side in high-Fowler's position Provide large basin, tissues, towels
Administer	1. 4-8 oz clear fluid (water, noncola carbonated drink, tea) 2. Follow with syrup of ipecac (30 ml for older children and adults; 15 ml for children). If there is no vomiting within 30 minutes, administer second dose. 3. After emesis administer activated charcoal* mixed in 8 oz water or 70% sorbitol† 50-100 g: adults 30-50 g: children 4. Follow charcoal with sodium sulfate, 250 mg/kg, to increase intestinal elimination if sorbitol is not used.

*Three of the most effective brands of charcoal are Merck, Norit, and Nuchar C. Amoco PX 21, which is in current clinical trial, is proported to be 3 times as effective (Manoguerra, 1981).

†Note: Sorbitol, an osmotic diuretic, decreases the bad taste of charcoal and increases rapidity of excretion through the intestines.

Table 4-4 Procedure for gastric lavage

Precautions	If airway is compromised, an endotracheal tube is inserted before lavage. Have functioning suctioning equipment readily available. Do not restrain combative patients on their backs because rapid turning may be necessary if patient vomits. Position oriented patient without airway protection in left lateral position with head lower than stomach.
Procedure	1. Select 34-36 Fr tube. Lubricate with water. Note: Water-soluble lubricants can invalidate gastric specimen toxicology testing. 2. Insert tube through mouth or nose, test for accurate placement, aspirate stomach contents, and place in labeled specimen container if toxicology screening is to be done. 3. Secure tube with paper tape. 4. Lavage until clear with: a. 200-250 ml warm saline per exchange for adults. b. 10 ml/kg warm saline for children. NOTE: Volumes exceeding this amount force stomach contents into small bowel (Manoguerra, 1981). 5. Administer: activated charcoal slurry 50-100 g: adults. 30-50 g: children. (Table 4-5 lists substances absorbed by charcoal.) 6. Follow with sodium sulfate 250 mg/kg to enhance excretion. 7. Remove tube rapidly. 8. Postlavage care: Provide oral hygiene for oriented patient. Position patient in a semi- or high-Fowler's position.

Table 4-5 Substances efficiently adsorbed by activated charcoal*

Amitriptyline	Ipecac	Phenobarbital
Amphetamine	Isoniazid	Phenol
Arsenic	Malathion	Phenolphthalein
Aspirin	Mefenamic acid	Phenytoin
Atropine	Meprobamate	Phosphorus
Camphor	Mercuric chloride	Primaquine
Chloroquine	Methyl salicylate	Propantheline
Chlorpheniramine	Morphine	Propoxyphene
Chlorpromazine	Nicotine	Quinidine
Cocaine	Nortriptyline	Quinine
Colchicine	Opium	Secobarbital
Digitalis	Oxalinic acid	Selenium
Ethchlorvynol	Parathion	Strychnine
Glutethimide	Penicillin	Sulfonamide
Imipramine	Pentobarbital	2, 4, D
Iodine		

*From Manoguerra, A.: Assessment and management of poisonings, Emergency Nursing Update **2**(3):2, 1981. Reprinted with permission from the author and *Emergency Nursing Update Series,* a publication of CPEC, Inc.

DEPRESSED LEVELS OF CONSCIOUSNESS

There are significant ranges in and multiple potential causes of depressed LOC. Minimally depressed LOC may be a result of boredom caused by a lack of mental stimulation or of brain hypoxia caused by immobility. Other potential causes include:

1. Use/abuse of prescribed or nonprescribed CNS depressants.
2. Endogenous disease such as kidney or liver dysfunction, diabetes, infections.
3. Exogenous poisonings, for example, by pesticides, insecticides.
4. Trauma.
5. Expanding lesions such as hematomas, neoplasms.
6. Vascular occlusions, that is, thrombi, emboli, vessel spasms, atherosclerosis.

Depressed LOC can range from a lack of ability to sustain concentration to totally nonresponsive, comatose states. To compound the problem, the patient with a depressed LOC can exhibit a concommitant depression of metabolic body functions, such as alterations in respiratory, circulatory, and neuromuscular functions as well as impairments of elimination and hydration status. Unfortunately, this generalized depressed state can facilitate a cyclical reaction: depressed LOC↔depressed body functions.

Because of their totally dependent status, nonresponsive, comatose patients present a challenge to care providers in both obtaining assessment data and initiating supportive and preventative homeostatic interventions. It is important to recognize that the LOC fluctuates. Therefore, continuing assessment and the provision of mental and sensory stimuli is imperative.

The unknowns of the situation, such as the length of time the depressed LOC will last and what the person will be like afterwards, can cause frustration for both the family and care providers. Unfortunately there are no pat answers. The duration of the coma and the outcome are dependent on numerous factors:

1. Cause: An uncomplicated, metabolic coma is more easily corrected than a trauma-induced vascular impairment with brain hypoxia.
2. Location and extent of damage to brain parenchyma: A brainstem dysfunction is most serious.
3. Complications: sepsis, vascular occlusion, hypercapnea, hypoxia.
4. Degree and duration of coma: Generally, the longer the nonresponsive status, the worse the prognosis.
5. Age of patient: Older patients have less potential for recovery than the young (Swartzman, 1981).

Because of the numerous causes of depressed LOC, accurate analysis of subjective and objective assessment data is essential to the development of a therapeutic plan of care. This section will identify the assessment data to be obtained, correlate them with the various potential causes, and suggest both general and specific interventions. The reader is advised to refer to the chapters on trauma, vascular insufficiency, neoplasms, and infections for more specific information.

Etiology

Causes of depressed LOC are numerous and they include:

1. Psychogenic causes
   Boredom or lack of mental stimulation
   Decreased self-concept as a result of alteration of body image
2. Inadequate cerebral perfusion
   Immobility
   Vascular insufficiency
3. Endogenous diseases
   Kidney
   Liver
   Pulmonary
   Diabetes
   Infection/sepsis
4. Trauma
   Contusions with subsequent parenchymal ischemia
   Intracerebral hemorrhage
5. Exogenous poisoning
   CNS depressant use/abuse
   Antipyretics/analgesics (salicylates, acetaminophen)
   Pesticides/insecticides

Table 4-6 illustrates important points in the differential diagnosis of causes of coma (Adams and Victor, 1981).

Table 4-6 Important points in the differential diagnosis of the common causes of coma*

General group	Specific disorder	Important clinical findings	Important laboratory findings	Remarks
Coma with focal or lateralizing signs of brain disease	Brain tumor	Stertorous breathing, neurologic signs dependent on location, papilledema	CSF pressure elevated; protein often >100 mg.	Steady progression of signs and symptoms
	Cerebral hemorrhage	Stertorous breathing, hypertension, flushed skin, hemiplegia	CSF grossly bloody and under increased pressure	Sudden onset, elderly patients

*From Principles of neurology by R. Adams and M. Victor. Copyright © 1981 McGraw-Hill Book Company, with the permission of McGraw-Hill Book Company.

Continued.

Table 4-6 Important points in the differential diagnosis of the common causes of coma—cont'd

General group	Specific disorder	Important clinical findings	Important laboratory findings	Remarks
	Cerebral thrombosis	Unilateral and bilateral paralysis of abrupt onset	CSF normal or protein modestly elevated	Stupor or coma
	Cerebral embolism	Sudden onset of paralysis	Same as above; occasionally up to 5000 RBC/mm^3	Evidence of heart disease
	Fracture or concussion	Signs of skin trauma	Skull fracture by x-ray; CSF bloody and under increased pressure	Bleeding from nose or ears; history of trauma
	Subdural hematoma	Slow respiration, rising blood pressure, hemiparesis, dilated pupil	Normal or increased CSF pressure; xanthochromia with relatively low protein	History of trauma; progressively severe headache and confusion
	Brain abscess	Neurologic signs depending on location; symptoms and signs of increased intracranial pressure	Fever, leucocytosis; increased pressure, protein and white cells, but normal glucose in CSF	Subacute evolution of headache and neurologic signs on background of sinus, ear, or lung infection or septicemia
	Hypertensive encephalopathy	Headache, severe hypertension, hypertensive retinopathy, convulsions	CSF pressure normal or increased; protein 50-200 mg	Confusion, stupor or coma; rapid evolution; duration several days
Coma without focal or lateralizing signs but with evidence of meningeal irritation	Meningitis	Stiff neck, positive Kernig's sign, fever, headache	Changes in CSF	Subacute or acute onset
	Subarachnoid hemorrhage	Stertorous breathing, hypertension, stiff neck, positive Kernig's sign	Bloody or xanthochromic CSF under increased pressure	Sudden onset with headache

Table 4-6 Important points in the differential diagnosis of the common causes of coma—cont'd

General group	Specific disorder	Important clinical findings	Important laboratory findings	Remarks
Coma without focal neurologic signs or evidence of meningeal irritation	Alcohol intoxication	Hypothermia, hypotension, flushed skin, alcohol breath	Elevated blood alcohol	
	Barbiturate intoxication	Hypothermia, hypotension	Barbiturate in urine	History of intake of intoxicating substance
	Opium intoxication	Slow respiration, cyanosis, constricted pupils		Administration of naloxone causes withdrawal signs
	Bromide intoxication	Hyperthermia, delirium	Blood bromides++	
	Carbon monoxide intoxication	Cherry-red skin	Carboxyhemoglobin	
	Anoxia	Rigidity, decerebrate postures, fever, seizures, involuntary movements	CSF normal; EEG may be isoelectric, or show high voltage delta	Abrupt onset following cardiopulmonary failure; damage permanent if anoxia exceeds 3-5 min
	Diabetic coma	Signs of extracellular fluid deficit, hyperventilation with Kussmaul respiration, "fruity" breath	Glycosuria, hyperglycemia, acidosis; reduced serum bicarbonate; ketonemia and ketonuria	History of polyuria, polydipsia, weight loss, or diabetes
	Hypoglycemia	Same as for anoxia	Low blood glucose; coeliac angiography may disclose insulinoma	Characteristic slow evolution through stages of nervousness, hunger, sweating, flushed face; then pallor, shallow respirations and seizures

Continued.

Table 4-6 Important points in the differential diagnosis of the common causes of coma—cont'd

General group	Specific disorder	Important clinical findings	Important laboratory findings	Remarks
	Uremia	Hypertension, sallow, dry skin, uriniferous breath, twitch-convulsive syndrome	Protein and casts in urine; elevated BUN and serum creatine; acidosis, hypocalcemia, etc.; anemia	Progressive apathy, confusion, and asterixis precede coma
	Hepatic coma	Jaundice, ascites and other signs of portal hypertension	Elevated blood NH_3 levels CSF yellow with normal protein	Onset over a few days or after hemorrhage from varices or paracentesis; confusion, stupor, asterixis and characteristic EEG changes precede coma
	Hypercapnia	Papilledema, diffuse myoclonus, asterixis	Increased CSF pressure; P_{CO_2} may exceed 75 mmHg; EEG theta and delta activity	Advanced pulmonary disease; profound coma and brain damage uncommon
	Severe infections; heat stroke	Extreme hyperthermia, rapid respiration	Vary according to cause	Evidence of a specific infection or exposure to extreme heat
	Idiopathic epilepsy	Episodic disturbance of behavior or convulsive movements	Characteristic EEG changes	History of previous attacks

Pathophysiology

Depressed LOC are caused by a disturbance or dysfunction in the ascending reticular activating system. The reticular activating system is an aggregate of nuclei in the brainstem that receive afferent (sensory) nerve impulses from the ascending spinal pathways, the retina of the eyes, and the auditory pathways from the inner ear. This column of nuclei projects to the thalamus, hypothalamus, cerebrum, and cerebellum. Physiologically, the ascending reticular activating system functions to facilitate, modify, or suppress transmission of neural information obtained through stimulation of sensory receptors. A lesion in the lower brainstem, supratentorial herniation causing pressure on the brainstem, or cerebral anoxia from extracerebral causes interferes with functioning of the reticular activating system resulting in progressive depression of the level of consciousness.

Classification

There are two accepted methods of classifying depressed LOC: causation and degree. The *degree* of a depressed LOC is classified in various ways:

- Glasgow Coma Scale (see Chapter 1)
- Stimulus/response method (see p. 115)
- Medical staging model:
  - Alert
  - Lethargic
  - Stupor
  - Light coma
  - Deep coma
  - Brain death

Causative categories include the classifications of functional (organic) or psychogenic (Plum and Posner, 1980).

- Psychogenic: caused by mental aberrations or illnesses (sometimes called functional)
- Organic: caused by structural, metabolic, or toxic causes
  - Structural: infarct, hemorrhage, hematoma, tumor
    - Supratentorial: causing secondary cerebral tentorial herniation, secondarily compressing the reticular activating system
    - Infratentorial: mass (cerebellar mass) directly compressing the reticular activating system or a blood vessel (basilar) obstruction
  - Metabolic: resulting from endogenous diseases (such as hepatic, renal, pulmonary dysfunction, diabetes)
  - Toxic
    - CNS depressant overdose:
      - Barbiturates
      - Opiates
      - Tranquilizers
      - Salicylates, acetaminophen
    - Pesticide/insecticide poisonings

Table 4-7 The characteristics of organic and functional coma*

Organic	Functional
No response to noxious stimuli	Response to noxious stimuli with manifestations such as withdrawal and grimacing
Loss of sphincter control	No loss of sphincter control
All reflexes are absent (pupils fixed, corneal reflexes absent, swallowing impossible)	Reflexes are present
Skin may be abnormal in color, texture, temperature, and moisture, depending on specific disease	Skin has normal characteristics
If a convulsion occurs and the client falls, invariably injury is sustained, and generally tongue biting is evident	No injury with falling; generally before an audience; no tongue biting
Eyelids may be elevated without difficulty; pupils are visible	Pronounced resistance to elevation of eyelids; eyeballs generally rotated upward; pupils not visible
May be pathological changes in blood pressure, pulse, respiration, and temperature	Pulse and respiration may be accelerated; temperature usually unremarkable
Paralysis of one or more extremities may be present	No true muscular paralysis

*From Conway-Rutkowski, B.: Neurological and neurosurgical nursing, ed. 8, St. Louis, 1982, The C.V. Mosby Co.

Table 4-7 delineates the distinguishing characteristics of functional and organic coma (Conway-Rutkowski, 1982). Another method sometimes used to differentiate functional from organic coma is to extend the victim's arm over his face. In an individual with an organic lesion, the flaccid arm will fall on the face when released. Persons with a functional disorder, however, retain a degree of muscle-tensing ability and generally will not allow their arms to fall directly on their faces.

Management of the unconscious patient

Because time is limited if permanent brain damage is to be prevented, a protocol for emergency management of the adult comatose patient is essential (Samuels, 1978). Initiation of this protocol precedes the neurological examination. A sample protocol is shown in Table 4-8.

The neurological assessment (see Chapter 1) must be modified somewhat in examining the unconscious patient. Because subjective data cannot be elicited from the patient, historical data must be obtained from other persons, commonly family members, friends, or rescue unit personnel. The following pertinent information should be obtained:

- Activity immediately preceding loss of consciousness
- Recent or chronic health problems: infections; kidney, liver, cardiovascular or cerebrovascular disease; arthritis; diabetes

Table 4-8 Emergency management of adult comatose patients

Goal	Intervention
Ensure airway	Insert nasotracheal or endotracheal tube
Ensure oxygenation	100% oxygen, 6-10 L/minute, by mask or ventilator
Ensure circulation	Following the drawing of blood specimens, initiate IV infusion of Ringer's lactate or 5% dextrose in water Administer vasopressor agent if systemic pressure is under 90
Provide glucose for neural metabolism	Administer 50% dextrose, 1 gm/kg, rapid IV push
Ensure neural transmission	Administer thiamine, 1-2 mg/kg, rapid IV push
If there are needle tracks or pupils under 1 mm with a history of narcotic abuse, antagonize depressant effects	Administer naloxone, 0.01 mg/kg, rapid IV push
Prevent and control seizures	Administer phenytoin, 250 mg, by IV push over 5 minutes

Occupation: farmer, crop duster, potter, chemical industry
Speech abilities
Vomiting without nausea
Progressive motor disabilities

General assessment data. A rapid survey assessment for the appearance and signs summarized in Table 4-9 should be completed and documented. Because of the necessity for frequent and continuing assessment (every 15 minutes till stable, then according to agency policy), use of an assessment flow sheet is practical in terms of recording and monitoring changes in status. The flow chart should be kept at the patient's bedside to increase accuracy in documentation and to decrease steps taken by the nurse. General objective assessment data include:

Level of consciousness: Stimulus/response method (see p. 115).

Vital Signs

Respiratory rate and pattern: See Fig. 4-3 for Anatomical correlations of altered patterns.

Pulse rate and dysrhythmias: If pulse rate is less than 70, pressure on the brainstem is suspected. If pulse rate is less than 60 and bounding, increasing intracranial pressure is suspected.

Blood pressure:

Less than 90/40 may indicate ischemic medulla, usually resulting from extracerebral causes.

Table 4-9 Correlation of appearance and signs with possible dysfunctional area or cause

Appearance and signs	Suggestive of
Stiff neck	Meningeal irritation
Jaundice	Hepatic disease
Bitten tongue/oral bleeding	Seizure
Needle marks/streaks	Drug abuse
Purpural/petechial hemorrhage	Renal/hepatic failure, leukemia
Miotic pupils	Insecticide/pesticide poisoning, drug abuse
Rhinorrhea/otorrhea	Frontal/basilar fracture
Incontinence	Seizure, cerebrovascular accident
Bradycardia with cold, clammy skin	Hypoglycemia
Tachypnea (40-60/min) with warm flushed skin	Poisoning
Vomiting: intermittent, projectile	Increased intracranial pressure
Position:	
Comfortable with occasional shifting	Lesser degree of coma
Uncomfortable, rigid	Greater degree of coma
Decorticate (Fig. 4-2, *A*)	Supratentorial lesion
Decerebrate (Fig. 4-2, *B*)	Brainstem damage
External rotation of leg	Pyramidal tract lesion or fractured/dislocated hip (Swartzman, 1981)

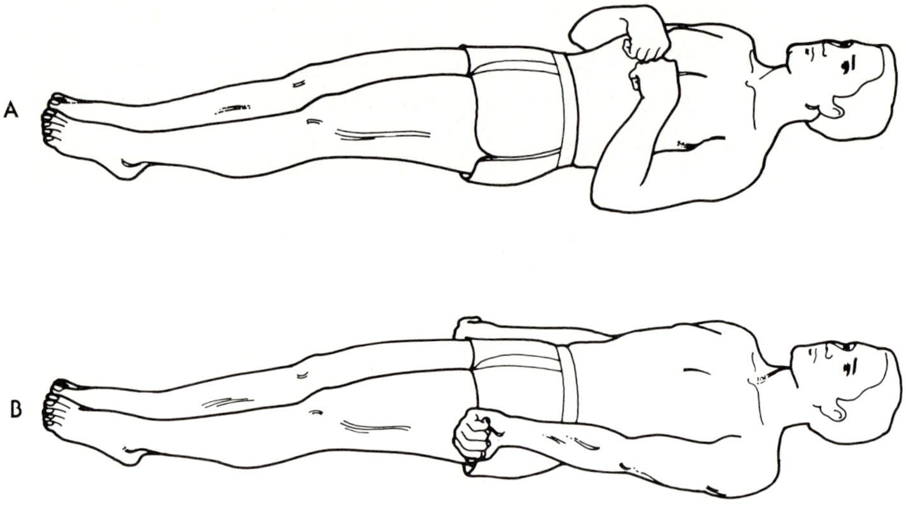

Fig. 4-2 **A,** Decorticate position indicates cerebral cortex lesion. **B,** Decerebrate position indicates brainstem lesion or pressure. (From Budassi, S.A., and Barber, J.M., Mosby's manual of emergency care, ed. 2, St. Louis, 1984, The C.V. Mosby Co.)

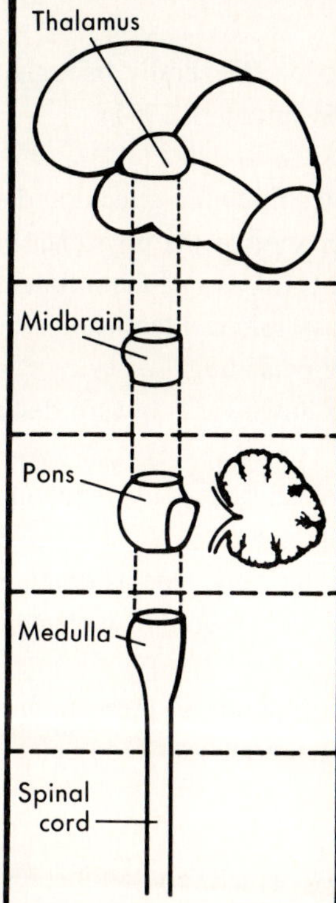

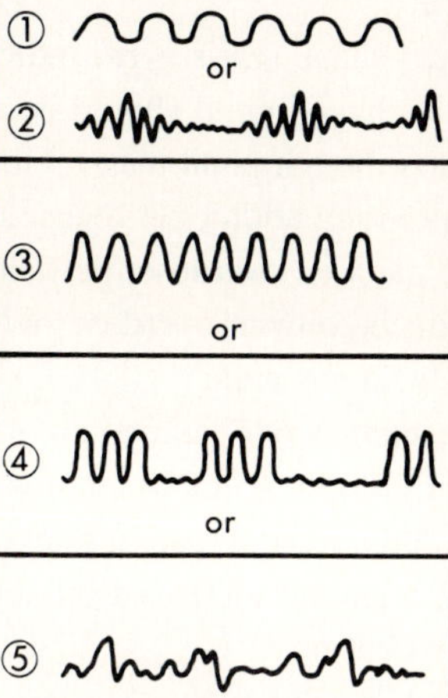

CNS level affected	Respiratory pattern	LOC	Pupils	Posture	Doll's eye
Thalamus	① or ②	Stupor Semi-coma	Small Reactive	Decorticate	−
Midbrain	③ or	Coma	Mid-position Nonreact	Decerebrate	+
Pons	④ or	Coma	"	Flaccid	+
Medulla	⑤	Coma	"	Flaccid	+
Spinal cord	1 Normal respiration 2 Cheyne-Stokes with decreased response to pain and decreased corneal reflexes				
	3 Neurogenic hyper-ventilation Not responsive to O_2 and "patterned"				
	4 Biot's respiration with regular periods of hyperventilation and irregular periods of apnea				
	5 "Apneustic" respiration with ataxic, gasping, shallow pattern				

Fig. 4-3 Altered respiratory patterns and neurological signs. (From Lanros, N.: Assessments and interventions in emergency nursing, Bowie, Md., 1978, Robert J. Brady Co.)

Greater than 130/70 with widening pulse pressure may indicate increased intracranial pressure.

Temperature (rectal or axillary because of increased potential for seizure):

Below 98.6° F indicates phenothiazine intoxication, hypoglycemia, cerebrovascular accident, or renal or hepatic disease.

Above 102° F indicates ruptured cerebral aneurysm, anticholinergic poisoning, or heat stroke.

Above 106° F indicates viral infection. Generally bacterial infections do not raise temperatures over 106° (Swartzman, 1981).

Pupil shape:

Elliptical shape (cat's eyes) indicates midbrain structural damage.

An oval-shaped pupil should be reported to the physician immediately.

Pupil size: Although pupil measurements may vary, the following sizes may assist in pinpointing additional focused assessments that should be made.

1 mm: narcotic overdose; pesticide poisoning

2-3 mm: barbituate overdose; with downward, inward deviation, hemorrhage in thalamus area.

3 mm, nonreactive: autonomic nervous system dysfunction

3-5 mm, elliptical: midbrain dysfunction

5 mm, unilateral: expanding lesion on same side as dilation

5 mm, bilateral: increased intracranial pressure (Swartzman, 1981)

Pupillary reaction:

Bilateral, slow: structural lesion in midbrain or pressure on oculomotor nerve.

Unilateral, slow: expanding supratentorial lesion on same side as slow reaction; drug overdose.

Eye movements:

Absent: brainstem lesions, overdose of tricyclic antidepressants, barbituates, alcohol, anticonvulsants.

Paresis of or abnormal eye movement: supratentorial lesions, hypoxia, endogenous metabolic disease, overdose of opiates or phenothiazines. Paresis of eye muscles results from pressure on or hypoxia of cranial nerves IV, VI, or III. Abnormal movements include upward, lateral or proximal rotation or deviation of one or both eyes or disconjugate gaze.

Nystagmus: brainstem infarction or, more commonly, exogenous poisoning with CNS depressants (Scott, 1975).

Motor abilities of extremities:

Spontaneous movement: symmetrical asterixis (flapping), myoclonic jerks, and tremors indicate metabolic or exogenous poisoning (Plum and Posner, 1980).

Arm and leg raising: also useful in assessing muscle tone and differentiating hemiparesis caused by contralateral supratentorial lesions.

If patient is responsive to verbal stimuli, test hand grasp equality, plantar flexion and extension.

Reflexes: gag, Babinski, Brudzinski, Kernig (see Chapter 1)

Diagnostic tests

Radiographs:

Skull x-rays: to visualize skull fracture, mastoid/sinus infection, midline shift of pineal gland,

Cervical spine x-rays: to visualize dislocated vertebral fractures compressing spinal cord,

CAT scan: identify space-occupying lesions causing compression of parenchyma, determine size and location of ventricles. Note: CAT scan with intravenous infusion of Reno M30 can be used to delineate vascular abnormalities.

Hematological tests:

Arterial blood gases: to determine Po_2, Pco_2, acidosis, alkalosis.

Electrolyte/chemistry profile: to determine status of:

Substance	Normal range
Glucose	80-120 mg/100 ml
Sodium	132-142 mEq/L
Potassium	3.5-5.5 mEq/L
Calcium	8.5-10.5 mg/100 ml
Phosphorus	3.0-4.5 mg/100 mg
Magnesium	1.5-2.5 mEq/L
Blood urea nitrogen	8-20 mg/100 ml
Creatinine	0.5-1.5 mg/100 ml

Screening toxicology tests: CNS depressants.

Coagulation studies: Prothrombin time (normal is 12-14 sec).
Partial thromboplastin time (normal is 35-45 sec).

Urine tests

Toxicology screening

Creatinine clearance (normal is 115-120 ml/min or 0.7-1.5 mg/ml). NOTE: Creatinine clearance is done to estimate glomerular filtration and thereby estimate the kidneys' ability to excrete waste products.

Lumbar puncture with cerebrospinal fluid examination: if CNS infection is suspected.

Specific assessment data. In addition to the general assessments discussed above, assessments to identify specific causes of the depressed LOC are prerequisite to accurate therapeutic, preventative, and supportive interventions. For specific assessments and interventions in trauma and vascular insufficiency see Chapters 9 and 13.

Psychogenic depression of LOC

Psychogenic depression of LOC may be a result of boredom, loneliness, decreased self-concept, or lack of mental stimulation.

Subjective assessment data

Feelings of loneliness, sadness
Apathy and drowsiness
Lack of energy and goal directedness
Inability to concentrate or use mental faculties
Loss of appetite with weight loss
Decreased feelings of self-worth
Self-blaming, guilty statements
Feeling of "lump in throat"
Frequent tearing, crying
Conversational focus on self
History of taking multiple medications

Objective assessment data

General appearance:
- Lack of eye contact
- Unkempt appearance
- Body odor, halitosis
- Slow motor movements

Low voice tone
Decreased pulse rate
Slow respirations with frequent audible sighs
Dehydrated skin and mucous membranes
Negative statements regarding self/others
Positioning: head lowered, facing away from people, stooped shoulders
Decreased urine and fecal elimination
Dysphagia
Increased sleeping
Ataxia, impaired dexterity

ENDOGENOUS DISEASES

Many nonneurological diseases can cause a metabolically induced depressed LOC. For example, the hyperglycemic state of the diabetic can progress to acidotic coma. Chronic pulmonary obstructive disease can cause brain hypoxia resulting in a depression in cerebral functioning. High blood urea nitrogen levels, indicative of advanced kidney disease, result in uremic poisoning with a concomitant depressed LOC. Hepatic coma in end-stage liver disease results in vascular retention of metabolic waste products. Infectious diseases such as meningitis or encephalitis as well as cardiac, respiratory, and severe urinary infections can cause a depression in the level of consciousness because of high fevers. A thorough assessment of the possible metabolic and infectious causes of depressed LOC is prerequisite to providing appropriate treatment. A high level of suspicion for the numerous endogenous causes of depressed LOC facilitates a definitive diagnosis. Careful examination of laboratory and diagnostic tests

Table 4-10 Correlation of laboratory tests with assessments corroborating endogenous disease states

Laboratory tests	Corroborative assessments	Dysfunction
Elevated BUN	Gastrointestinal upsets Dehydration; skin, mucous membranes Polyuria progressing to oliguria Drowsiness with headache Muscle fasciculations Seizure activity Foul breath/body odor	Kidney disease
Elevated SGOT, SGPT, bilirubin	Mentation changes Drowsiness progressing to disorientation Motor incoordination Tremors, particularly of hands Jaundice Musty body odor Headache Clay-colored stools Musty breath odor	Liver disease
Elevated CO_2, decreased O_2	Excessive tenacious mucous Hacking productive cough Dyspnea during exertion or at rest Variable disorientation and apprehension Excessive fatigue Pallor progressing to cyanotic color	Pulmonary disease
Elevated blood sugar	Thirst though fluid intake high Polyuria Drowsiness Anorexia, nausea, vomiting Abdominal cramps Headache and weakness Visual disturbances Deep slow respirations	Glucose imbalance
Elevated lymphocytes and/or segmented neutrophils	Fever with chills Drowsiness with increased shallow respirations Decreased concentration Fatigue Gastrointestinal upsets	Infection

facilitates a focused physical assessment. Table 4-10 summarizes the correlation of significant laboratory test data with focused physical assessments.

Exogenous poisonings

The number of potentially toxic agents in the home, industry, and in health care has increased dramatically in the past 10 years. Use and abuse of prescription, over-the-counter, and illicit drugs is increasing. Likewise, chemicals used in industry have increased. In some cases, CNS depressants are prescribed but are then taken inaccurately by the patient or they are sometimes administered incorrectly by care providers. In other instances, illegally obtained agents, commonly a mixed variety, are ingested, inhaled, or injected by drug abusers. Some people are at risk because of their occupations, such as farmers, crop dusters, potters, and factory workers. Others are at risk because of their age, that is, young children and the elderly. Because specific antidotes are available for some types of poisonings, an accurate history is essential. Because of this "chemical explosion," health care providers must be familiar with the assessments and interventions necessary to prevent death and to reduce morbidity. In this section we will discuss specific assessments necessary to detect CNS depressant drug overdoses, salicylate or acetaminophen overdoses, and pesticide/insecticide poisonings.

CNS depressants

CNS depressants are classified as opiates, hypnotics/sedatives, psychotropic agents, or analgesic/antipyretic agents.

- Opiates:
  - Narcotics: morphine, codeine
  - Synthetic narcotics: meperidine, methadone
- Hypnotics/sedatives:
  - Barbiturates: phenobarbital (Luminal), pentobarbital (Nembutal), secobarbital (Seconal)
  - Nonbarbiturates: Ethchlorvynol (Placydyl), methyprylon (Noludar), flurazepam (Dalmane)
- Psychotropic agents (tranquilizers):
  - Phenothiazines: chlorpromazine (Thorazine), thioridazine (Mellaril), prochlorperazine (Compazine)
  - Benzodiazapines: Diazepam (Valium), chlordiazepoxide (Librium)
- Analgesic/antipyretic agents:
  - Salicylates (aspirin)
  - Acetaminophen (Tylenol, Apamide)

Opiates. Opiates depress the cortical and some subcortical areas, thus inhibiting mental, gastrointestinal, and genitourinary activities. Subcortically, opiates depress the cough reflex and respirations and cause miosis and hypothermia. Their primary use is as an analgesic for acute pain.

Subjective assessment data

History of taking analgesics for chronic pain
Abdominal cramps
Inability to concentrate and make decisions
Drowsiness
Nausea with dry mouth
Vertigo
Decreased elimination: urine and feces

Objective assessment data

Difficult to arouse
Depressed respiration rate and depth
Dyspnea
Constipation
Ataxia with decreased muscle tone
Slurred, incoherent speech
Constricted pupils with decreased reaction to light
Warm, flushed skin with diaphoresis
Decreased urinary output
Disoriented to time, person, and place
Needle/track marks
Vomiting
Positive toxicology screening: urine and thin layer chomatography

Barbiturates. Barbiturates depress neural and synaptic activity in the reticular activating systems, thus decreasing cortical stimulation. In large doses, respiratory and vasomotor depression occurs, resulting in hypotension and respiratory distress.

Subjective assessment data

History of taking medication for insomnia, seizures, short-term pain following surgery, mental illness
Drowsiness and lethargy
Thick tongue and fumbling extremities with uncoordinated movements
Memory impairment
Impaired decision-making abilities
Muscle weakness
Feelings of dizziness, ''dazed''

Objective assessment data

Slurred speech
Impaired motor dexterity
Nystagmus
Ataxia
Loss of memory

Indecisiveness
Decreased muscle tone
Decreased pulse, respirations, and blood pressure (NOTE: If not corrected, circulatory collapse and respiratory arrest can occur)
Disorientation

Diagnostic tests:

EMIT screen and thin layer chromatography: positive for barbiturates
Serum level: over 5 mg/100 ml

Tranquilizers. These agents are used to alter the affective or behavioral state from anxiety to tranquility, thus permitting more normal interaction by the person with other people in the environment. Tranquilizers are classified as major or antipsychotic agents and as minor or antianxiety agents.

Subjective assessment data

History of anxiety, agitation, mental illness
Taking pills to decrease anxiousness, to prevent and control seizure disorders, or for mental illness
Feelings of physical and mental fatigue
Nasal congestion
Dry mouth, blurred vision
Constipation and urinary retention
Loss of libido
Vertigo and syncope
Delayed or lack of menstruation
Weight gain with increased appetite
Dysphagia
Dysphasia
Lack of perspiration
Edema of extremities
Urticaria

Objective assessment data

Lack of and/or incoordinated motor activities
Tremors of face and extremities
Dry oral mucosa
Decreased blood pressure, pulse, respirations
Decreased urinary and fecal elimination
Postural hypotension
Cardiac dysrhythmias
Skin discoloration: blue to purple spots on arms, neck, and face
Dyskinesias of legs and face (Fig. 4-4) with long-term use or overdosage with major (antipsychotic) agents
Pupils constricted

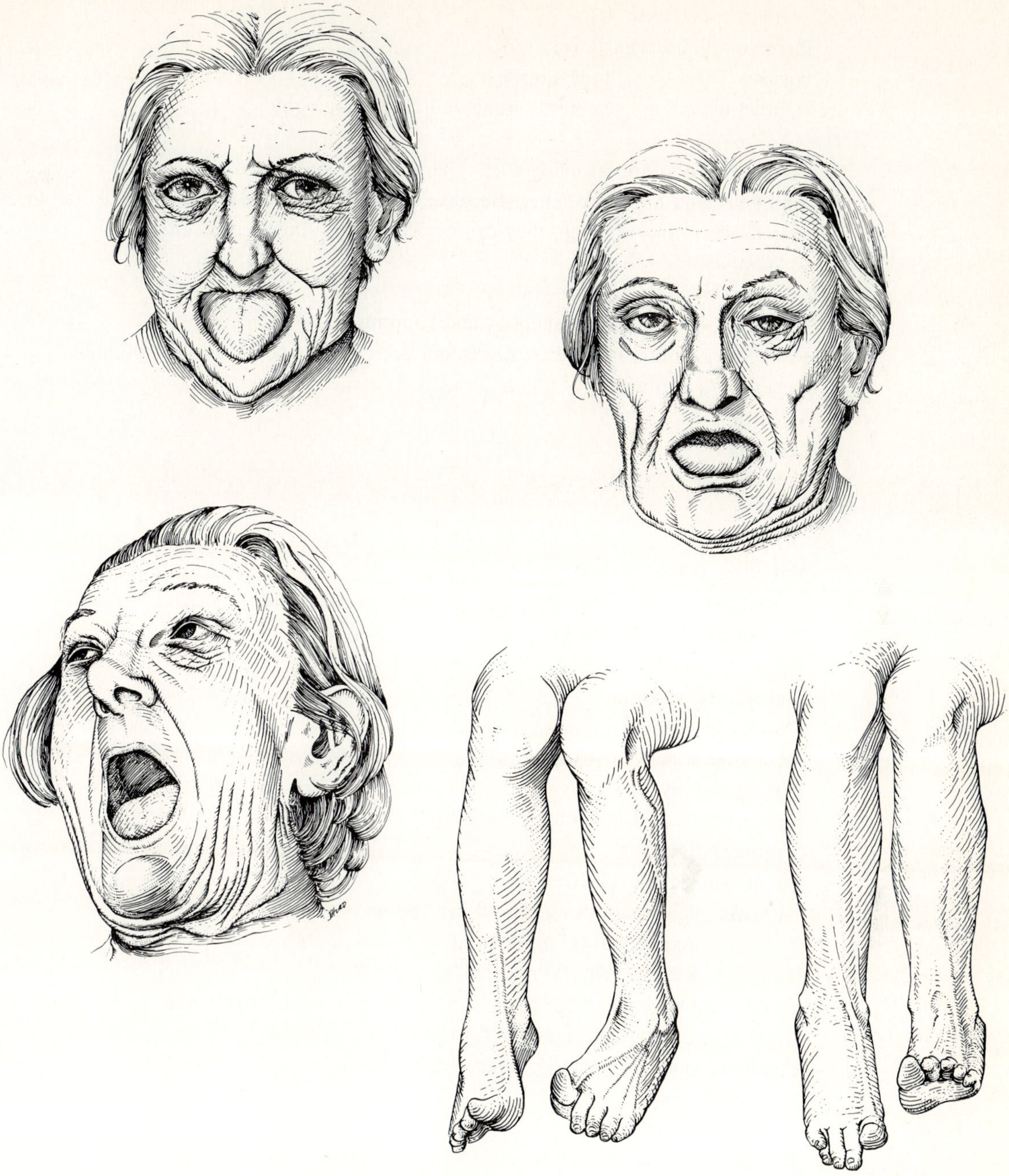

Fig. 4-4 Dyskinesias caused by long-term use or overuse of tranquilizers. (From Hahn, A.B., Barkin, R.L., and Oestreich, S.: Pharmacology in nursing, ed. 15, St. Louis, 1982, The C.V. Mosby Co.)

Diagnostic tests

Increased blood sugar level

Positive Tes-Tape, clinitest/acetest

Positive toxicology screening: urine and chromatography

Nonnarcotic analgesics/antipyretics. These agents are used to relieve head or muscle/joint pains and to reduce fever. Because of the frequent use of these agents and their availability in most homes, they can be accidentally ingested by children.

Salicylates

SUBJECTIVE ASSESSMENT DATA

Gastric upsets: nausea, dyspepsia, and vomiting

Restlessness followed by drowsiness and decreased responsiveness to stimuli

Generalized itchiness

Tinnitus

Dyspnea

OBJECTIVE ASSESSMENT DATA

Fever

Dehydration

Vomiting and diarrhea

Disorientation with slow response to stimuli (verbal/tactile)

Increased respirations initially, followed by respiratory depression (under 12/minute)

Rales

Red skin rash, hives

Petechiae

Decreased urine output

Seizure activity

Signs of increased intracranial pressure

DIAGNOSTIC TESTS

Blood salicylate level: over 30 mg/100 ml

NOTE: therapeutic level: 20-40 mg/100 ml
toxic level: 60 mg/100 ml
lethal level: 100 mg/100 ml

Complete blood count (CBC): decreased red blood count (RBC), hemoglobin, platelets

Adult blood pH: alkalosis, over 7.45 pH

Children blood pH: acidosis, under 7.35 pH

Acetaminophen

SUBJECTIVE ASSESSMENT DATA

History of ingestion of toxic dose: 24 to 30 tablets (325 mg/tablet)

Nausea

Anorexia

Upper right quadrant pain

Generalized weakness

Drowsiness

Table 4-11 Signs and symptoms of acetaminophen toxicity related to stages

Stage	Signs and symptoms
First 24 hours	Nausea and vomiting Anorexia Pallor Increased perspiration
24-72 hours	All the above signs and symptoms plus Upper right quadrant pain Decreased urinary output
72-120 hours	Signs of renal failure Cardiac failure Hepatic failure

OBJECTIVE ASSESSMENT DATA

Vomiting
Pallor with diaphoresis
Liver enlargement
Right upper quadrant tenderness
Fever
Decreasing response to verbal or painful stimuli
Jaundice
Rales
Decreased urine output

DIAGNOSTIC TESTS

Blood:

Plasma level of acetaminophen: over 200 μm produces hepatic toxicity
SGOT and SGPT: elevated
Prothrombin time: prolonged
Bilirubin: increased
Blood sugar: decreased
Platelets: normal (a differential between salicylate and Acetaminophen overdose)

Urine:

Toxicology screening: Acetaminophen present in urine

The differentiation of the signs and symptoms related to early, intermediate, and late stages of acetaminophen toxicity is illustrated in Table 4-11.

Pesticides/insecticides

A focused interview to determine the patient's occupation is essential in determining the potential of pesticide/insecticide poisoning. Farmers, crop dusters, pest control persons, and industrial workers in pesticide production plants are all likely suspects. These chemical substances can be ingested or inhaled as well as absorbed through the skin. The initial signs and symptoms are related to the method of exposure. When the pesticides/insecticides are ingested, gastric signs and symptoms appear first. Bronchial signs occur initially following inhalation. Dermatological and ophthalmic signs and symptoms correlate with topical exposure. Muscarinic signs and symptoms result from an inhibition or blocking of cholinesterase with an accumulation of acetylcholine at cholinergic neuroeffector sites. The vasoconstrictive nicotinic effects affect autonomic ganglia. The CNS signs and symptoms result from impaired neural transmission in the brain causing depressed LOC and alterations in behavior as well as a depressed respiratory drive and depressed voluntary motor function (Morgan, 1982).

Subjective assessment data

Nausea and anorexia
Abdominal cramps
Blurred vision
Sore, red, tearing eyes
Increased urination
Generalized itchiness
Chest pain
Drooling
Excessive perspiration
Generalized weakness
Restlessness followed by extreme drowsiness
Headache, dizziness
Muscle twitching in face and arms

Objective assessment data

Muscarinic signs

Vomiting
Diarrhea
Hyperactive bowel sounds
Increased salivation and lacrimation
Conjunctivitis
Diaphoresis
Involuntary micturition and defecation
Miosis (diagnostically significant indicator of pesticide poisoning in the presence of gastric flu signs)

Nicotinic and CNS signs

Depressed respirations, pulse, blood pressure
Pallor
Diaphoresis
Decreased muscle tone progressing to flaccid paralysis
Uncoordinated movements
Decreasing orientation progressing to nonresponsiveness to verbal/painful stimuli
Muscle fasciculations when specific areas are tapped. NOTE: To elicit tap muscles over cheek bones, upper arm, and thorax and observe for fasciculations.

Mnemonic for signs and symptoms: SLUDGEM

Salivation
Lacrimation
Urination
Defecation
GI upsets
Emesis
Miosis

Laboratory data

Blood

Increased blood sugar
Plasma cholinesterase screening test (Acholtest): positive
Decreased RBC cholinesterase level: $<0.5\ \mu g$
Decreased potassium level (<3.0 mg)

Urine

Urinary pesticide metabolites present: phenol or alkyl phosphate
Glycosuria with ketones negative (Morgan, 1982).

Nursing care plan: **DEPRESSED LEVEL OF CONSCIOUSNESS**

NURSING DIAGNOSIS	EXPECTED OUTCOMES	NURSING INTERVENTIONS
Ineffective airway clearance due to: **1. Paresis of tongue** **2. Nonresponsive status**	Patent airway	Position in left lateral semi-Fowler's position to prevent airway occlusion by tongue. Maintain tracheal alignment. Insert oral airway. Prepare for and assist with endotracheal intubation. Hyperventilate patient, then aseptically suction endotracheal tube for no longer than 15 seconds.
Ineffective breathing pattern due to: **1. Supratentorial herniation with pressure on pneumotaxic centers in brainstem** **2. Direct pressure on brainstem from infratentorial lesions** **3. Lack of CO_2 stimulation of pneumotaxic centers or decreased hypoxic drive from carotid sinus interference** **4. Decreased pH** NOTE: Glucose and O_2 are essential for neural activity	Eupneic respiratory pattern pH 7.35-7.45	Observe for altered respiratory patterns. (see Fig. 4.3) Demonstrate and continue deep breathing or sustained maximal inspiration procedures every 2 hours at minimum. Monitor ICP readings (see Chapter 2) for altered waves. Monitor blood pH. If pH is lower than 7.35, administer prescribed sodium bicarbonate to correct acidosis. Administer prescribed 50% glucose to correct hypoglycemia. NOTE: Most protocols for care of unconscious patients include immediate administration of 50 ml of 50% glucose and oxygen (10 L/min) to prevent brain damage. Apply prescribed thigh-high antiembolism stockings. NOTE: Change stockings daily.

Continued.

Nursing care plan: **DEPRESSED LEVEL OF CONSCIOUSNESS—cont'd**

NURSING DIAGNOSIS	EXPECTED OUTCOMES	NURSING INTERVENTIONS
Impaired gas exchange due to ineffective breathing patterns. NOTE: Constant oxygen requirement for neural functioning is 20%	Po_2 80-100%	Initiate 100% humidified oxygen at 6-10 L/min per mask, cannula, or mechanical ventilator. Monitor arterial blood-gas tests. Observe for signs of hypoxia. Monitor rectal temperature every 4 hours. NOTE: Oxygen requirements increase by 10% for every degree centigrade increase in temperature (Swatzman, 1981).
Decreased cardiac output due to acid base imbalance and/or hypoxia, resulting in decreased perfusion of blood to brain and periphery	Blood pressure 120/80; capillary refill time: 2 sec	Monitor blood pressure for (1) increases due to increased intracranial pressure; (2) decrease due to ineffective ventricular contraction. Monitor capillary refill time: fingernails, toenails, and forehead. Monitor for dysrhythmias. Initiate prescribed IV infusion using microdrip. Rate of infusion is titrated to maintain 30 ml/hour urinary output and blood pressure of 90/50.
Potential for systemic poisoning due to ingestion or injection of CNS depressant agents	Negative toxicology test Normal vital and neurological signs	If substance was ingested within 4-8 hours: 1. Induce vomiting (Table 4-3). 2. Initiate gastric lavage (Table 4-4). Administer prescribed antidotes (see Table 4-12).
Impaired cognitive functioning in nonresponsive state due to organic lesions, CNS depressants, or sensory deprivation	Oriented to time, person, place Responsive to verbal and environmental stimuli	Monitor and record orientation and arousal level and other neurological assessment signs on flow sheet. Continue orientation measures: verbal reminders of person, place, and time; visits from significant others; calendars, clocks, personal pictures, intermittently turn on favorite radio station or TV program; open window coverings during day; turn off lights at night. Provide verbal and tactile stimuli: visit patient regularly to prevent isolation; converse with patient about favorite topics: sporting events, theater, family community; explain rationale for and methods used in care procedures; encourage family and friends to visit with patient; keep significant persons informed as to progress or regression of status; express caring concern verbally and through touch.
Potential for physical injury	No injury	Provide a safe, nonisolative environment: padded side rails in up position; judicious use of soft restraints to prevent falls, self-injury. For partially oriented, mobile patients: keep light on in bathroom at night; place furniture to prevent tripping or falls.

Continued.

Table 4-12 Pharmacologic antidotes*

Antidote	Use
Acetylcysteine (Mucomyst)	Acetaminophen poisoning
Antivenin (Crotalidae), polyvalent	Pit viper snakebites
Antivenin, Lactrodectus mactans	Black widow spider bites
Atropine injection	Organophosphate and carbamate poisonings
Calcium disodium edetate (EDTA) (Versenate)	Lead and other types of heavy metal poisoning
Deferoxamine (Desferal)	Iron poisoning
Dimercaprol (BAL)	Arsenic, gold, lead, mercury poisoning
Ethanol (for oral and IV use)	Methanol and ethylene glycol poisoning
Methylene blue	Methemoglobinemia
Naloxone (Narcan)	Narcotic poisoning
Oxygen	Carbon monoxide poisoning
Penicillamine	Copper, lead, mercury, and arsenic poisoning
Physostigmine (Antilirium)	Anticholinergic and tricyclic antidepressant poisoning
Pralidoxime (2-PAM) (Protopam)	Organophosphate poisoning
Cyanide antidote kit	Cyanide poisoning
Contains: Amyl nitrite inhaler	
Sodium nitrite	
Sodium thiosulfate	

*From Manoguerra, A.: Assessment and management of poisonings, Emergency Nursing update **2**(3):3, 1981. Reprinted with permission from the author and *Emergency Nursing Update Series,* a publication of CPEC, Inc.

Nursing care plan: **DEPRESSED LEVEL OF CONSCIOUSNESS—cont'd**

NURSING DIAGNOSIS	EXPECTED OUTCOMES	NURSING INTERVENTIONS
Nutritional deficiency due to inadequate intake of nutrients	Normal muscle mass and tone Maintenance of weight	If gag and swallowing reflexes are present, provide nutritious diet including patient's preferred foods and fluids. If patient is comatose, initiate prescribed enterotherapy slowly via nasogastric or gastrostomy tube using an intermittent schedule. Monitor daily weights.
Potential skin breakdown	Integrity of skin	Change position every 2 hours. Remember that patients should not be positioned on red skin areas. Skin breakdown will occur within 20 minutes. Provide daily baths with warm water. Use soap sparingly to prevent dryness. Initiate passive range of motion exercises to increase peripheral skin circulation. Inspect skin for pressure areas, abrasions, or rashes. Provide eye hygiene: Instill artificial tears every shift. If eyelids do not close to cover cornea, butterfly tape lids closed. Change tape every shift, at minimum. Provide oral hygiene every shift: Use tongue blades covered with moistened 4 × 4's to swab oral cavity. Brush teeth and tongue every shift.
Altered bowel elimination due to immobility and decreased food and fluid intake	Normal bowel evacuation	Initiate digital stimulation or daily suppository procedure. Place in Fowler's position to enhance normal gravity evacuation.
Impaired urinary elimination	Output of 30 ml/hr	Aseptically insert prescribed retention catheter if urine is retained or patient is incontinent. Remove within 3-4 days on males and replace with external catheter. Monitor CBC for increased WBC indicative of infection. Monitor urinary output: NOTE: Minimum output to sustain kidney function is 30 ml/hour. Inspect urine for color, sediment. Measure specific gravity. NOTE: Urine dipsticks are available to qualitatively test for pH, glucose, ketone, protein, and blood. Initiate bladder training program as soon as possible (see Chapter 11 on rehabilitation).

Continued.

Nursing care plan: DEPRESSED LEVEL OF CONSCIOUSNESS—cont'd

NURSING DIAGNOSIS	EXPECTED OUTCOMES	NURSING INTERVENTIONS
Potential for joint contractures due to malpositioning and spastic paralysis consistent with upper motor neuron dysfunction	No joint contractures	Position in alignment: Trochanter rolls at hips when supine; high top tennis shoes or footboard to prevent plantar flexion; hand rolls, nerf balls, or plastic splints to prevent finger and wrist flexion. NOTE: A nerf ball is a sponge ball available in toy departments. Position changes (supine and lateral) (see Fig. 4-5) Transfer to recliner chair at intermittent (3-4 times daily) intervals as soon as condition is stable.

Continued.

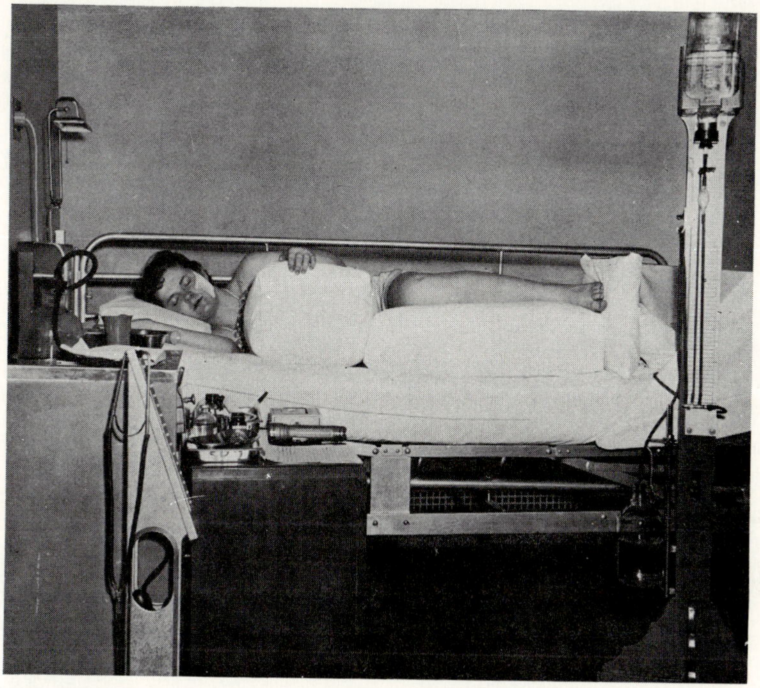

Fig. 4-5 Unconscious client in optimal position with necessary equipment at bedside to expedite nursing care. (One side has been removed temporarily.) (From Conway-Rutkowski, B.L.: Carini and Owens' neurological and neurosurgical nursing, ed. 8, St. Louis, 1982, The C.V. Mosby Co.)

Nursing care plan: **DEPRESSED LEVEL OF CONSCIOUSNESS—cont'd**

NURSING DIAGNOSIS	EXPECTED OUTCOMES	NURSING INTERVENTIONS
Self-care deficit requiring reliance on family or others for assistance in home setting	Family member demonstrates skills required in physical care and knowledge of resources available	Encourage family partication in care in early stages. Demonstrate physical care measures including: Body hygiene methods Respiratory hygiene methods: Deep breathing Yawning Sighing Tracheostomy care Position changes: Joint mobility exercises Transfer techniques Gastric lavage Discuss: Nutrition and hydration needs and methods Need for diversion and physical and mental stimulation Depending on cause of depressed LOC, inform family of resources for information and referral: Poison control centers Environmental protection agencies Public/community health services Mental health inpatient and outpatient facilities Chemical dependency rehabilitation centers and programs Voluntary agencies such as stroke clubs, diabetes association
Knowledge deficit: ways to prevent poisonings	Decreased incidence of poisonings, the use of preventive measures.	Discuss the prevention of poisonings: Medications: Safe storage of medications Correct methods of taking prescribed medications Methods of keeping track of medications taken: calendars, muffin tins. Pesticides/insecticides: The use of protective clothing covering entire body, goggles for eyes, masks with charcoal trap changed every 2 hours during mixing and application. Showering thoroughly after use. Washing clothes separately from family wash. Safe storage and disposal of containers: Storage: Store in containers labeled poison in a location not accessible to children. Disposal: Rinse container three times in Clorox water, replace lid, and bury in land fill or return to store where purchased. Name and phone number of local environmental protection agency

Suggested readings

Adams, R., and Victor, M.: Principles of neurology, New York, 1981, McGraw-Hill Book Co

Bergersen, B.: Pharmacology in nursing, ed. 14, St. Louis, 1979, The C.V. Mosby Co.

Conway-Rutkowski, B.: Carini and Owen's neurological and neurosurgical nursing, ed. 8, St. Louis, 1982, The C.V. Mosby Co.

Jaffe, J.: Drug Addiction and drug abuse. In Goodman, L., and Gilman, A., editors: Pharmacological basis of therapeutics, ed. 6, New York, 1980, Macmillan Publishing Co., Inc.

Manoguerra, A.: Assessment and management of poisonings, Emergency nursing update, Vol. 2, No. 3, Princeton, 1981, Continuing Professional Education Center, Inc.

Mauss-Clum, N.: Bringing the unconscious patient back safely, Nursing '82 **12:**34-43, Aug. 1982.

Morgan, D.: Recognition and management of pesticide poisonings, ed. 3, Washington, D.C., 1982, U.S. Environmental Protection Agency.

Pisarcik, G.: Psychiatric emergencies. In Budassi, S., and Barber, J.: Emergency nursing: principles and practice, St. Louis, 1981, The C.V. Mosby Co.

Plum, F., and Posner, J.: Diagnosis of stupor and coma, ed. 3, Philadelphia, 1980, F.A. Davis Co.

Scott, R.: The challenge of coma, Emergency Med. **6**(7):179, Oct. 1975.

Swartzman, R.: Neurological evaluation of the unconscious patient, Postgraduate course No. 237, Sept. 1981, ACEP Scientific Assembly.

Audiovisual resources

Samuels, M.: Emergency management: the first 30 minutes—coma, I.C.P.E., Minneapolis, 1978, McGraw-Hill Publications Co.

Silver, M.: The comatose patient, AMA Video Clinic, Los Angeles, 1979, UCLA-AMA.

CHAPTER 5

Congenital and developmental disorders

This chapter focuses on three developmental disorders that may affect the infant or young child. Each will be discussed in relation to the disease process itself with an emphasis on nursing care. The disorders to be included are spina bifida, hydrocephaly, and cerebral palsy.

SPINA BIFIDA

Spina bifida is a term used to describe a group of congenital deviations of the spine. It is the second most frequent handicap of children after cerebral palsy. This condition results when the neural tube does not close and this failure to close results in brain or spinal cord malfunction. These patients may display deviations ranging from no symptoms to severe neurological, urological, or orthopedic manifestations. The exact etiology is unknown.

Classifications

Spina bifida occulta. This type occurs most frequently but is rarely symptomatic. At times there is no physical evidence or there may be a slight indentation or tuft of hair in the area of the fifth lumbar to first sacral vertebral segment. For a small number of children, there may be evidence of a slight gait disturbance. Others may develop urinary impairment or pain radiating to the legs.

Spina bifida cystica. This type occurs in approximately 0.2 to 4.0 per 1000 births and is subdivided into two further types.

Meningocele: a cystic lesion along the midline of the back through which only the meninges protrude. This is relatively rare.

Meningomyelocele: results when meninges and a malformed spinal cord protrude through an opening in one or more vertebrae. Meningomyelocele most commonly occurs in the lumbosacral area. (Fig. 5-1)

If there is a family history of neural tube defects, amniotic fluid can be obtained with an amniocentesis (before 18 weeks) and examined for alpha fetoprotein (AFP). The level of this protein is elevated if the fetus has anencephaly (absence of the cerebrum, cerebellum, and the flat bones of the skull), meningomyelocele, encephalocele, and omphalocele (herniation of the abdominal contents into the base of the umbilicus).

When a baby is born with meningomyelocele, it is apparent immediately at the time

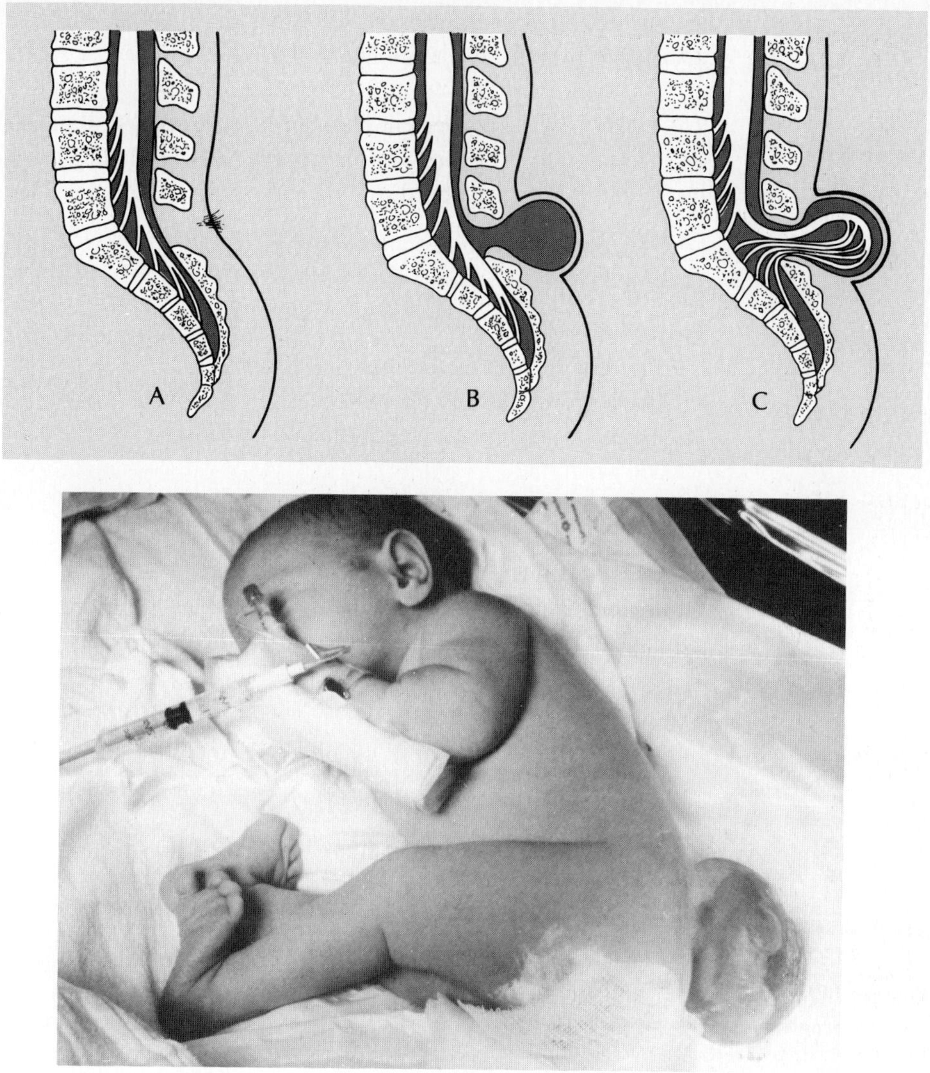

D

Fig. 5-1

Midsagittal view of spinal column with various degrees of neural defect. **A,** Spina bifida occulta. Note posterior vertebral arches have not fused. There is no herniation of the cord or meninges. **B,** Meningocele. Meninges protrude through the spina bifida forming a saclike cyst visible on the infant's back. **C,** Meningomyelocele. Meninges, elements of the cord with its nerves, and spinal fluid protrude through the spina bifida. This defect resembles a meningocele externally. **D,** Infant with lumbar myelomeningocele. (Courtesy of Dr. Paul Winchester. Reprinted from Maternal-Newborn Nursing: A Family-Centered Approach by Sally Olds, Patricia Ladewig, Marcia London. Copyright © 1984 by Addison-Wesley Publishing Company, Inc., Medical-Nursing Divison.)

of birth. It is crucial that the parents quickly become aware of what this defect involves and the outcome for their infant. Decisions regarding treatment of the infant must be made during the first 24 to 48 hours of life.

Nursing assessment

The extent of the involvement may not be accurately determined at birth. The baby must be carefully examined by a team of specialists including the pediatrician, neurologist, urologist, and orthopedist. The nursing assessment includes subjective and objective data.

Subjective data (from parents)

Prenatal history
- Any diseases the mother may have had
- Medications taken by the mother
- Family history related to congenital anomalies

Objective data

Is the sac closed, open, macerated? An open sac would require emergency surgery to close it immediately.
Bowel and bladder function: Is there a continuous wet diaper and a leakage of stool?
Assess the infant for accompanying orthopedic defects such as congenital hip, knee, foot, or spine deformities.
Assess motor and sensory functions. The lower extremities particularly should be assessed for response to painful stimuli and for the presence of flaccid or spastic paralysis.
Observe for the presence of hydrocephalus.
Assess the family's coping abilities.

Nursing care plan: SPINA BIFIDA

NURSING DIAGNOSIS	EXPECTED OUTCOMES	NURSING INTERVENTIONS
First few days: Potential for impairment of skin integrity	The sac will remain intact. The sac and incision area will be free from infection.	Position on side or abdomen only. Avoid pressure on back when holding. Immediately in the delivery room cover the sac with sterile towel or dressing. After surgical closure keep incision clean, uncontaminated from urine and feces. Observe the sac for pus or drainage, redness, or edema. Monitor vital signs for evidence of localized or systemic infection.
Alterations in patterns of urinary elimination	There will be absence of urinary tract infection as evidenced by lab values within normal limits and by absence of elevated temperature and pulse.	Use Credé maneuver to ensure complete emptying of bladder. Routine urinalysis.

NURSING DIAGNOSIS	EXPECTED OUTCOMES	NURSING INTERVENTIONS
Impaired mobility	The child will maintain optimal range of movement of all extremities.	Change position at least every 2 hours. Passive range of motion for all joints.
Observe for development of hydrocephalus	The child will be assessed for signs of hydrocephaly.	Measure head circumference daily. Observe for signs and symptoms of increased intracranial pressure such as lethargy, irritability, vomiting. Check fontanelle with infant sitting upright.
Potential impairment of significant others in their adjustment to illness	Parent-infant interactions will be enhanced and maintained by providing for closeness and touching.	Encourage family to hold infant even if he has to be kept prone. Include family in care-giving activities such as feeding and bathing.
As the child gets older: Alterations in nutrition	As the child grows older, he will maintain a balance between nutritional intake and energy expenditure.	If the child shows the ability to use braces to learn to walk, there is a need to increase the caloric intake, but when that child becomes older and starts using a wheelchair, the energy expenditure may decrease and the child may become obese if caloric intake remains increased. Obtain nutritional intake records. Record height and weight. Consult with a dietician if necessary.
Impaired mobility	The child will achieve and maintain his optimal level of mobility.	With flaccid paralysis proper positioning and passive range of motion exercises are initiated at birth and continued as part of playtime as the child becomes older. Use coasters or wagons for those children able to utilize upper extremities. Braces for standing can be introduced at 18-24 months. Eventually, crutches may be used for short periods of time, and a wheelchair for community ambulation.
Alterations in self-esteem, self-concept, role performance, personal identity, and/or body image Infant	The child will develop and maintain a good self-concept.	The lesion itself, braces, or other equipment inhibits the usual touching and cuddling by the mother. Encourage parents to touch and hold their infant.
Young child		Provide the child positive experiences to increase acceptance of self and prepare him for peer interactions. Family must be encouraged to show acceptance of the child and an understanding of his problems yet set consistent, firm limits.
Preadolescence and adolescence through adulthood		Allow for ventilation of feelings regarding problems of urinary and bowel incontinence, immobility, lack of sensation below lesion. Recognize that the adolescent identifies the problems of urinary incontinence and the establishment of a daily bowel regimen as frustrating or embarrassing. Sexual counseling and evaluation should be available. (The amount of sexual sensation depends on the level of the lesion and whether there is partial or complete involvement.) Recognize concerns involved with architectural barriers, schooling, and establishment of close friendships and marriage.

HYDROCEPHALUS

Hydrocephalus literally means "water head" and is almost always the result of an interference in the circulation of cerebrospinal fluid (CSF) in the system (Fig. 5-2). This interference may result from an alteration in the absorption or the production of CSF. The incidence of hydrocephalus is 4 per 1000 births through the age of 3 months, and it may develop at any time during this period.

Classifications

Hydrocephalus is classified as communicating or noncommunicating. Communicating hydrocephalus involves excessive accumulation of CSF within the ventricular system. The fluid accumulates as a result of an alteration of absorptive capacity from the subarachnoid space. In noncommunicating (obstructive) hydrocephalus CSF accumulates as a result of the obstruction of the normal flow at some point in the ventricular system.

Most obstructions to the flow of CSF are the result of congenital abnormalities. In fact, 70% are the result of the narrowing of the aqueduct of Sylvius (Olds, 1980) (Fig. 5-3). Another congenital deviation closely associated with hydrocephaly is meningomyelocele. The hydrocephalus associated with meningomyelocele is usually the result of an Arnold-Chiari malformation (herniation of the lower brainstem and cerebellum through the foramen magnum with fixed attachment of the spinal cord at the site of meningomyelocele).

Etiology

Obstruction of the flow of CSF may be the result of one of a variety of causes. Posttraumatic or postinflammatory obstruction can result from intracranial bleeding at birth and from meningitis or other infections. Brain tumors, particularly gliomas of the third or fourth ventricles, can also cause obstruction. Choroid plexus tumors are rare in childhood.

Even though signs and symptoms of hydrocephalus may be evident at birth, it is necessary to perform diagnostic tests such as the following to confirm hydrocephalus and to identify the etiology:

1. Lumbar puncture. The CSF should be analyzed for cell count, glucose, protein, and particulate matter. Caution must be taken because of the usual presence of increased intracranial pressure (ICP).
2. Computerized axial tomography (CAT). The CAT scan provides a more comprehensive view of the skull. The pictures show variations of the ventricular system, tissue density, and the presence of masses. This examination is most beneficial when used with other radiological tests.
3. Skull x-ray films
4. Angiogram
5. Pneumoencephalogram
6. Ventriculogram
7. Subdural and ventricular taps

Pathophysiology

The CSF is produced in the choroid plexuses in each of the ventricles and within the brain itself. The fluid flows from the lateral ventricle through the foramen of Luschka

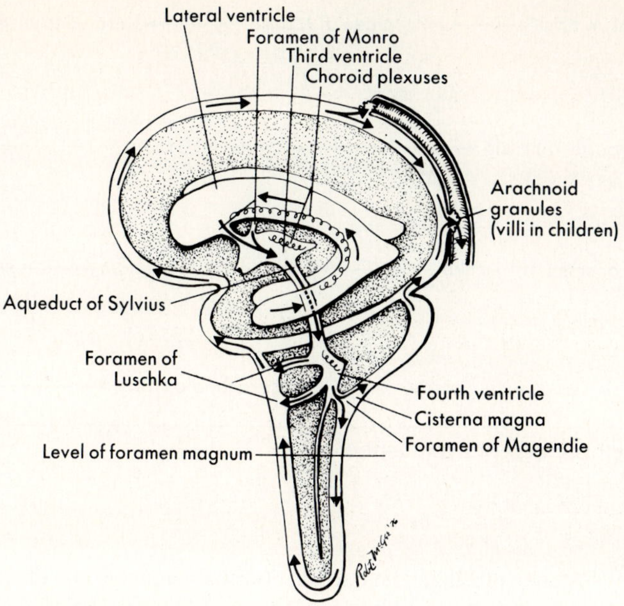

Fig. 5-2 Cerebrospinal fluid circulation. (From Whaley, L., and Wong, D.: Nursing care of infants and children, ed. 2, St. Louis, 1983, The C.V. Mosby Co.)

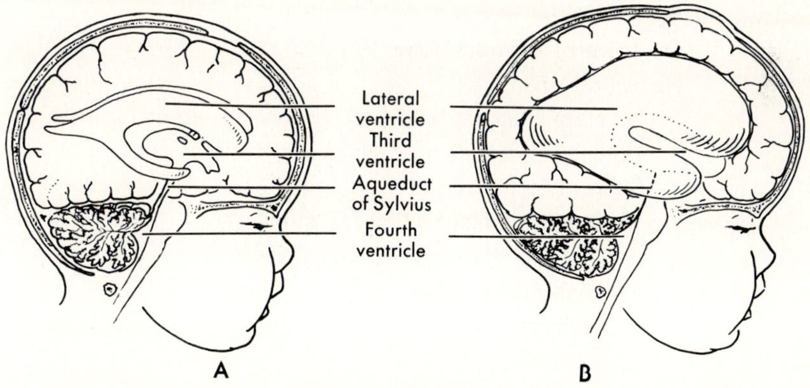

Fig. 5-3 Hydrocephalus: a block in the flow of cerebrospinal fluid. **A,** Patent cerebrospinal fluid circulation. **B,** Enlarged lateral and third ventricles caused by obstruction of circulation-stenosis of aqueduct of Sylvius. (From Whaley, L., and Wong, D.: Nursing care of infants and children, ed. 2, St. Louis, 1983, The C.V. Mosby Co.)

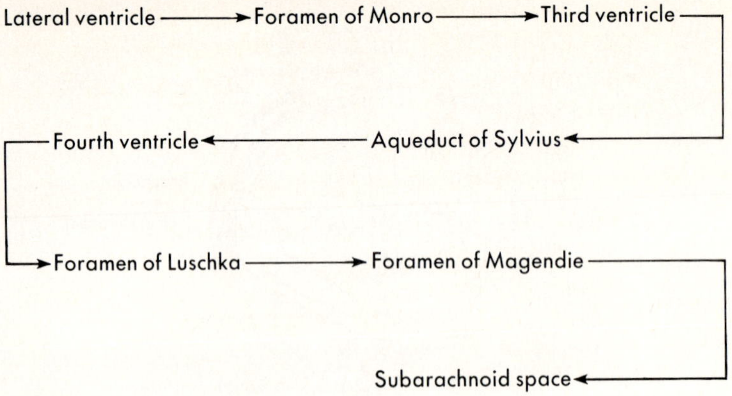

Fig. 5-4 Pathophysiology of hydrocephalus.

and the foramen of Magendie into the cisterna magna. Some of the CSF then flows into the subarachnoid space around the spinal cord, upward to the anterior surface of the cord, and around the anterior of the brain. As the CSF passes through the subarachnoid space, a large part of it is absorbed into the venous sinuses by way of the arachnoid villi. When this flow is obstructed, hydrocephalus results (See Fig. 5-4).

Nursing assessment

Successful treatment for hydrocephalus has been achieved only within the last 30 years through:

- Medical treatment: to control the quantity of CSF secreted.
- Surgical treatment: to implant extracranial shunting devices. Most commonly, the shunt drains the CSF into either the peritoneal cavity or the right atrium.

Objective assessment data

Neonates, infants

- Severely enlarged head (well beyond the normal growth curve)
- Downward deviation of the eyes: ''sunset'' gaze
- Signs of increased ICP
  - Bulging fontanels that fail to pulsate
  - Clearly visible and distended veins of the scalp and forehead
  - High-pitched cry
  - Lethargy
  - Irritability
  - Vomiting, anorexia
- Transillumination of the head. Normally in a full-term infant, the light forms a halo extending 1 to 2 cm from the rim of the light source. Varying degrees of localized glowing may be seen in abnormal fluid accumulations in various areas of the head.

Older children (onset symptoms are related to increasing ICP)
- Vomiting
- Irritability
- Papilledema
- Vital sign changes as a result of the older child's lack of ability to increase head size as the pressure increases
- Seizures, focal or general
- Behavioral changes
  - Change in feeding patterns
  - Lethargic, yet irritable when stimulated

Nursing care plan: HYDROCEPHALUS

NURSING DIAGNOSIS	EXPECTED OUTCOMES	NURSING INTERVENTIONS
Potential alteration in internal regulatory functions (production and circulation of CSF)	The child will be assessed for manifestations of hydrocephaly such as increased head circumference, seizure activity, signs and symptoms of increased ICP.	Measure head circumference daily (particularly important for premature infants because of their greater tendency for intraventricular or subdural hemorrhages. Head measurement is routinely done during developmental checkups. Monitor for and record any seizure activity.
IF SURGICAL INTERVENTION IS REQUIRED: Preoperative period: Potential alterations in growth and development patterns	The child will attain optimal levels of growth and development.	Assess growth and developmental milestones. Record height and weight gains. Compare with norms.
Alterations in skin integrity	The skin will remain intact without evidence of redness or breakdown.	Proper positioning with frequent turning. Good skin care.
Potential impairment of parents' and child's adjustment to illness	The child and parents will show adjustment to and acceptance of the illness process.	Encourage parental involvement with care of the child such as with bathing, feeding. Promote a clear understanding of what is to come. Provide auditory, visual, tactile environmental stimulation that is appropriate for age. Recognize that parents may need to verbalize and actually grieve the loss of the "ideal" child. Emphasize progress being made by the individual child.

Continued.

Nursing care plan: HYDROCEPHALUS—cont'd

NURSING DIAGNOSIS	EXPECTED OUTCOMES	NURSING INTERVENTIONS
Postoperative period: Potential alteration of regulatory functions Infection	The child will show no evidence of infection at the shunt site or systemically.	Observe for signs and symptoms of infection such as elevated temperature, redness at the shunt site, warmth. Monitor appropriate laboratory values for signs of an infectious process (CBC, blood cultures, CSF cultures).
Shunt obstruction	The child will show maintenance of normal cerebral pressures.	Observe for signs and symptoms of increased ICP. (Preoperative irritability from the hydrocephalus itself may persist for several days so this symptom cannot be used conclusively as a sign of increased ICP.) Pumping of the shunt as per physician's orders. Monitor vital signs and record.
Postanesthesia complications	The child will be free of complications associated with receiving anesthesia: Atelectasis Allergic reactions Aspiration	Reposition child frequently. Stimulate infant to cry. The older child is encouraged to take deep breaths and cough. IV fluids given only proportionate to weight to avoid possible circulatory overload and cardiac failure. Introduce fluids slowly observing for nausea. Listen for lung sounds. Suction if necessary. Observe for allergic reactions to anesthesia such as: Rash. Respiratory difficulties. Fluctuations of vital signs. Change in level of consciousness.
Understanding of preventive health measures	The child and parents will understand the shunt and what to observe for in the event of malfunction.	Review function and care related to the shunt: "pumping" signs and symptoms of infection signs and symptoms of increased ICP: Increased head size Irritability Lethargy Change in behavior Vomiting
	The child and parents will be aware of care necessary to: Prevent lesions. Maintain mobility.	Teach parents the importance of passive exercises, frequent turning, cleanliness, and observation for pressure areas. Reassess parent's ability to perform above measures.
	Increase self-esteem	Provide a list of toys suitable for the child's physical and mental capabilities. Encourage parents to take the child out in baby stroller as soon as possible.

Long-term care

1. Involve parents in the care of the child.
2. Teach them the signs of increased ICP.
3. As the child grows older, intellectual functioning should be evaluated.
4. Make the parents aware that the National Spina Bifida Association provides parent groups and health information for the parents.

The prognosis for the hydrocephalic child is difficult to predict. If a shunting procedure is performed before 3 months of age, there is an increased likelihood of complications and the need for shunt revisions. If the shunting is done after 3 months of age with periodic follow-ups, neurological examinations, CAT scans, and elective revisions of the shunts as the child grows, the prognosis improves.

CEREBRAL PALSY

Cerebral palsy (CP) is a nonspecific term used to describe a chronic, nonprogressive disorder caused by damage to some portion of the brain. It is the most frequent cause of permanent physical disability in children. The American Academy for Cerebral Palsy has arbitrarily defined 5 years as the upper age limit for brain damage to occur (Davis, 1980).

Cerebral palsy is typically characterized by motor disorders but may also involve sensory deficits. If sensory deficits are involved, then virtually all body processes may be affected—intellectual development, perception, nutritional intake, or mobility.

Classifications

The most widely used classification is based on the clinical manifestations presented (Davis, 1980).

Spastic cerebral palsy. This type of cerebral palsy involves pyramidal fibers, which extend from the cortex, come together in the medulla, cross from one side to the other, and then extend down the cord to synapse with anterior horn cells. It is the type that occurs most frequently (more than half of all cases) and it results from a lesion of the motor neurons. This classification is characterized by:

- Hypertonicity of muscles
- Exaggerated stretch reflex
- Presence of primitive reflexes (moro, tonic neck, grasp) beyond the time at which they would normally disappear
- Contractures of affected muscle groups

Areas of dysfunction are:

- Hemiplegia—one side of body is affected
- Quadriplegia (tetraparesis)—involvement of all four extremities
- Diplegia—involvement of all four extremities, but with more pronounced dysfunction and spasticity of lower extremities (used interchangeably with quadriplegia)
- Monoplegia—involvement of only one extremity (rarely occurs)
- Triplegia—involvement of three extremities (rarely occurs)

Athetoid cerebral palsy. This type of cerebral palsy affects the extrapyramidal system, which is a network of motor neurons that comprise relays between motor areas of the cortex, basal ganglia, thalamus, cerebellum, and brain stem. Athetoid cerebral palsy is rarely diagnosed in early infancy. The infant usually presents with opisthotonos progressing on to hypotonia or rarely rigidity. The involuntary movements that typify the athetoid classification are rarely apparent before 18 months and possibly not before the child is 3 years of age or older. Characteristics of this classification are:

- Involuntary, unpurposeful movements
- Initially infant may be limp or flaccid
- Presence of primitive reflexes (moro and tonic neck reflexes may persist throughout lifetime)
- Opisthotonic postures (arching of neck and back)
- Poor sucking, feeding, tongue control
- All four extremities usually involved
- Hearing often impaired

Ataxic cerebral palsy. This occurs in less than 10% of all cases. Ataxic cerebral palsy results from a defect of the cerebellum and cerebellar pathways. It is characterized by:

- Poor balance
- Unsteady, wide-based gait
- Poor diagnosis until child is walking

Mixed cerebral palsy. The mixed classification is a combination of forms occurring in 20% to 40% of all cases. It is characterized by:

- A variety of symptoms characteristic of any or all other classifications
- Developmental lags
- Full extent of the disability is not diagnosed until child is older

Pathophysiology

The cause of cerebral palsy is often unidentifiable or complex, but etiological factors may be classified according to a time period in which the insult occurs.

- Prenatal factors (10%)
  - Maternal illnesses: infection, anemia, toxemia
  - Any process that causes hypoxia such as separation of the placenta, hemorrhage, maternal trauma, maternal drug ingestion
  - Maternal and fetal blood incompatabilities
  - Genetic factors
  - Fetal brain anomalies
- Perinatal factors (75%)
  - Prematurity
  - Birth trauma
  - Cerebral hypoxia, such as from the use of analgesics
  - Jaundice
  - Metabolic disturbances of neonate

Postnatal factors (15%)
- Head trauma, such as falls
- Infection
- Cerebrovascular accidents
- Other neurological conditions

Nursing assessment

Diagnosis is often difficult, particularly in early infancy. A thorough pediatric physical and neurological examination is essential and should include:
- Vision and hearing testing
- EEG
- Skull x-ray
- Urine screening for metabolic disorders

A comprehensive nursing assessment should include prenatal, natal, and postnatal history and the child's growth, developmental and nutritional histories. To be most effective the evaluation and treatment should incorporate a multidisciplinary approach with involvement by audiology, psychiatry, psychology, special education, speech therapy, and social services.

Nursing care plan: **CEREBRAL PALSY**

NURSING DIAGNOSIS	EXPECTED OUTCOMES	NURSING INTERVENTIONS
Potential alterations in nutrition The child with cerebral palsy may have a hyperactive gag reflex, poor sucking and swallowing reflexes, and lack of control of tongue movements.	The child will receive adequate nutritional intake appropriate to the child's age, developmental status, and dietary requirements with minimal evidence of feeding problems.	Offer food and liquids slowly and in small amounts. Use rehabilitative devices such as dual-handled cups, dishes with suction cups on the bottom and lipped sides. Use straws to facilitate fluid intake. Use "finger foods" and regular food finely chopped or blenderized. Keep environment quiet and free from distractions during mealtimes. Provide positive reinforcement to reduce frustrations for all involved. Replace strained foods with other mixtures as soon as the child demonstrates that he can tolerate it.
Impaired mobility (especially common in the child with spastic cerebral palsy)	The child will remain free from contractures and maintain an optimal level of motor function.	Constant passive and active stretching exercises. Proper application of short leg braces to prevent footdrop and heel cord tightening if appropriate. Teach parents about the appliances and braces. Encourage the child's mobility even when at times it would be easier to carry the child. Surgical intervention may be used to correct deformities such as for the lengthening of tendons or correction of a dislocated hip.

Continued.

Nursing care plan: CEREBRAL PALSY—cont'd

NURSING DIAGNOSIS	EXPECTED OUTCOMES	NURSING INTERVENTIONS
Potential poor adjustment to illness: Infant/child	The parent will allow the child to explore his environment and to establish his own self-esteem.	Parent teaching: Allow time for play and relaxation. Encourage parents not to be overprotective. Assist the parents to set limits and provide discipline as necessary. Give the child an opportunity to explore his environment and to learn to solve his own problems.
Adolescent/adult	The adolescent and later the adult with cerebral palsy will express his feelings and will strive toward development of a strong self-esteem.	Psychological and neurological counseling and evaluation. Allow for verbalization regarding feelings of inadequacy and lack of self-assurance. Provide for opportunities for success. Set realistic goals.

The prognosis for the individual with cerebral palsy is variable depending on the clinical type. Generally the prognosis is favorable for children with hemiparesis, but poor when the presenting symptom is either rigidity or severe permanent hypotonia. Usually, hemiplegic children will eventually walk unless there are also intellectual deficiencies. Milestones of growth and development are generally delayed by 4 to 6 months. Children with the rigid and atonic types of cerebral palsy may have both severe physical and intellectual deficiencies. These children may remain functionally dependent, even into adulthood.

Suggested readings

Bleck, E.: Musculoskeletal examination of the child with cerebral palsy, Pediatr. Ann. **8**(10):58-71, Oct. 1979.

Burton, B.: Recurrence risks for congenital hydrocephalus, Clin. Genet. **16**:47-53, 1979.

Capute, A.: Identifying cerebral palsy in infancy through study of primitive-reflex profiles, Pediat. Ann. **8**:34-42, Oct. 1979.

Davis, G., and Hill, P.M.: Cerebral palsy, Nurs. Clin. North Am. **15**:35-50, March 1980.

Holt, K.: Medical examination of the child with cerebral palsy, Pediatr. Ann. **8**:20-32, Oct. 1979.

Hook, E., Albright, S., and Cross, P.: Use of bernoulli census and log-linear methods for estimating the prevalence of spina bifida in live births and the completeness of vital record reports in new york state Am. J. Epidemiol. **112**:750-758, 1980.

McAndrew, I.: Adolescents and young people with spina bifida Dev. Med. Child Neurol. **21**:619-629, 1979.

McElroy, D.B.: Hydrocephalus in children, Nurs. Clin. North Am. **15**:23-24, March 1980.

Molnar, G.: Cerebral palsy: prognosis and how to judge it, Pediatr. Ann. **8**:44-56, Oct. 1979.

Olds, S., et. al.: Obstetric nursing, Cambridge, Mass., 1980, Addison-Wesley Publishing Co., Inc.

Papile, L., et. al.: Posthemorrhagic hydrocephalus in low birth-weight infants: treatment by serial lumbar punctures, J. Pediatr. **97**(2):273-277, 1980.

Penn, R.: The neurosurgical treatment of cerebral palsy, Pediatr. Ann. **8**:73-78, Oct. 1979.

Sternfeld, L.: The pediatrician's role, Pediatr. Ann. **8**:14-18, Oct. 1979.

Vigliarolo, D.: Managing bowel incontinence in children with meningomyelocele, Am. J. Nurs. **80**:105-107, Jan. 1980.

Whaley, L.F., and Wong, D.: Nursing care of infants and children, St. Louis, 1979, The C.V. Mosby Co.

CHAPTER 6

Seizure disorders

A seizure is not a disease in itself but a symptom of a disease. When a seizure chronically reoccurs, it is termed epilepsy. The resulting clinical symptoms may include alterations in mental functioning, level of consciousness, sensations, coordination, and convulsive movements in a variety of combinations depending upon the cause, location, and manner of spread of electrical activity. There are three main phases involved in a seizure. The preictal phase occurs immediately preceding a seizure. The ictal phase occurs during a seizure, and the postictal phase follows a seizure.

ETIOLOGY

Based on their etiology, seizures may be divided into two broad categories: (1) idiopathic or primary and (2) symptomatic or secondary.

Idiopathic (primary)

In this category the cause of the seizure cannot be determined. Idiopathic seizures and epilepsy most commonly occur during early adulthood. Recurrent seizures in children older than 3 years of age are most commonly idiopathic. Also included in this category are those seizures that may have genetic influences as contributing factors (for example, the seizures such as febrile seizures, that begin in childhood but diminish with age). Some research has shown that there is an inherited tendency for cerebral dysrhythmias in some families; however, this is not to say that the actual seizure disorder is inherited.

Symptomatic (secondary)

In this category cerebral changes can be found that are caused by a number of conditions or injuries. These conditions include but are not limited to:

Genetic and birth factors: hydrocephalus; infections (German measles); poisonous substances (drugs and alcohol); brain injury during the prenatal, perinatal, or postnatal periods (for example, anoxia, exposure to x-rays, congenital syphilis); and prematurity.

Degenerative disorders: leukoencephalopathy, tuberous sclerosis, lobar atrophy, Alzheimer's disease, Jakob-Creutzfeldt disease, and multiple sclerosis.

Infectious disorders: meningitis, encephalitis, abscesses (brain, epidural, subdural), and fever.

Circulatory disorders: cerebrovascular accidents (thrombosis, embolus, hemorrhage), aneurysm, hypertensive encephalopathy, arteriosclerosis, vasospasm, and arteriovenous malformations.

Toxic factors: carbon monoxide, lead and mercury poisonings, alcohol and drugs, uremia, water intoxification, and protein shock.
Trauma: acute cerebral injuries (contusions, lacerations, depressed skull fractures).
Metabolic and nutritional disturbances: excess fluid intake, hypoglycemia, hypocalcemia, hypomagnesemia, supernatremia or hyponatremia, phenylketonuria, vitamin B_6 deficiency, and neoplasms.

Age groups. The major causes of seizures do vary when considering different age groups. During the newborn and infant periods, seizures are most apt to be caused by birth injuries, congenital defects, or metabolic disturbances. Between the ages of 2 and 25 most commonly the cause of seizures is unknown or idiopathic. From ages 25 to 50, the main causes are trauma, tumors, and alcohol. After the age of 50, the most common causes of beginning seizures are cerebrovascular disease and tumors (Adams and Victor, 1977; Hawken, 1979).

Stimuli. Sometimes a seizure may be triggered by very specific stimuli such as flickering lights, television, video games, certain odors, music, reading, startling noises, and sleep. Other stimuli may possibly lower the threshold for seizures in susceptible persons. These include but are not limited to the lack of sleep, hunger, stress, menstruation, pregnancy, alcohol, and emotional disturbances (Conway-Rutkowski, 1982; Taylor and Ballenger, 1980).

PATHOPHYSIOLOGY

A seizure occurs when there is an abnormal and excessive electrical discharge of neurons within the brain. This electrical activity may be confined to one specific location or may spread to other areas of the brain.

CLASSIFICATION

Historically, epileptic seizures have been classified by terms such as grand mal, petit mal, and psychomotor. These are very familiar terms to most people and should not be discarded. However, a more detailed international classification of epileptic seizures was adopted in 1969, which classifies the types of seizures in relation to the area of the brain involved. This helps differentiate etiology, sites, and manner of spread (Gastaut, 1970).

Partial or focal seizures

These seizures originate in one localized area of the cerebral cortex. Clinical symptoms correspond to the location of the lesion. Partial seizures consist of two general forms: (1) those of simple symptomatology resulting in no impairment of consciousness and (2) those of complex symptomatology usually resulting in an alteration or loss of consciousness.

Partial seizures with simple symptomatology. Partial seizures with simple symptomatology consist of motor, sensory, or autonomic symptoms or combinations of the three:

So-called jacksonian or jacksonian march seizures consist of mainly motor symptoms. The focus is the prerolandic gyrus or posterior frontal lobe. The symptoms are characterized by a localized onset with convulsive twitching in an upper extremity or the face (distal portion of hand or side of face contralateral to site of lesion). There may be versive movements such as turning of the eyes and head, an ability or inability to talk, and sensory symptoms. Typically the symptoms spread or "march" to involve the entire limb, side of the face, and lower extremity, and they may also become secondarily generalized (grand mal). Jacksonian seizures occur most often in adults.

Epilepsia partialis continua seizures consist of motor symptoms. The focus is the prerolandic gyrus or posterior frontal lobe. The symptoms are characterized by a localized convulsive twitching confined to one area of the body but continuing for a prolonged length of time (such as hours or a day).

Seizures involving only sensory symptoms include:

Focus	Symptoms
Parietal lobe	The patient experiences feelings of numbness and tingling sensations in the affected area (such as a hand), which may spread similarly to jacksonian seizures.
Occipital lobe	The patient experiences disturbances in the visual field opposite the side of the lesion (such as seeing bright lights or spots).
Temporal lobe	The patient experiences disturbances in hearing, which may be reported as an abnormal intensification of sound or as unrecognizable words.
Posterior temporal lobe of dominant hemisphere	The patient experiences difficulty speaking or a total inability to speak.
Infratemporal	The patient experiences a disturbance in smell.

Seizure activity involving only autonomic symptoms has the focus in the diencephalon. Symptoms may include flushing of the face, nausea, vomiting, fever, tachycardia, diaphoresis, hypotension, hypertension, or pupillary changes. These symptoms are also often seen with other types of seizures.

Partial seizures with complex symptomatology. Partial seizures with complex symptomatology are also known as psychomotor seizures. The focus is the anterior temporal lobe. The seizure activity often starts with an aura, which reflects the site where the seizure activity first begins. The aura may include a variety of symptoms. They may be cognitive feelings of déjà vu (that the event now being experienced occurred before), jamais vu (the unfamiliarity with an event), or the ability to recall past memories in detail; psychosensory (visual, auditory, olfactory, or epigastric hallucinations and illusions such as distortions of objects, people, or one's own body; or affective (feelings of great anxiety or fear—the patient may have a very fearful look on his face). The patient experiences an altered level of consciousness (is in an awake but dreamy state and is not aware of activities during the seizure) and conducts psychomotor activities, automatisms (purposeless and repetitive activities such as patting a part of the body, lip smacking, walking up and down a flight of stairs) or may run away to hide or cry during the seizure. The patient may appear aggressive and violent, but never is it a directed or purposeful aggression. The seizure may become secondarily generalized however. It usually lasts 2 to 3 minutes, ending abruptly with the person being confused and drowsy or possibly experiencing a headache.

Generalized seizures

These seizures have no local onset. The symptoms begin bilaterally and are symmetric because both hemispheres of the brain are involved.

Absence seizures. Absence (petit mal) seizures occur mainly during childhood and are rarely seen after adolescence. They consist of a very brief and sudden loss of consciousness, which is noticed as a "blank stare." There is usually little or no motor activity and no loss of muscle tone. There may be some fluttering of the eyes or minor mouth movements. The majority of these seizures last for less than 10 seconds but they may last for 30 seconds. The person may experience only one seizure a day or may have as many as one hundred. At the cessation of the seizure, the child will continue with activities as if nothing had happened. The seizure is not harmful unless it interferes with learning ability. The child may also experience brief myoclonic jerks or a tonic-clonic seizure (grand mal).

Myoclonic seizures. Myoclonic seizures are characterized by violent jerking contractions of major muscles which throw the individual to the ground. The seizure may be focal or generalized and may involve only one side of the body or the whole body. There is usually no loss of consciousness. In infants myoclonic seizures may be seen with developmental disabilities and they may disappear as the child matures. When seen in later childhood, they are usually indicative of a hereditary degenerative disease that results in a severe dementia. They may be seen in later middle life as a symptom of Creutzfeldt-Jakob disease. Often, these seizures are sensitive to stimuli, worsening when the person is disturbed. Myoclonic seizures may be seen with or may become secondarily tonic-clonic.

Infantile seizures. Infantile spasms begin in infants from 3 to 9 months of age and usually disappear by the age of 3 years to be replaced by other types of seizures. The symptoms consist of the "salaam" posture, which is a sudden and violent flexion of the trunk, drawing up of the legs, extension of the arms, and jerking of the head, which last only a few seconds. Mental retardation is characteristically present.

Clonic seizures. Clonic seizures are found mainly in early childhood. There is a sudden loss of consciousness, a sudden loss of muscle tone, or a brief generalized tonic spasm.

This is followed by several minutes of bilateral jerking movements of the muscles. A postictal period is similar to the tonic-clonic (grand mal) seizure type.

Tonic seizures. Tonic seizures usually occur between 1 and 7 years of age. There is a loss of consciousness after which the muscles become very rigid and the arms and legs are extended. Postictal confusion is also present.

Tonic-clonic seizures. Tonic-clonic seizures (grand mal) may occur at any age. They may be preceded by an aura or warning. An aura may include brief sensory changes such as smelling an unpleasant odor, a feeling of weakness, dizziness, numbness of an extremity, or gastrointestional pain. There is a loss of consciousness because of the rapid spread of electrical activity. A tonic phase occurs in which the total body stiffens. The individual falls to the floor uncontrollably if standing. An ''epileptic cry'' may be heard, caused by the thoracic and abdominal spasm forcing air out the glottis. Respirations are temporarily interrupted. Hands and jaw are clenched shut, which may cause the person to bite his tongue. Pupils may be dilated and nonreactive. There may be incontinence of urine or stool. A clonic phase follows with violent rhythmic contractions of all muscle groups. Respirations are jerky and stertorous. The person may appear to be frothing at the mouth because of the increased salvation and expulsion of air. The total seizure lasts for 2 to 4 minutes after which the individual totally relaxes, remaining unresponsive for a short period of time while gradually reawakening. There may be neurological residual deficits or Todd's paralysis (for example, weakness of an arm or aphasia), which might last for a few hours. Confused and tired, the individual will sleep if left alone (postictal phase). Upon awakening, the individual may experience a throbbing headache, fatigue, sore muscles, and no memory of the seizure.

Of special note are febrile seizures. These occur as a symptom of an acute febrile illness in an infant. The temperature is characteristically greater than 102° F and the seizure occurs at the onset of the fever. It is usually similar to a tonic-clonic seizure, lasting less than 4 minutes.

Atonic seizures. Atonic (''drop'') seizures are characterized by a total loss of muscle tone causing the person to fall. This lasts only a few seconds and there is no loss of consciousness.

Akinetic seizures. Akinetic seizures are difficult to differentiate from atonic seizures. There is a sudden loss of muscle movement lasting only a few seconds with no detectable loss of consciousness.

Status epilepticus

Status epilepticus refers to seizure activity that is constant without any periods of consciousness. It is a medical emergency as brain damage may result. Tonic-clonic seizures are the main type of activity that is involved in status epilepticus; however, it may be composed of other forms of seizures. Status epilepticus occurs mainly in children.

NURSING ASSESSMENT

Subjective assessment data

Previous neurological disorders
Unusual events preceding the seizure, such as head traumas, falls
Diet, sleep, work habits
Recent acute illnesses
Alcohol and drug ingestion (purposeful or accidental)
Medications
Time of day seizure occurred
Activities before seizure
Preictal symptoms: aura (special feeling or sensation before the seizure)
Postseizure symptoms: visual problems, decreased coördination, muscular soreness, stiffness, twitching, weakness, bruises, numbness or tingling, bitten tongue, incontinence, decreased attention span, mental confusion, headache
For infants and children, additional information is needed:
- Events related to birth such as prolonged delivery or cord around neck
- Events related to perinatal period
- Childhood diseases

Objective assessment data

Activity before the seizure
Patient's behavior before the seizure
Presence of an aura
Responsiveness of patient such as loss of consciousness or verbalization during the seizure
Patency of airway
Initial movements
Progression and characteristics of movements
Length and duration of each phase (tonic, clonic) of the seizure
Vital signs (particularily the respirations and pulse)
Reaction of the pupils
Incontinence, deviated tongue
Injuries acquired
Postictal period
Electrolytes
Signs of status epilepticus

Nursing care plan: **SEIZURE DISORDERS**

NURSING DIAGNOSIS	EXPECTED OUTCOMES	NURSING INTERVENTIONS
Ineffective breathing pattern **Ineffective airway clearance**	Respirations only temporarily interrupted during the tonic phase of a generalized seizure Patent airway immediately established and maintained No signs of an airway obstruction such as Stertorous respirations Tachypnea Dyspnea Tachycardia Cyanosis Apnea Arterial blood gases within normal limits	Observe patient for signs or symptoms of an airway obstruction. If the tongue blocks the pharnyx: Turn the patient onto the back Hyperextend the patient's jaw. If this doesn't bring the tongue forward, insert an oral airway. If the patient is vomiting: Turn the patient's head to the side. Suction the patient. Ventilate patient using a bag-mask device if necessary. Call for assistance. Notify the physician immediately. Have arterial blood gases determined. Obtain an order for oxygen therapy. Monitor vital signs.
Potential fluid volume deficit and electrolyte imbalance during status epilepticus	Fluid and electrolyte imbalances are identified and treatment begun immediately Mucous membranes are moist and pink Urine output within normal limits	Assess patient for signs of dehydration. Monitor urine output. Obtain an order for initiation of an intravenous infusion. Have blood electrolytes determined. Monitor vital signs.
Potential for physical injury	Patient is free of injury Patient demonstrates knowledge of precautions	NOTE: Any seizure may become secondarily generalized. Establish seizure precautions including the following: Poorly controlled patients should not: Smoke in bed if unattended. Have their temperature taken orally. Take tub baths. Showers are preferred. Side rails should be up at all times. Padded side rails for those patients prone to tonic-clonic contractions. An oral airway and padded tongue blade should be kept at the bedside. NOTE: Do not try to place anything in the patient's mouth once the tonic phase of a generalized seizure begins because this may cause more injury to the patient. Rarely is there sufficient time to place a soft object between the teeth before the tonic phase since no one is usually either aware of the seizure activity or immediately at hand. An oral airway may be of assistance in establishing a patent airway if necessary after the clonic phase.

Continued.

Nursing care plan: SEIZURE DISORDERS—cont'd

NURSING DIAGNOSIS	EXPECTED OUTCOMES	NURSING INTERVENTIONS
Potential for physical injury—cont'd		During a seizure: Remain with the patient. Remain calm. Assist the patient to the bed or to the floor if he is prone to generalized seizures. Put all side rails up. Loosen constrictive clothing. Place a folded blanket, towel, or pillow under the patient's head. Do not restrain the patient's movements. Do not lift the patient during a seizure. Move away objects that are in the immediate environment. Protect limbs during tonic-clonic contractions by padding the environment.
Fear and knowledge deficit following a seizure	Patient's verbal and nonverbal behavior indicates relaxation Patient oriented to person, place, and time	Remain calm. Assess the patient's level of consciousness, memory, pupillary responses, vital signs, coordination, muscle strength and symmetry, and deep tendon reflexes. Reorient the patient. Provide an explanation as to what has just occurred in terms appropriate to the patient's developmental level. A more detailed explanation can be given at a later time when appropriate. Allow patient time to sleep.
Knowledge deficit: What is a seizure?	Patient and/or family verbalizes understanding of what a seizure is Verbalizes fears and concerns Cooperates with procedures	Give an explanation appropriate to the patient and family's level of comprehension and emotional state. Give encouragement and the opportunity to ask questions. Provide psychological support. Make appropriate referrals (such as to a psychiatric nurse) NOTE: When diagnosed as having epilepsy, an individual may experience feelings of guilt, hostility, depression, or a poor self-image. The patient may fear the loss of a job and friends. Family members may become overprotective. Parents of children may experience guilt, blaming themselves for their child's disorder.

Nursing care plan: **SEIZURE DISORDERS**—cont'd

NURSING DIAGNOSIS	EXPECTED OUTCOMES	NURSING INTERVENTIONS
Knowledge deficit: diagnostic procedures	Verbalizes understanding of procedures Verbalizes fears and concerns Cooperates with procedures	See Chapter 2 for a detailed description of diagnostic procedures and of specific nursing interventions. NOTE: The most useful diagnostic procedure is the electroencephalogram (EEG). Other procedures that may be performed include skull x-rays, computerized axial tomography (CAT), arteriography, and lumbar puncture. Anticipate and prepare patient for the possibility that blood samples will be collected to test therapeutic medication levels, arterial blood gases, alcohol levels, blood sugar, calcium and phosphate, electrolytes, magnesium, and blood urea nitrogen (BUN). Anticipate and prepare patient for the possible collection of throat, blood, urine, stool, and cerebrospinal fluid cultures if the patient is febrile.
Knowledge deficit: surgery	Verbalizes understanding of surgery Verbalizes fears and concerns	See Chapter 10 for a description of preoperative and postoperative neurosurgical nursing care. NOTE: The use of surgery as an intervention for epileptic patients is very infrequently done. However, surgery is indicated when (1) there is a space-occupying lesion such as a brain abscess, neoplasm, or cyst; (2) the use of various antiepileptic drugs has not controlled the seizures. Surgical procedures include removal of the specific lesion, stereotactic surgery, cortical resection, and hemispherectomies. A stereotactic procedure involves the placing of discrete lesions to destroy foci and interrupt the spread of electrical activity. A cortical resection involves the removal of a portion of a lobe and is done when the focus of abnormal electrical activity is accessible and located within a somewhat dispensable lobe. This is mostly used when the focus is located in the anterior portion of the temporal lobe. Hemispherectomies are rarely performed. They are done mainly in children when the seizure activity involves the entire hemisphere and the patient is severely hemiplegic and has a complete visual field defect.

Continued.

Nursing care plan: SEIZURE DISORDERS—cont'd

NURSING DIAGNOSIS	EXPECTED OUTCOMES	NURSING INTERVENTIONS
Knowledge deficit: nutrition	Verbalizes understanding of proper nutrition	NOTE: The diet should be well balanced. Some individuals may have seizures because their diets are high in salt or there is a deficiency in vitamin B_6. For them a referral to a nutritionist would be vital. In premenstrual women seizures may be precipitated by the retention of fluids, thus requiring a limitation of fluid intake before menstruation.
Knowledge deficit: alcohol	Verbalizes understanding of limited alcohol intake Verbalizes understanding of interaction between alcohol and antiepileptic drugs	NOTE: If one drink precipitates a seizure, alcohol should not be taken. For other individuals an occasional social drink may be permitted. Excessive drinking is prohibited. Antiepileptic drugs and alcohol should not be used together because of the cumulative effects that may occur.
Knowledge deficit: bathing	Verbalizes understanding of preferred bathing	NOTE: Showers are recommended over tub baths
Knowledge deficit: physical activity	Verbalizes understanding of possible need to limit physical activity	NOTE: It is important to stress the importance of a daily routine of physical activity and rest. The patient should not become too fatigued or overexhausted. As long as the seizures are in good control, sports should be encouraged. Swimming and boating should obviously not be done alone. If seizures are poorly controlled, the two previously mentioned sports and also contact sports should be avoided.
Knowledge deficit: driving	Verbalizes understanding of driving laws	NOTE: State laws and the patient's seizure control determine when the patient may drive. This varies from state to state.
Knowledge deficit: employment	Verbalizes fears and concerns	NOTE: Patients may fear the loss of their jobs because of societal stigmas that still exist in certain sectors of the population in relationship to epilepsy. This is just another added burden on the patient with epilepsy. Many employers need educational programs to have a better understanding of epilepsy. Certain precautions should be understood by the patient with epilepsy. If their seizures are poorly controlled they should not drive, operate potentially dangerous equipment, or work at heights. Frequent changes from day to night shifts may also initiate seizures. Referrals for vocational rehabilitation programs may be made to the State Vocational Rehabilitation Agency or to programs of the Epilepsy Foundation of America.

Nursing care plan: SEIZURE DISORDERS—cont'd

NURSING DIAGNOSIS	EXPECTED OUTCOMES	NURSING INTERVENTIONS
Knowledge deficit: marriage and pregnancy	Verbalizes fears and concerns	NOTE: Researchers have found a strong history of seizures in some families. However, the exact role of heredity in epilepsy has not yet been determined. The marriage partner or prospective partner should be informed of the situation. There is usually no reason why the person with epilepsy should not marry; however, this must be decided on an individual basis. Genetic counseling should be considered. Before becoming pregnant, the patient with epilepsy should consult her physician. Medication doses may have to be changed to maintain therapeutic plasma levels. Also, the fetus may be affected by the antiepileptic medications. The patient needs to be advised about the potential risks by the physician.
Knowledge deficit: avoidance of precipitation factors	Verbalizes understanding of precipitating factors	NOTE: As mentioned earlier in this chapter, seizures in some individuals may be triggered or precipitated by very specific stimuli. For these individuals, it is important to avoid such stimuli in order to reduce the frequency of seizures.
Knowledge deficit: identifications	Verbalizes understanding of carrying proper identification	NOTE: The person with epilepsy should wear a Medic Alert bracelet. Information should also be carried in the wallet giving the name and telephone number of the physician, medication schedule, allergies, and the name and number of the person to be notified in case of an emergency.
Knowledge deficit: recording of seizure activity at home	Verbalizes understanding of proper recording of seizure activity	Instruct patient and family to identify and collect information pertaining to the objective data base found on page 174.
Knowledge deficit: medications **Proper administration of medications**	Seizure activity is under control Early recognition and treatment of untoward effects Patient and family verbalize understanding of dosage, administration, and possible untoward effects of drug therapy	NOTE: Once the diagnosis is made, the physician will then determine what antiepileptic drug or combination of drugs to initiate. This is a very individualized process. Therapy usually begins with a small dose of a single drug. Dosage is increased until seizure control is accomplished or drug toxicity occurs. Many times one single drug will decrease the frequency of seizures but will not completely prevent them. Then a second drug is added and given concomitantly with the first drug. Inform the patient that drug therapy will start slowly and the physician will adjust dosage or drugs appropriately.

Continued.

Nursing care plan: SEIZURE DISORDERS—cont'd

NURSING DIAGNOSIS	EXPECTED OUTCOMES	NURSING INTERVENTIONS
Proper administration of medications—cont'd		Remind the patient to take the medication until the physician prescribes otherwise. Assess the patient for psychological problems before initiation of medications. Assess the elderly for confusion and agitation before and after initiation of medications. Caution the patient against working with potentially hazardous machinery, working at unguarded heights, or driving while taking medications. Observe for signs of hypersensitivity (rash, fever, headache, rhinitis). Stress importance of frequent blood studies. Instruct the patient on signs of hematological (sore throat, petechiae, easy bruising) and liver (jaundice, dark urine, abdominal pain) toxicity. Administer medications at the same times each day, such as at mealtimes and at bedtime. A written schedule will help the patient remember when and how to take medications. Advise the patient about potential changes in drug dosage that may be required if there is trauma or emotional stress. If necessary, administer tablets in applesauce or other fruit sauces for children or elderly patients. Observe infants who are nursed by epileptic mothers for signs of toxicity NOTE: See Table 6-1 for major antiepileptic drugs and their usual maintenance doses, indications, untoward effects, and specific nursing interventions.

Table 6-1 Major antiepileptic drugs

Drugs	Indications	Usual maintenance dose	Untoward effects	Nursing interventions
Phenytoin (Dilantin)	Tonic-clonic Complex partial Elementary partial Static epilepticus	4.8 mg/kg/day IV/PO in children; 300-400 mg/day, IV/PO in adults Loading dose: 50 mg/min IV, 15 to 20 mg/kg total in children; 1000 mg in adults	Ataxia Exfoliative dermatitis Drowsiness Fever Gingival hyperplasia Hirsutism Tremor Mental confusion Nystagmus Leukopenia Cardiac arrthymias Cardiac arrest	Promote good oral hygiene and frequent dental visits. Gum massage to minimize gum problems. May benefit from an electric toothbrush. Administer with meals or with at least two glasses of water to minimize gastrointestinal disturbances. Promote good skin care to help prevent acne formation. Observe for motor incoordination. Report to physician excessive facial and body growth. When administered intravenously it *must* be given slowly to prevent cardiac complications. Phenytoin must also be given with a sodium chloride solution to prevent precipitation. Intramuscular administration of phenytoin is not recommended because absorption is unpredictable.
Phenobarbital	Tonic-clonic Complex partial Elementary partial Status epilepticus	5-10 mg/kg/day IM, PO in children; 90-180 mg/day IM/PO in adults. Loading dose: Over 5 to 10 minutes give 10 to 20 mg/kg IV in children; 2 g in adults	Ataxia Drowsiness Physical dependence Mental dullness Hyperexcitability in children Excitability or depression in elderly. Nausea Postpartum hemorrhage Hemorrhage disease in newborns	Observe for motor incoordination. Observe for psychic changes, especially in children and the elderly. Administer with meals or with at least two glasses of water to minimize gastrointestinal disburbances. Anticipate vitamin K administration to pregnant mothers 1 month before delivery to prevent bleeding in the newborn.

Continued.

Drugs	Indications	Usual maintenance dose	Untoward effects	Nursing interventions
Primidone (Mysoline)	Tonic-clonic Complex partial Elementary partial	10-20 mg/kg/day PO in children; 750 mg-1.5 g/day PO in adults	Ataxia Drowsiness Rash Nystagmus Megaloblastic anemia Alopecia Impotence Hyperexcitability in children Postpartum hemorrhage Hemorrhage disease in newborns Nausea	Observe for motor incoordination. Note excessive hair loss. Observe for psychic changes especially in children. Question the patient as to whether the drug has made him impotent. Anticipate vitamin K administration to pregnant mothers 1 month before delivery to prevent bleeding in the newborn.
Carbamazepine (Tegretol)	Complex partial Tonic-clonic Elementary partial	400-1000 mg/day PO in children; 400-1200 mg/day PO in adults	Ataxia Dizziness Drowsiness Nausea Vomiting Bone marrow depression Acne Liver dysfunction Urinary retention or frequency Blood dyscrasias such as aplastic anemia and leukopenia	Observe for motor incoordination. Administer with meals or with at least two glasses of water. Observe for early signs of bone marrow depression such as fever, sore throat, mouth ulcer, and easy bruising. Watch lab values closely for signs of bone marrow depression, blood dyscrasias, and abnormal liver function test results. Observe for signs of abnormal renal function. Do not administer with monoamine oxidase (MAO) inhibitors.
Valproic acid (Depakene)	Absence	15-60 mg/kg/day PO	Nausea Vomiting Ataxia Drowsiness Rash Tremor Alopecia Depression Hepatic toxicity Platelet aggregation Dysfunction	May cause a false-positive urine test for acetone. Valproic acid syrup contains sodium. Do not administer to patients on a sodium-restricted diet. Do not open the capsule or mix with food as it is irritating to the mucous membranes. Observe for motor incoordination.

Drugs	Indications	Usual maintenance dose	Untoward effects	Nursing interventions
				Note excessive hair loss. Observe lab studies for signs of hepatic toxicity and the inhibition of platelet aggregation.
Ethosuximide (Zarontin)	Absence	250 mg twice a day PO in children; 750-1500 mg/day PO in adults	Dizziness Anorexia Nausea Vomiting Headache Transient personality changes Blood dyscrasias such as leukopenia and aplastic anemia May increase incidence of grand mal seizures	Observe for changes in personality. Administer with meals or with at least two glasses of water. Observe lab studies for signs of blood dyscrasias. Report increase in grand mal seizure activity.
Clonazepam (Clonopin)	Absence Atypical absence Myoclonic Akinetic	0.1-0.2 mg/kg/day PO; 20 mg/day PO maximum in adults	Drowsiness Ataxia Nystagmus Tremor Increased libido Alopecia Rash Anorexia Blood dyscrasias such as leukopenia and thrombocytopenia Behavior problems	Observe lab studies for blood dyscrasias. Observe for motor incoordination. Note excessive hair loss.
Diazepam (Valium)	Absence Complex partial Elementary partial	0.15-2 mg/kg/day PO in children; 8-40 mg/day PO in adults	Ataxia Drowsiness Confusion Depression Hypotension Rash Blurred vision	Have the patient rise slowly. Monitor vital signs closely. Note personality change.
	Status epilepticus	Loading dose: 5 mg/min IV, 2.5 mg total in children, 35 mg in adults. May repeat in 15 min	Respiratory depression and arrest	

Suggested readings

Adams, R., and Maurice, V.: Principles of neurology, ed. 2, New York, 1981, McGraw-Hill Book Co.

Alpers, B.J., and Elliot, L.M.: Clinical neurology, ed. 6, Philadelphia, 1971, F.A. Davis Co.

Bindler, R., and Howry, L.: Nursing care of children with febrile seizures, Am. J. of Maternal Child Nurs. **3**(5):270-273, 1978.

Chee, C.M.: Seizure disorders. In McElroy, D.B., and Davis, G.T., editors: Nurs. Clin. North Am. **15**(1): 71-82, March 1980.

Conway-Rutkowski, B.L.: Carini and Owens, neurological and neurosurgical nursing, ed. 8, St. Louis, 1982, The C.V. Mosby Co.

Freeman, S.W.: The epileptic in home, school and society: coping with the invisible handicap, Springfield, Ill., 1979, Bannerstone House.

Gastaut, H.: Clinical and electroencephalographical classification of epileptic seizures, Epilepsia **11:** 102-113, 1970.

Hawken, M.: Seizures: etiology, classification, intervention, J. Neurosurg. Nurs. **11**(3):166-170, Sept. 1979.

Litel, G.R.: Neurosurgery and the clinical team, New York, 1980, Springer Publishing Co.

Loebl, S., and Spratto, G.: The nurses' drug handbook, ed. 2, New York, 1980, John Wiley & Sons, Inc.

Lovely, M.P.: Identification and treatment of status epilepticus, J. Neurosurg. Nurs. **12**(2):93-96, June 1980.

Merritt, H.H.: A textbook of neurology, ed 6, Philadelphia, 1979, Lea & Febiger.

Muehl, J.N.: Seizure disorders in children: prevention and care, Am. J. Maternal Child Nurs. **4**(3): 154-160, May/June 1979.

Newmark, M.E., and Penry, J.K.: Photosensitivity and epilepsy: a review. New York, 1979, Raven Press.

Newmark, M.E., and Penry, J.K.: Genetics of epilepsy: a review. New York, 1980, Raven Press.

Norman, S.E., and Browne, T.R.: Seizure dsorders, Am. J. Nurs. **81**(5):984-1000, May 1981.

Oppenheimer, E.Y., and Rosman, N.P.: Seizures in childhood: an approach to emergency management. In Alpert, J.J., and Reece, R., editors: Pediatr. Clin. North Am. **26**(4):837-856, Nov. 1979.

Riechert, T.: Stereotactic brain operations: methods, clinical aspects, indications, Vienna, 1980, Hans Huber Publisher.

Sands, H., and Minters, F.C.: The epilepsy fact book, ed. 3, Philadelphia, 1979, F.A. Davis Co.

Smith, R.R.: Essentials of neurosurgery, Philadelphia, 1980, J.B. Lippincott Co.

Sutherland, J.M., and Eadie, M.J.: The epilepsies: modern diagnosis and treatment, ed. 3, New York, 1980, Churchill Livingstone.

Taylor, J.W., and Ballenger, S.: Neurological dysfunctions and nursing intervention, New York, 1980, McGraw-Hill Book Co.

Trekas, J.: Managing epilepsy: don't forget the patient, Nursing, **82:**63-65, Oct. 1982.

Tyrer, J.H., editor: Current status of modern therapy. Vol. 5. The treatment of epilepsy, Philadelphia, 1980, J.B. Lippincott Co.

CHAPTER 7

Infections and inflammations

ANATOMICAL AND PHYSIOLOGICAL PROTECTIVE MECHANISMS

With the exception of influenzal meningitis in children, primary infection of the nervous system are rare. This is because of several anatomical structures and physiological mechanisms protecting the central nervous system (CNS) and the peripheral nerves.

Central nervous system

Anatomically, the CNS (brain and spinal cord) is protected by:

Bone (skull and vertebral).

Meninges (pia, arachnoid, dura).

Cerebrospinal fluid (CSF).

Physiologically, the CNS is protected by the blood-brain barrier, which prevents or inhibits access of foreign substances to the CNS. The components of the blood-brain barrier are:

Capillary walls.

Pia glial membrane (pia mater surrounding blood vessels entering the CNS parenchyma).

Astroglial cells (CNS phagolytes) (Gilroy and Meyer, 1975).

In spite of the protection afforded by these protective mechanisms and structures, when an organism reaches the CSF, the organism flourishes. Two components of CSF, glucose and protein, provide an excellent growth medium. The CSF-brain barrier is much less effective than the blood-brain barrier in preventing infections. This is because the endothelial cells lining the capillaries in the pia mater are less tightly joined than the larger blood vessels supplying the dura and arachnoid mater, thus permitting a freer flow of therapeutic or foreign substances into the brain parenchyma. Therefore, an organism reaching the CSF has easy access to the CNS when it reaches the CSF-brain barrier. When this occurs, parenchymal inflammation and infection result. To further complicate CNS infections, few antibodies produced outside the CNS can cross the tightly knit blood-brain barrier (Adams and Victor, 1981).

Peripheral nerves

Peripheral nerves are protected by:

Nerve coverings (myelin and myelin sheath).

Location (surrounded by muscle mass and proximity to bony structures).

DIFFERENTIATION

Infection versus inflammation

Infection is a condition in which a microorganism has gained entrance into body tissue and grows in or on the tissue, producing a clinical reaction. Common symptoms include fever, chills, nausea, and headache (Frobisher, Sommermeyer, and Fuerst,

1980). The extent and acuity of the infectious process is dependent on (1) the number and virulence of the organism; (2) the type of toxin produced; (3) the resistance capacity of the host, such as through mechanical barriers and immune responses; (4) the disease-causing capacity of the organism.

Inflammation is a defensive response to an irritating or injurious agent. The inflammatory response involves redness, heat, swelling, and pain. Inflammations range from mild to severe, from acute (Reye's syndrome) to chronic (leprosy), from localized (Bell's palsy) to systemic (influenzal meningitis).

Classification

CNS infections
- Meningitis: infection of the meninges
- Encephalitis: infection of the brain parenchyma
- Myelitis: infection of spinal cord parenchyma
- Abcess: localized collection of infective materials

Peripheral or cranial nerve infections or inflammations
- Guillian-Barré syndrome
- Bell's palsy
- Herpes zoster
- Leprosy (Hansen's disease)

CNS INFECTIONS AND INFLAMMATIONS

Meningitis

Meningitis is an infection of the pia and arachnoid mater as well as of the subarachnoid space through which the CSF flows. Typically, the person with meningitis complains of headache, fever, neck pain and stiffness, and drowsiness or irritability.

Etiology. Rapid identification of the causative organism is prerequisite to definitive treatent. Recognition of incidence factors can help differentiate the causative organisms (Merritt, 1979).

Causative organisms	Incidence
Meningococci	Crowded, unhygienic conditions; winter season
Pneumococci	Infants, the elderly
Streptococci	Present or recent ear, sinus, mastoid infection
Haemophilus influenza	Infants and children with recent upper respiratory infections
Gram-negative organisms *(Escherichia coli, Pseudomonas, Proteus)*	Neonates
Staphylococci	Infants or elderly persons with recent penetrating wounds
Tubercle bacillus	History of or contact with tubercular person.
Fungi *(Cryptococcus, coccidioides immitis)*	Residents of areas with (1) high bird population (sparrows, pigeons); (2) high temperatures and low humidity

Generally, persons at risk for developing meningitis include:

- Infants, children, and the elderly.
- Malnourished individuals.
- Immunosuppressed persons, such as from radiation or cancer chemotherapy, long-term steroid therapy.
- Persons with debilitating diseases such as tuberculosis, heart or lung disease, cancer, alcoholism.
- CNS trauma victims.

Pathophysiology. The causative organism and the resultant pus formation are antigens to the CNS. Therefore, the antigen-antibody process follows the CNS infiltration resulting in:

- Hyperemia of meninges.
- Infiltration and degeneration of segmented neutrophils in the CSF.
- Vasculitis with microthrombi resulting in localized infarction (sterile abscesses) with fibrin surrounding the pus pocket.
- Rupture of pus pockets causing yellow discoloration of the CSF.
- Sterile abscesses adhering to meninges causing:
  - Thickening and focal destruction of pia and arachnoid mater.
  - Impeded flow of CSF, particularly over the convexity of the brain and at the base of the brain.
  - Adherence to the roots of cranial nerves resulting in cranial nerve palsies especially involving cranial nerves II, III, and VIII (Merritt, 1979).

Classification. There are two methods of classifying meningitis: (1) severity of symptoms or organism and (2) source of the infection.

Source

Direct extension from:

- Existing sinus, ear, or mastoid infection
- Depressed skull or vertebral fractures
- Penetrating trauma, such as from a bullet, sharp object, septic lumbar or ventricular puncture

Metastasis through the vascular system from the heart, lungs, or viscera

Severity of symptoms or organism

Acute purulent:

- Bacterial
- Viral

Subacute, secondary to:

- Tuberculosis
- Fungal infections

See Table 7-1 for information on differentiating between oranisms causing meningitis with relation to their incidence, history, and signs.

Table 7-1 Differentiating between organisms causing meningitis based on incidence, history, and signs

Causative organisms	Incidence	History	Signs
Meningococci	Children, young adults Rare over 50 years of age Crowded living conditions	Recent/concomitant respiratory infection with sore throat and joint pains	Cold sores Rapid, sharp rise in temperature Vomiting Petechial rash (spotted fever)
Pneumococci	Very young and elderly persons with alcoholism	Concomitant heart, lung, ear, sinus infection	Decreased lung sounds Heart murmur Meningeal signs
Haemophilus influenzae	Children 2 months to 6 years of age (90%)	Upper respiratory ear, sinus infection Skull fracture	Abrupt onset of meningeal signs Rhinorrhea, otorrhea Hydrocephalus and cranial nerve palsies occur within 7 to 10 days
Staphylococci streptococci	Persons with concomitant staphylococcal or streptococcal infection	Recent upper respiratory infection Facial boils/furuncles	Meningeal signs Heart murmur Petechial/pustular body rash Positive PPD, chest lesion
Gram-negative organisms (*E. coli, Pseudomonas*)	Neonates, elderly	Premature/traumatic birth Head injury Urinary infection	Low-grade fever, hallucinations (adults) Low-grade fever, bulging fontanelles, seisures (infants)
Tubercle bacillus		Primary tuberculosis	Positive PPD, chest lesion

Nursing assessment. In addition to the causative organism, the major differentiation between acute and subacute meningitis is the severity of the symptoms and the rapidity of onset. Distinguishing characteristics of the various types of meningitis are summarized in Table 7-1.

Subjective assessment data

History of:
- Sinus, ear, mastoid, or upper respiratory infection
- Penetrating trauma or basal skull fracture
- Tuberculosis
- Residence in unhygienic, crowded areas
- Environment with high temperatures and low humidity

Fever with chills
Nausea, vomiting
Alternating, variable level of consciousness ranging from irritability and drowsiness to coma
Stiff neck
Headache
Sensitivity to light or loud noises
Difficulty in breathing
Skin rash, itchiness
Focal or generalized seizures
Infants and children: meningeal cry (sharp, shrill), convulsions

Objective assessment data

Fever over 102° F
Increased pulse and respiratory rate
Dyspnea with decreased base lung sounds
Vomiting
Positive Kernig's (Fig. 7-1) or Brudzinski's (Fig. 7-2) sign
Decreased tendon reflexes
Seizure activity (focal or generalized)
Conjunctivitis
Hypersensitivity to light, noise, touch
Decreased responsiveness to stimuli
Skin rash (caused by coagulation of capillaries):
- Petechial, facial rash: meningiococcal meningitis
- Petechial/pustular total body rash: staphylococcal meningitis

Facial furuncles or herpes simplex: staphylococcal meningitis
Nystagmus with visual field defects, ptosis, papilledema
Heart murmur: staphylococcal or pneumococcal meningitis
Infants and children: bulging fontanelles, increased head circumference (Fig. 7-3), meningeal cry, opisthotonos (extreme extension) position, generalized seizures

Laboratory data:
- Blood: Increased white blood cells(10,000-40,000/mm^3), culture of causative organism
- Urine: Albumin, casts red blood cells (RBCs) and white blood cells (WBCs) present
- Nasopharynx and skin lesions: organism cultured
- CSF examination: See Table 7-2 for a comparison between normal CSF and CSF in meningitis.

Radiographs: taken to determine the primary source of infection or trauma

Skull and spine:
- Fractures and/or osteomyelitis
- Sinus or mastoid infection

Chest:
- Pneumonia
- Lung abcesses
- Tubercular lesions
- Granulomas caused by fungal infections

Brain scans: radioisotope concentration noted in areas of infection

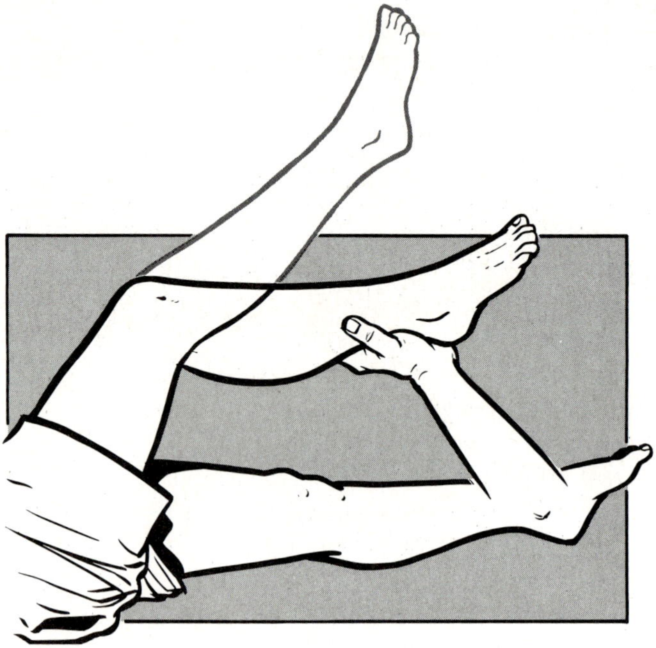

Fig. 7-1 Testing for Kernig's sign. (From Snyder, M., and Jackle, M.: Neurologic problems: a critical care nursing focus, Bowie, Md., 1981, Robert J. Brady Co.)

A

B

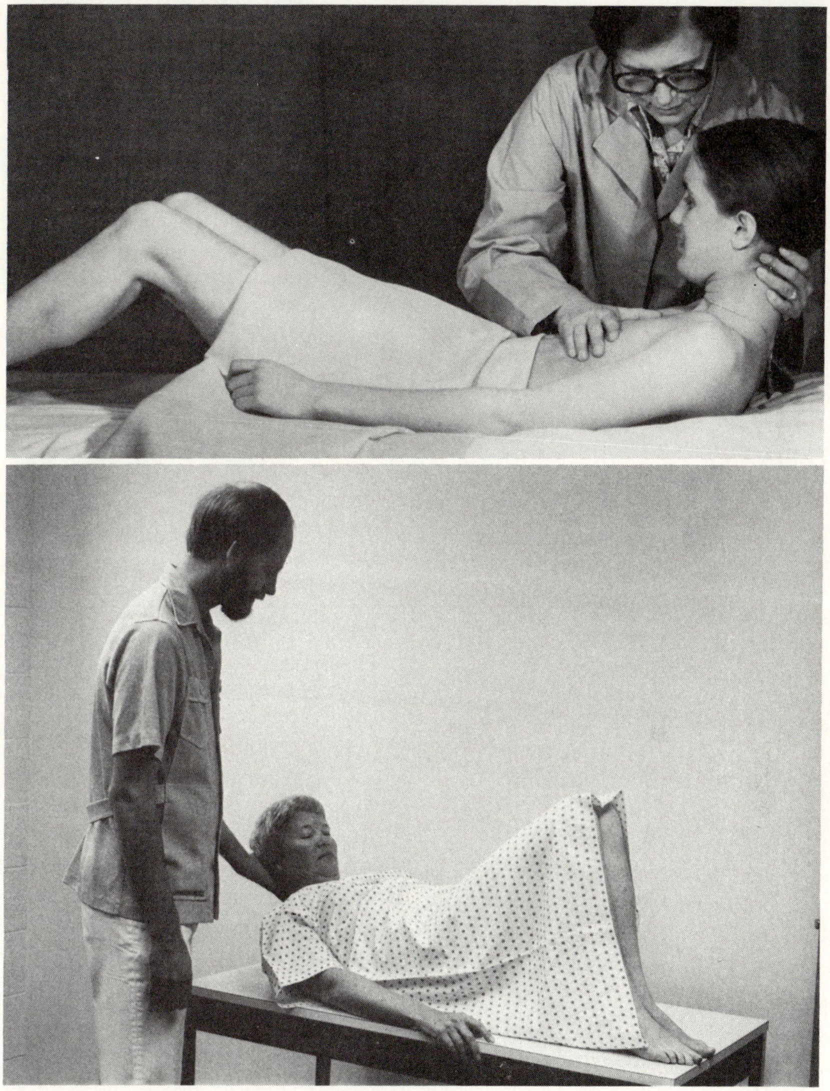

Fig. 7-2 **A,** Elicitation of Brudzinski's sign. **B,** Brudzinski's sign. Knees and hips flex when head is lowered to chest. (**A** from Malasanos, L., and others: Health assessment, ed. 2, St. Louis, 1981, The C.V. Mosby Co.)

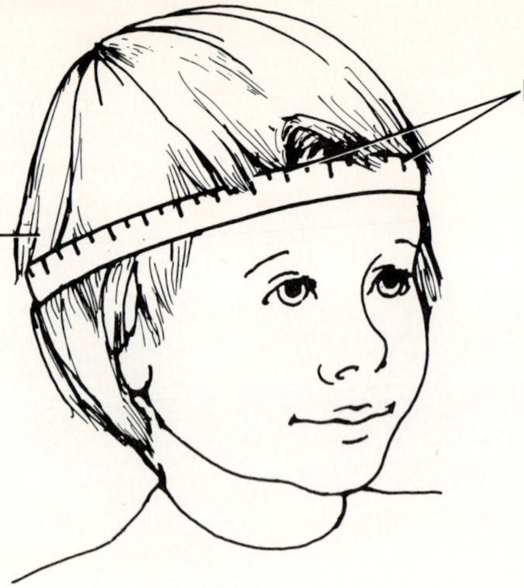

Fig. 7-3 Measuring circumference of child's head.

Table 7-2 **Comparison between CSF normally and in meningitis**

CSF characteristic	Meningitis	Normal
Pressure	200-500 mm H_2O	80-180 mm H_2O
Appearance	Cloudy, turbid, yellow	Clear
Cell count (polymorphonuclear or segmented neutrophils)	2000-25,000/mm^3	0-8/mm^3
Protein*	70 mg	15-45 mg
Glucose†	20 mg/100 ml	45-75 mg/100 ml
Chloride‡	700 mg/100 ml	118-132 mEq/L (adult) 120-128 mEq/L (children)
Smears for culture	Infective organism	Negative
Antigens	*H. influenzae*	None
	D. pneumoniae	None
	N. meningitidis	None

*Increased protein is caused by diffusion of albumin from serum.

†Glucose level is normal or slightly decreased in viral meningitis. Glucose that passes the blood-brain barrier is used by leukocytes in phagocytosis, which is increased in meningitis. Hence, the rise in CSF glucose levels.

‡Decreased chloride content is indicative of tubercular meningitis (Gilroy, 1975).

Nursing care plan: **MENINGITIS**

NURSING DIAGNOSIS	EXPECTED OUTCOMES	NURSING INTERVENTIONS
Inadequate body response to infective agent	No infection	Administer prescribed antimicrobial agents (Table 7-3). Monitor for side effects (Table 7-4).
Ineffective airway potential or actual due to increased intracranial pressure or depressed cerebral function	Patent airway	Endotracheal intubation with mechanical ventilation for nonresponsive, comatose patient. Gentle oropharyngeal or endotracheal suctioning. Observe for dyspnea/obstruction.
Impaired gas-gas exchange NOTE: Oxygen requirements, increase by 7% for each degree of fever (Shea, 1981)	Maintain Po_2 at 80-100 mm Hg to prevent brain hypoxia	Administer oxygen, 6-10 L/min, by cannula/mask as prescribed by physician or protocol. Provide nasal hygiene: Cleanse nares with damp wash cloth. Cleanse nasal prongs with soap and water every 8 hours. Do not use alcohol because it disintegrates plastic. Change nasal prongs every 24 hours. Assess and record: 1. Respiratory rate and depth. 2. Lung sounds. 3. Level of orientation. Elevate head of bed 15 to 30 degrees. Monitor arterial blood gases. Initiate bed rest to conserve energy and decrease metabolic requirements. Initiate hypothermic measures according to agency protocol: 1. Cooling blanket 2. Tepid sponges 3. Prescribed antipyretic agents 4. Monitor temperature every hour 5. Cool environment
Fluid volume deficit	Volume sufficient to ensure hydration and tissue perfusion: Central venous pressure (CVP): Adults: 7.5-15 cm Children: 2.5-4.5 cm Blood pressure sufficient to ensure 30 ml/hr urinary output	Initiate prescribed volume sustenance therapy: Ringer's lactate or dextrose in one quarter strength saline with potassium supplement, 1000 ml/24 hr for adults. Monitor and record: 1. Blood pressure. 2. Pulses 3. CVP 4. Intake/output record. Assess for: 1. Overhydration: extremity or pulmonary edema; decreased specific gravity. 2. Dehydration: fever, decreased skin turgor, dry mucous membranes, oliguria, increased specific gravity. Monitor serum electrolytes for imbalances.

Continued.

Nursing care plan: **MENINGITIS—cont'd**

NURSING DIAGNOSIS	EXPECTED OUTCOMES	NURSING INTERVENTIONS
Alteration in tissue perfusion	No emboli, venous stasis Normal capillary refill (2 sec)	Apply prescribed elastic hose. Institute passive/active range-of-motion exercises. Monitor capillary refill in extremities and forehead.
Potential for nutritional deficit	Nutritional balance supportive of healing	Provide small servings of easily digested foods and fluids. Consider patient preferences. Gavage for comatose patients. Weigh patient.
Altered urinary elimination	Output equates with intake. Minimum 30 ml/hour	Monitor and record urinary output. Initiate prescribed intermittent catheterization, voiding schedule, or retention catheter.
Altered bowel elimination	No impaction, constipation	Commode at bedside. Administer prescribed suppositories to reduce need for valsalva maneuver. Provide fluids.
Impaired mobility	No contractures Normal muscle mass Normal joint mobility	Position in correct alignment. Initiate active/passive range-of-motion exercises every 4 hours. Maintain hourly turning schedule.
Altered sensory perception	Oriented to time, person, and place	Reorient minimally every 4 hours. Monitor and record neurological status (see Chapter 1). Limit light and noise stimuli. Explain diagnostic tests and therapeutic measures.
Potential for physical injury	Prevention of accidents	Low bed position. Side rails up and padded. Call light or bell accessible.
Potential for complications:	Prevention of complications	
Thromboplebitis		Adequate dilutent for antibiotics. Slow push for bolus doses (1 ml/min). Use aseptic technique for intravenous infusions, CVPs, catheterizations, lumbar punctures. Change intravenous sites and dressings according to agency policy.
Hydrocephalus (infants/children)		Measure head circumference daily. Observe for bulging fontanelles. Report changes to the physician immediately.

Nursing care plan: MENINGITIS—cont'd

NURSING DIAGNOSIS	EXPECTED OUTCOMES	NURSING INTERVENTIONS
Increased intracranial pressure		Monitor and record neurological status every 15 minutes till stable. Notify the physician of changes.
Seizures		Administer prescribed antiseizure medications. See Table 6-1 for dosage, untoward effects, and nursing interventions. Institute safety precautions.
Hypotension		Monitor blood pressure. Administer prescribed antihypertensive medications. NOTE: Isoproterenol is effectively used to reverse septic shock caused by H. influenzae.
Vascular coagulation		Administer prescribed anticoagulants and observe for side effects.
Spread of infection		Isolate patients with meningococcal meningitis according to agency protocol.
Knowledge deficit: status, diagnostic tests, therapies, and home care	Family informed and/or included in care	Communicate patient's status and diagnostic and treatment measures initiated. Use humane, empathetic, supportive approach. Teach family range-of-motion methods.
	Patient/family comprehend preventive, therapeutic, and supportive measures	Initiate patient/family teaching plan including information about: Prevention or prompt attention to sinus, ear, and upper respiratory infections. Prophylactic rifampin for all contacts with patient with meningococcal meningitis. Immunizations available: group A and C vaccine. Inform family of: Signs and symptoms of meningitis. Maintenance of medication schedule. Signs and symptoms of possible sequelae requiring contact with the physician such as: Diminished hearing. Ocular palsies. Decreased visual acuity. Seizure activity. Care during seizures (See Chapter 6).

Table 7-3 Antibiotic therapy in meningitis

Causative organisms	Antibiotic	Method of administration	Monitor
Meningococci	Aqueous penicillin G Ampicillin Choramphenicol (for allergic persons)	IV for 7-10 days	Skin for rash Tongue for glossitis CBC Platelet count
	For exposed persons prophylactic: Rifampin Minocycline	Orally for 14 days	
Pneumococci	Aqueous benzyl penicillin	IV for 7-10 days	
Streptococci	Ampicillin	IV for 12-15 days	
Staphylococci	Methicillin Nafcillin	IV for 2-4 weeks	
Haemophilus influenzae	Moxalactam	IV for 10-14 days Loading dose for children: 100 mg/kg, then 50 mg/kg q5h. Never exceed 200 mg/day	Hematuria Vertigo Tinnitis Hearing loss CBC Protrombin time
E. coli, Pseudomonas	Gentamicin or Moxalactam (Rodman, 1982)	IV for 14 days, then 3 times weekly for 2 years (children: 20-30 mg/kg)	
Tuberculosis bacillus	Streptomycin Isoniazid daily	Adults: 1 g daily IM, 400 mg orally for 10-14 days	Hearing loss
Coccidioides immitis *Cryptococcus*	Amphotericin B	IV, 0.25-1 mg/kg Mix well in 500 ml dextrose (5%) in water. Administer every other day over 6 hr period for 6 weeks	BUN Serum creatinine CBC Headache Vomiting

Table 7-4 Untoward effects of antibiotics

Medication	Untoward effects
Penicillin	Fever, skin eruptions Anaphylactic reactions Super infections Convulsions (rarely) Oral/vaginal fungus
Ampicillin	Same as above, plus leukopenia
Chloramphenicol	Gastric upsets Bone marrow depression Glossitis Anaphylactic reactions
Cephalothin	Pain during infusion Thrombophlebitis Superinfections
Gentamicin	Renal impairment Eighth cranial nerve dysfunctions: hearing loss, vertigo, tinnitis Convulsions
Amphotericin B	Renal impairment Phlebitis at injection site Bone marrow depression Fever, chills, headache Gastric upsets
Streptomycin	Renal impairment Eighth cranial nerve dysfunctions Anaphylactic reactions
Tetracycline	Skin rash/eruptions Gastrointestinal irritation Discoloration of teeth in children Phlebitis at injection site
Methicillin	Same as penicillin plus hematuria and bone marrow depression
Moxalatam	Prolonged prothrombin time Leukopenia Phlebitis at injection site Diarrhea Hypersensitivity reactions

Encephalitis

Encephalitis is an inflammation of brain parenchyma resulting from infective agents, viral or bacterial. Bacterial encephalitis usually results from depressed skull fractures or septic penetrating instruments. Viral encephalitis generally results from the bite or sting of an infected arthropod or secondary to viral infections. Environmental controls and prophylactic immunizations have decreased the rate of incidence. However, increasingly sophisticated diagnostic methods have resulted in more accurate diagnoses.

Etiology

Arthropod-borne viruses (arboviruses):

- Equine
- St. Louis
- Rabies
- Rocky Mountain fever

Table 7-5 identifies the types, carriers, areas of concentration, incidence, and symptoms of arthropod-borne viral encephalitis.

Organisms present in the person (host organisms):

- Measles viruses
- Herpes simplex virus

Table 7-6 identifies causative organisms and symptoms for host-acquired viral encephalitis.

Pathophysiology. Arboviruses are transmitted to humans through the bite of an infected animal or insect. Specific carriers have been identified for the varius types of encephalitis. The virus infiltrates the perivascular areas of the brain. Leukocytes and glial cells proliferate extensively, giving the appearance of an abscess. Vascular congestion and petechial hemorrhage cause degeneration of neurons. Host viruses, such as measles and herpes simplex, are transmitted systemically to the CNS.

Some viruses have predilection for specific areas of the brain. For example, equine viruses concentrate in the cerebrum and brainstem; St. Louis infections concentrate in the thalamus and midbrain. Others, such as rabies and Rocky Mountain, are characterized by diffuse infiltration of brain parenchyma.

Nursing assessments

Subjective assessment data

Bite by animal
Recent or present viral infection: measles, mumps, cold sores
Drowsiness, lethargy, weakness
Headache and fever
Nausea, anorexia, vomiting
Visual/hearing disturbances
Skin rash, itchiness
Sensitivity to light, noise

Table 7-5 Arthropod-borne viral encephalitis

Type	Carrier	Areas of concentration	Incidence	Symptoms
Equine	Horse mosquito	Cerebrum and brainstem	Adults over 50 years of age Occupational exposure to horses	Sudden onset of: Drowsiness progressing to coma Convulsive seizures Meningeal signs Cranial nerve palsies* Hemiplegia Nausea, vomiting
St. Louis	Mosquito	Blood vessels in thalamus and midbrain	Late summer	Recent "flu": Meningeal signs Intention tremors (fingers, lips, and tongue)* Constricted pupils* Absent abdominal reflex*
Rabies	Rabid animal (skunk, dog, bat, rodent, cat)	Diffuse throughout brain parenchyma	Persons at risk: Farmers Veterinarians/animal workers Children under 4 years of age	Pain, numbness at bite site* Decreasing level of consciousness Anorexia, nausea, vomiting Lethargy followed by hypersensitivity Generalized convulsions Hallucinations Increased saliva* Spasms of pharynx and larynx* Dehydration and fever Flaccid paralysis
Rocky Mountain	Tick, reservoir in squirrels and rodents	Diffuse CNS and localized in skin	Rural, mountainous terrain Late spring to early autumn	Fever Decreased consciousness Measleslike rash on third or fourth day. Rash fades and is followed by maculopapular rash on ankles and wrists spreading to legs, arms, trunk* Tremors Convulsions Muscle rigidity

*Differentiating signs.

Table 7-6 Host-acquired viral encephalitis

Type	Causative organism	Symptoms
Measles	Measles virus	Symptoms 4 to 5 days after rash appears: Fever, headache Cranial nerve palsies Dystonic movements (twisting)* Ataxia and incoordination Forgetfulness* Restlessness
Herpes simplex	Herpes virus Type I: cold sores, conjunctivitis Type II: genitalia	Meningeal signs Sore throat Stomatitis (oral sores)* Myoclonic jerks of extremities* Memory deficits Vaginal, penile sores/drainage* Disorientation Personality changes Hemiparesis/paralysis

*Differentiating signs.

Irritability
Seizures

Objective assessment data

Skin puncture (bite, tick)
Skin rash
Enlarged parotid glands (mumps)
Meningeal signs
Myoclonic jerks of extremities
Nystagmus, motor visual defects
Tremors of extremities
Depressed level of consciousness ranging from difficulty in arousal or disorientation to a comatose state
Dysphagia and dysphasia (rabies)
Hypersensitivity to stimuli
Oral sores
Laboratory tests:
- Blood:
  - Increased WBC with lymphocytes predominating
  - Isolation of virus
  - Increased antibody titer

CSF:
- Elevated protein (80-100 mg/mm)
- Normal glucose and chloride
- Immunofluorescent examination: virus present

Urine: Increased albumin

Smears (oral, throat, vaginal, penile): organism visible

Radiologic examination:

CAT scan:
- Congested vasculature
- Concentration of contrast materials in:
  - Cerebrum/brainstem: equine
  - Thalamus/midbrain: St. Louis
  - Diffuse: rabies, Rocky Mountain
  - Frontal/temporal lobes: herpes simplex
  - Cranial nerves II, VIII: measles

Interventions. During the acute phase, nursing care involves maintenance of vital functions and promotion of homeostasis. Systematic ongoing neurological assessment is necessary to detect changes in patient status. Deteriorating signs indicating increasing intracranial pressure such as, altered level of consciousness, pupillary changes, seizure activity, and vital sign alterations should be reported immediately to the physician. Medical treatment is supportive and symptomatic. General nursing care is as outlined for the patient with meningitis (pp. 193 to 195). Specific interventions follow:

Nursing care plan: **ENCEPHALITIS**

NURSING DIAGNOSIS	EXPECTED OUTCOMES	NURSING INTERVENTIONS
Disturbed sleep pattern: commonly a reversal of normal night/day pattern	Sleep at night Awake during day	Provide activities during day hours to maintain wakeful state.
Knowledge deficit: regarding preventive and treatment measures	Comprehension of preventive and treatment measures	Equine Advocate mosquito control and vaccination of horses. St. Louis: Advocate mosquito control. Explain use of insect repellents and protective clothing Rabies: 1. Wound care: Cleanse bite wound thoroughly with soap and water. Disinfect with benzalkonium (Zephirin) (2%), which inactivates the virus (Adams and Victor, 1981). Administer prescribed tetanus prophylaxis. 2. Report to the county health agency and to the Humane Society. The Animal is quarantined 10 days or is killed and the brain examined)

Continued.

Nursing care plan: **ENCEPHALITIS—cont'd**

NURSING DIAGNOSIS	EXPECTED OUTCOMES	NURSING INTERVENTIONS
Knowledge deficit: regarding preventive and treatment measures—cont'd		3. Administer prescribed a. Immune globulin (Hyperrab), Cutter Biological (312-595-3620) Dosage: 2 ml per 33 pounds. Method: One half of the dosage is injected into the bite (exceptions: face, ear, shin). One-half of the dosage is given intramuscularly. Immune globulin can be given up to 8 days after the first dosage of vaccine. b.. Human diploid cell vaccine (Merieux Institute and Wyatt Laboratory). Dosage: 1 ml on days 1, 3, 7, 14, and 28 after bite. Method: Intramuscularly administration. NOTE: In some states human diploid cell vaccine is available from the state health department. 4. Follow-up care. A serum antibody response test should be administered 2 weeks following the last dose of the vaccine (day 28). If there has been no increase in the antibody level, a 1 ml booster dose of vaccine is administered. 5. This method of protection replaced the use of duck embryo vaccine as of October 1981. Rocky Mountain: Explain to the patient about (a) wearing protective clothing (b) examining the body for ticks. Tick removal: (1) apply gasoline or ether to tick; (2) wait 10 minutes for disengagement; (3) remove dead tick; (4) thoroughly cleanse tick bite area with antiseptic. Herpes simplex: Administer prescribed: 1. Vidarabine (Vira-A), 15 mgm/kg/day IV dissolved in 2.2 ml of fluid added to IV fluid and infused over a 24-hour period. Monitor patient for (a) increased intracranial pressure, (b) kidney function, (c) bone marrow depression, (d) side effects such as gastrointestinal upset, tremors, hallucinations, dizziness, ataxia, disorientation. 2. Dexamethasone and mannitol to prevent decrease cerebral edema. 3. Phenytoin and phenobarbital to prevent/control seizures (Swisher, 1981).

Reye's syndrome

Reye's syndrome is an acute disease occurring primarily in infants, children, and adolescents. The acute brain edema is secondary to fatty infiltration of the liver, occurring 3 to 7 days after an upper respiratory infection, flu, chicken pox, or measles (Adams and Victor, 1981). Because of the rapid evolution of cerebral edema causing cerebellar herniation, early detection and prompt treatment is essential to decreasing the fatality rate. In an effort to increase awareness of Reye's syndrome, the National Reye's Syndrome Foundation will supply posters upon request to emergency departments and pediatric clinics (Fig. 7-4). Because of increased awareness and the prompt aggressive treatment currently used, the mortality rate has decreased from 40% to approximately 5% nationally (NIH Consensus Development Conference Summary, 1981).

Etiology. Reye's syndrome is secondary to viral infection, commonly influenza or varicella. Use of salycilates as antipyretic therapy during these viral infections has been implicated in the development of the encephalopathy associated with Reye's syndrome.

Pathophysiology. While the specific pathophysiology is unclear, fatty infiltration of the liver without signs of inflammation or necrosis following a viral infection is a consistent finding (Adams and Victor, 1981). The dysfunctioning liver is unable to convert protein to urea, which results in the systemic circulation of ammonia (NH_4), which interferes with cerebral function. Cerebral edema is another consistent finding. If not decompressed this causes cerebellar herniation.

Classification. Table 7-7 delineates the stages of Reye's syndrome developed by the NIH Consensus Development Conference in 1981. The full report is available without cost from the Office for Medical Applications of Research, Bldg I, Room 216, NIH, Bethesda, MD 20505.

Nursing assessments

Subjective assessment data

History elicited from parents of an upper respiratory infection, flu, measles, or chicken pox 3 to 7 days previously.

Aspirin given during illness

Protracted vomiting without nausea or diarrhea

Change in behavior from normal

Excessive staring into space

Alternating drowsiness and screaming progressing to nonresponsive coma

Weakness accompanied by tenseness of leg and arm muscles

Extreme sensitivity to light, sounds, and touch

Generalized seizures

Objective assessment data

Vomiting without diarrhea

Disturbed cerebral functioning with alternating screaming and lethargy

CONSIDER REYE'S

Reye's syndrome is a disease of infants and children through age 19.

SUSPECT REYE'S IN A PATIENT WITH:

1. Unexpected VOMITING following a prodromal flu-like upper respiratory infection or chickenpox (usually no diarrhea)
2. Signs of DISTURBED BRAIN FUNCTION
   Characterized by lethargy • staring • stupor • agitated delirium and screaming • drug reaction-like behavior • extensor spasms • decerebrate rigidity • aspirin poisoning-like symptoms • coma
3. Elevated SGOT-SGPT (usually 200 or more units) in the absence of jaundice

FOR EARLY DIAGNOSIS

1. Vomiting, think Reye's syndrome
2. Emergency SGOT-SGPT
3. Elevated blood NH_3
4. Hypoglycemia and hepatomegaly may be present

INITIAL TREATMENT

1. Give 10% glucose in maintenance salt solution.
2. Maintain airway and brain oxygen.
3. Consult a special treatment center.

EARLY DIAGNOSIS AND TREATMENT WILL PREVENT
DEATH IN 4 OUT OF 5 CASES

Fig. 7-4 Poster from the National Reye's Syndrome Foundation. (Courtesy National Reye's Syndrome Foundation, Bryan, Ohio.)

Table 7-7 Staging of Reye's syndrome*

Stage	I	II	III	IV	V
Level of consciousness	Lethargy: follows verbal commands	Combative/stupor; verbalizes inappropriately	Coma	Coma	Coma
Posture	Normal	Normal	Decorticate	Decerebrate	Flaccid
Response to pain	Purposeful	Purposeful/nonpurposeful	Decorticate	Decerebrate	None
Pupillary reaction	Brisk	Sluggish	Sluggish	Sluggish	None
Oculocephalic reflex (doll's eyes)	Normal	Conjugate deviation	Conjugate deviation	Inconsistent or absent	None

*Developed by the NIH Consensus Development Conference, 1981. Reprinted with permission.

Extensor spasms of legs and arms progressing to decorticate or decerebrate posturing
Tachycardia and tachypnea with mild fever or normal temperature
Bilateral dilated pupils, nonresponsive to light
Lack of corneal and vestibuloocular reflexes
Hepatomegaly without jaundice (in some cases)
Diagnostic tests (Merritt, 1979):
- SGOT: elevated over 250 u
- SGPT: over 225 u.
- Blood glucose: subnormal, particularly in infants
- BUN: elevated
- Blood ammonia: elevated over 350 ng/100 ml. NOTE: This test takes longer and is more expensive than SGOT (Richmond and Stair, 1982)
- PPT: prolonged (thought to be related to administration of salycilates)
- Arterial blood gases: NOTE: Respiratory acidosis usually precedes respiratory alkalosis
  - $pH > 7.50$
  - $P_{CO_2} < 28$
- Lumbar puncture: (used primarily to rule out sepsis):
  - Pressure over 160 mm H_2O
  - Protein: normal
- Urine: protein and RBCs present
- CAT scan: small ventricles
- EEG: diffuse, arrhythmic waves

Interventions. Aggressive, therapeutic interventions are aimed at sustaining vital functions, reducing the metabolic rate, decreasing the cerebral edema, and correcting the basic metabolic dysfunctions.

Nursing care plan: REYE'S SYNDROME

NURSING DIAGNOSIS	EXPECTED OUTCOMES	NURSING INTERVENTIONS
Ineffective gas exchange due to respiratory alkalosis	Arterial P_{O_2}: 80-100 mm Hg P_{CO_2}: 35-45 mm Hg	Initiate prescribed hyperventilation procedures to decrease ICP by decreasing CO_2 level 1. If patient is oriented, demonstrate rapid breathing technique; 2. If patient is comatose; use endotracheal intubation with positive pressure ventilatory assistance.
Impaired cognitive functioning due to cerebral edema and metabolic dysfunctions: hypoglycemia and hyperammonemia	ICP: 4-15 mm Hg 50-200 mm H_2O without plateau waves Blood glucose: 70-110 mg/dl Blood ammonia: 80-110 ug/dl BUN: 8-25 mg/dl	Orient patient to person, place, and time. Assess and record neurological data every 15 minutes. Promptly report changes. Prepare for and assist with insertion of intracranial catheter or screw. Initiate prescribed hypothermia measures.

Continued.

Nursing care plan: REYE'S SYNDROME—cont'd

NURSING DIAGNOSIS	EXPECTED OUTCOMES	NURSING INTERVENTIONS
Impaired cognitive functioning due to cerebral edema and metabolic dysfunctions: hypoglycemia and hyperammonemia—cont'd		Initiate measures to decrease metabolic rate: 1. Reduce environmental stimuli. 2. Provide cool quiet environment. 3. Stagger patient care procedures. Maintain patency of ICP monitoring line. When suctioning endotracheal tube, hyperventilate with 100% oxygen and allow 30-60 seconds minimally between catheter insertions. Assist with CSF removal through catheter and record amount and fluid characteristics. Insert nasogastric tube and connect it to low-grade intermittent suction to prevent vomiting and aspiration.
	ICP: 4-15 mm Hg	Administer prescribed medications to: 1. Decrease brain edema: mannitol; dexamethasone.
	Serum osmolality under 310	2. Correct or prevent hypoglycemia: Administer glucose (10%) in normal saline with insulin sufficient to move glucose into cells as prescribed (Richmond and Stair, 1981).
	BUN: 8-25 mg/dl	3. Decrease ammonia levels by administering prescribed acetohydroxamic acid, which inhibits bacterial action on proteins in the gastrointestinal tract (Conomy, 1982). Prepare patient for peritoneal dialysis or hemodialysis.
	Normal ICP and pattern	Initiate protocol for pentobarbital coma: Procedure: Administer pentobarbital (Nembutal), 5-15 mg/kg IV push over 30 minutes. Maintain with 1-3 mg/kg every 2 hours. Constantly monitor neurological signs. Expect depressed neurological signs consistent with comatose status (Budassi and Barber, 1981). NOTE: EKG changes are lost as a parameter when this procedure is used.
Altered cardiac output to metabolic depression and altered electrolyte balance	Blood pressure of 90/50 minimum Urinary output 30 ml/hour No dysrhythmias	Initiate prescribed cardiac monitoring. NOTE: Loss of potassium from damaged cells causes hyperkalemia. Assist with insertion of CVP line and monitor pressure every 15-30 minutes. Monitor and record vital signs every 15 minutes. Regulate intravenous infusions to maintain 30 ml/hour urinary output.
Nutritional deficit due to vomiting; vitamin K deficit and inability to catabolize and excrete urea due to liver dysfunction	Prothrombin time: 12-14 seconds Normal electrolyte profile	Administer prescribed vitamin K (Mephyton) to prevent/control cerebral bleeding. Insert nasogastric tube to decompress stomach and prevent aspiration of vomitus. Limit protein intake until blood ammonium level is normal. Monitor serum electrolytes and ammonia; after acute stage gradually increase nutritional intake.

Nursing care plan: REYE'S SYNDROME—cont'd

NURSING DIAGNOSIS	EXPECTED OUTCOMES	NURSING INTERVENTIONS
Impaired physical mobility resulting in pneumonia and loss of muscle tone	No lung consolidation/infection	Aseptic endotracheal suctioning. Initiate prescribed chest physiotherapy. Monitor vital capacity. Report values under 10 ml/kg immediately.
	No loss of muscle mass; retention of muscle tone	Initiate passive/active range-of-motion exercises on all four extremities. Maintain 2-hour turning schedule.
Potential joint contractures	No joint contractures	Position in normal body alignment.
Anxiety of parents	Reduced anxiety	Keep parents informed about patient's condition and treatment measures.
Knowledge deficit: use of salycilates in viral infections	Parents comprehend Centers for Disease Control (CDC) recommendations.	Explain current CDC recommendations: No child with flu, chicken pox, measles should be given aspirin for fever. Acetaminophin (Tylenol) is recommended when fever is 39° C or over. Under 39° C increase fluids, remove clothes, and sponge (CDC, 1981). Inform parents of Reye's Syndrome Foundation. Teach home care and rehabilitative procedures.

Myelitis

Myelitis is an inflammation of the spinal cord that is most commonly secondary to an infectious process elsewhere in the body, such as influenza, measles, or meningitis, and it results in necrosis of the spinal cord parenchyma. The primary sign is a rapidly developing flaccid paralysis with loss with urinary and fecal control without a subjective complaint of back pain (Merritt, 1979). Although the incidence of poliomyelitis has decreased substantially, it will be used to delineate the nursing assessments and interventions used for persons with an inflammation of the spinal cord.

Etiology. The most common etiological agents are:

- Viruses
  - Poliomyelitis.
  - Herpes.
  - Influenza.
  - Varicella (postinfections or postvaccinal).
- Bacteria
  - Pneumococci.
  - Meningococci.
  - Tuberclebacilli.
  - *Treponema pallidum*.

Pathophysiology. The infective organism gains access to the spinal cord through the lymphatic system, causing a localized inflammatory response. Some organisms have a predilection for particular areas of the cord parechyma: for example, polio virus for anterior motor horn cells, herpes for the dorsal root ganglion, tubercle bacilli and *Treponema* for ascending tracts. The inflammed area becomes edematous, resulting in a pressure necrosis of cord parenchyma. This phase is followed by vascular congestion caused by the presence of leukocytes and the glial activity required for the removal of the necrosed tissue (Adams and Victor, 1981).

Classification. Myelitis is classified in various ways including by the infective agent, the type of inflammatory process, and the location and type of involvement (Adams and Victor, 1981).

- Infective agent:
  - Viral
  - Bacterial
  - Fungal/parasitic
- Type of process:
  - Acute (symptoms evolve within days)
  - Subacute (symptoms evolve over 2 to 6 weeks)
  - Chronic (symptoms slowly evolve over more than 6 weeks)
- Location (in descending order of incidence):
  - Thoracic
  - Cervical
  - Lumbosacral
- Type of involvement:
  - Gray matter: poliomyelitis
  - White matter: leukomyelitis
  - Both: diffuse or disseminated
  - Both and meninges; meningomyelitis

Poliomyelitis

The incidence of polio has drastically diminished since 1953 when immunization procedures, initially the injected Salk vaccine and later in 1960 the more effective oral Sabin vaccine, were initiated in the United States. However, sporadically cases are seen when immunization has not been carried out (Merritt, 1979). Poliomyelitis is characterized by destruction of motor cells in the anterior horn of the spinal cord and brainstem, resulting in a flaccid paralysis of the muscles innervated by the destroyed neurons.

Etiology. Poliomyelitis is caused by one of three viruses that invade the CNS from the pharynx or gastrointestinal tract entering, the blood stream by way of the regional lymph nodes. Polio viruses can be spread by:

- Droplet inhalation.
- Ingestion of fecally contaminated foods.

Pathophysiology. The polio viruses generally enter the host through the oropharynx or gastrointestinal tract and enter the circulation through the lymphatic system. Polio viruses have a predilection for the motor cells in the spinal cord (anterior horn) and brainstem. The initial inflammation, with an increase in segmented neutrophils, is followed by an increase in lymphocytes and monocytes, which attempt to engulf and destroy the virus. If the virus infiltrates the neurons, the nissel substance and nucleus disintegrate and glial cells proliferate to ingest the necrosed neurons (Adams and Victor, 1981). This causes scarring and shrinkage of the anterior horn.

Classification

Spinal: anterior horn of the spinal cord
Bulbar: motor cells of the brainstem (cranial nerves IX, X, and XII)

Nursing assessment

Subjective assessment data

Recent acute respiratory or gastrointestinal infection followed by recovery and a subsequent rise in temperature
Malaise with gastrointestinal upsets and generalized weakness
Nonthrobbing headache and stiff neck
Muscle aches and pains particularly in the neck, back, and legs
Alternating irritability and drowsiness
Difficulty in walking
Muscle weakness progressing to paralysis of extremities
Difficulty in swallowing, speaking, breathing, and hiccoughs (indicative of bulbar involvement)
Noncurrent or inadequate immunization status

Objective assessment data

Fever and chills
Excessive perspiration
Nuchal rigidity with positive Kernig's and Brudzinski's signs
Muscle tenderness, especially back, neck, and legs
Irritability and apprehension
Convulsive seizures
Cerebellar-type ataxia
Progressive asymmetrical flaccid paresis of extremities and trunk (spinal)
Dysphagia, dysphasia, and dyspnea (bulbar involvement)
Laboratory data:
- Blood: Moderate increase in WBC
- CSF: 10-200 WBC
  - Increased segmented neutrophils in the early stage
  - Increased lymphocytes/monocytes after 6 to 24 hours
  - Elevated protein content (150 mg/100 ml)
  - Normal glucose and chloride levels

Tissue culture:
- Oropharynx: polio virus present for first 24 hours
- Feces: polio virus present for months

Complement fixation:
- Four-fold rise in antibody titer in serum, CSF, or fecal specimens

Nursing care plan: MYELITIS, INCLUDING POLIOMYELITIS

NURSING DIAGNOSIS	EXPECTED OUTCOMES	NURSING INTERVENTIONS
Impaired gas exchange	Respiratory sufficiency Po_2 80-100 mm Hg	Observe for respiratory distress. NOTE: Anxiety in a previously calm patient indicates cerebral hypoxia. Administer oxygen when hypoxia is evident. Monitor respiratory rate, pattern, and muscles used. Auscultate chest for consolidation. Bed rest is prescribed to conserve energy. Explain prescribed pulmonary function tests such as vital capacity. Have intubation and ventilatory assistance equipment readily available. Provide pulmonary toilet: deep breathing with sustained maximal inspiration, yawning, removal of excessive or thickened oral/pharyngeal secretions.
Fluid volume deficit	Fluid/electrolyte balance	Ensure adequate fluid intake: oral, enteral, or parenteral. Assess for fluid and electrolyte imbalances: physical assessment and monitor electrolyte studies. Maintain accurate intake/output records.
Altered elimination: due to immobility or flaccidity of bladder	Urine output correlates with fluid intake	Maintain accurate intake/output records (urine and fecal) Catheterize patients with flaccid bladder.
Altered bowel elimination (such as constipation) due to immobility and/or loss of intestinal muscle tone	Normal fecal elimination	Insert prescribed rectal suppositories. Administer enemas as prescribed. Provide roughage foods. Increase fluid intake. Assess for bladder/bowel distention.
Impaired physical motility with potential for joint contractures and loss of muscle mass/tone	No joint contractures Maintenance of muscle mass	Institute passive and active range-of-motion exercises every 4 hours. Gently massage muscles following acute phase. Administer prescribed muscle relaxants. Apply corrective or preventive appliances: sand bags or trochanter rolls at hips; splints; footboard or high-top tennis shoes. Consult the physical therapist in cooperatively designing individualized long-term goals and approaches. Position in correct alignment on regular or rocking bed. Assist with physical therapy program: whirlpool, strength-building exercises.

Nursing care plan: MYELITIS, INCLUDING POLIOMYELITIS—cont'd

NURSING DIAGNOSIS	EXPECTED OUTCOMES	NURSING INTERVENTIONS
Potential for impaired skin integrity	Skin integrity without excoriation	Initiate hourly turning schedule. Maintain dry, clean skin. Massage skin over bony prominences. Use soap sparingly to prevent skin dryness. Provide Roto-rest bed, kinetic bed or water/air mattress.
Body-image disturbance due to loss of mobility and dependence on others	Positive self-image	Encourage verbalization of feelings. Solicit aid of professional counselors, social services, occupational therapists. Discuss patient problems with family members to solicit their assistance in the resolution of the problems. Encourage realistic goal-setting.
Knowledge deficit: immunization and home care measures	Comprehension of preventive and rehabilitative measures	Preventive measures: Explain and encourage immunization procedures. The Sabin vaccine (oral) is usually given in 3 doses, 2 months apart, during the first year of life and booster doses are given at 15 months and 5 years of age. Rehabilitative measures: Demonstrate: 1. Respiratory hygiene measures. 2. Progressive exercise and muscle-retraining program. 3. Application of splints. 4. Positioning methods. 5. Transfer techniques. 6. Skin care. Explain: 1. Nutritional needs. 2. Psychosocial needs.

Abscess

Abscesses in the CNS are typically secondary to infections in other parts of the body, most commonly the ear, mastoid, sinus, heart, respiratory tract, or bone. They can also be caused by septic surgical or diagnostic procedures or penetrating trauma. The abscess formation mimics a space-occupying lesion, exerting pressure on the brain or spinal cord, resulting in focal neurological signs.

Etiology

Direct extension of bacterial infections (staphlococcal, streptococcal) from the frontal or sphenoid sinuses, the ear, mastoid, or bone

Secondary to infections such as from *Streptococcus, Proteus, Bacteroides, E. Coli, Klebsiella* existing elsewhere in the body

Pathophysiology. There are three phases in abscess development:

1. Free liquid pus without boundaries, causing focal encephalitis with edema and vascular congestion

2. Thin layer, irregular encapsulation of the pus by fibroblasts.
3. Thickening of the pus with granular glial encapsulation and formation of supportive capillaries surrounded by hyperemic, edematous parenchyma (Wing, 1981)

Because of the soft, freely movable substance of the cerebrum, cerebral abscesses are generally quite large before neurological deficits occur. However because of the relative stability of the brainstem and the small circumference of the spinal cord, abscess formation in these areas results in rapidly evolving objective signs.

The encapsulated abscess mimics an expanding lesion, causing outward displacement of brain or spinal cord tissue, thus inhibiting the normal flow of CSF. In some cases, the signs of increasing intracranial pressure are the initial signal of the presence of an abscess. The encapsulation of the abscess results in a normal or subnormal temperature unless the primary infection is still active. Focal neurological signs are dependent on the size and location of the abscess. See Table 7-8. The classification of abscesses is based on the location and the primary source.

Classification

Brain

Type	Mode of infection
Extradural	extention of skull osteitis
Subdural	extension of sinus infection
Intracerebral	extension of ear/mastoid infection

Spinal cord

Type	Mode of infection
Epidural	extension of skin infection or vertebral osteitis
Intramedullary	secondary to lung or genitourinary infection

Brain abscess

Nursing assessment. The variability of the presence and the degree of patient complaints presents a real problem in the nursing assessment.

Subjective assessment data

History of:

- Recent ear, sinus, mastoid, or upper respiratory infection
- Chronic heart disease, bacterial endocarditis, rheumatic fever
- Recent course of antibiotic therapy or of taking over-the-counter sinus or cold medications

Headache (frontal or suboccipital) NOTE: This is the most frequent initial symptom
Chills and malaise
Neck stiffness
Scalp tenderness
Visual disturbances
Difficulty in speaking/comprehension
Facial and particularly eye tics or lack of facial muscle tone
Lethargy, apathy

Table 7-8 Abscess and signs and symptoms related to abscess location and source

Location	Signs and symptoms	Source
Brain		
Frontal lobe	Scalp tenderness Localized frontal headache Lethargy, apathy, disorientation Contralateral hemiparesis/paralysis High fever Seizures Dysphasia (motor)	Paranasal sinuses
Temporal lobe	Dysphasia (sensory) Visual field disturbances Palsies of cranial nerves III and VI Contralateral facial paresis	Ear infection
Cerebellum	Ipsilateral ataxia Nystagmus and gaze toward lesion Dystonia Nuchal rigidity Suboccipital headache Dysfunction of cranial nerves III, IV, V, VI	Middle ear or mastoid infection
Spinal cord		
Epidural (thoracic area is the most common site)	Pain in thoracic area; exacerbated by movement Rapid onset of paraparesis/paralysis Loss of sensation below abscess Urinary retention with overflow incontinence	Staphylococcal skin infection
Intramedullary	High fever Rapidly progressive paraplegia Sensory loss below abscess Bladder paralysis	Systemic from an existing or inadequately treated lung of genitourinary infection

Inability to concentrate
Unilateral weakness
Difficulty in walking and balance
Decreased dexterity
Nausea, vomiting, anorexia
Convulsions, focal or generalized

Objective assessment data

Fever over 101° F with chills. NOTE: Temperature returns to normal following abscess encapsulation
Decreased pulse rate
Increased systolic blood pressure with widening pulse pressure
Papilledema (late sign)
Hemiparesis/paralysis (flaccid)
Visual defects: hemianopsia, paralysis of conjugate gaze toward lesion
Dysphasia; motor and/or sensory
Ataxia
Nystagmus
Positive Kernig's and Brudzinski's signs
Bulging tympanic membrane
Ptosis of eyelids
Hypotonia; face and extremities
Sinuses full or draining
Child: holds head, tugs at ear
Diagnostic tests:
- CSF:
  - Elevated pressure: 200-300 mm of water
  - Elevated WBC count with lymphocytes predominating
  - Protein elevated
  - Glucose normal
- CBC: increased WBC and sedimentation rate
- Skull x-ray:
  - Shift of pineal gland
  - Consolidation in sinuses or mastoid
- Chest x-ray: consolidation
- EEG: slowing around abscess site
- CAT scan: sharply delineated ring around lesion with displacement of midline parenchyma and surrounding tissue (Fig. 7-5)
- Brain scan: high uptake of radioactive material around abscess
- Angiography: increased vasculature surrounding abscess (vascular blush)

NOTE: A lumbar puncture is not advisable because of the potential for herniation

Nursing interventions. General nursing interventions are aimed at maintenance of vital and homeostatic functions.

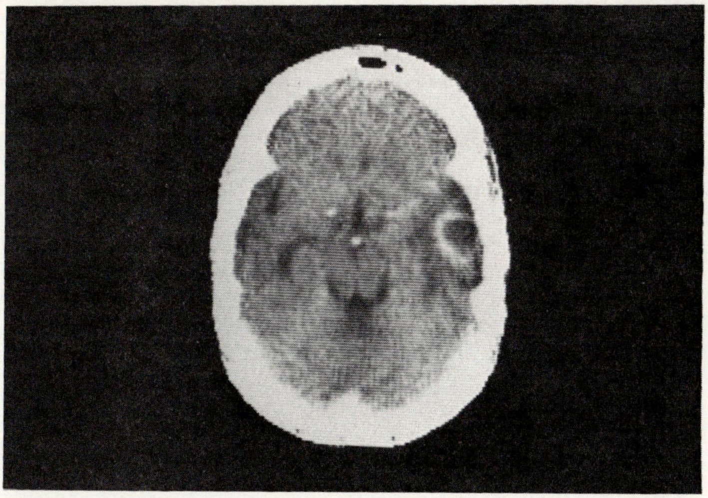

Fig. 7-5 CAT scan: brain abscess.

Nursing care plan: ABSCESS

NURSING DIAGNOSIS	EXPECTED OUTCOMES	NURSING INTERVENTIONS
Inadequate body response to lyse infective agent or inadequate autoimmune response	Infection-free	Monitor and record neurological status. Administer prescribed systemic antibiotics that pass blood-brain barrier: chloramphenicol, methicillin (Staphcillin), penicillin. NOTE: Antimicrobial agents are administered preoperatively and postoperatively for 10 to 14 days to sustain antibiotic blood levels high enough to effect bacteriocidal action. Intravenous drip administration decreases seizure potential caused by the high dosages of antibiotics administered. Monitor 1. CBC for depression of WBC or platelets. 2. For phebitis at intravenous insertion site. 3. Sensitivity/allergic responses. 4. Seizure activity caused by high antibiotic dosages. 5. Output: check for hematuria. 6. Specific gravity for increase indicataive of nephrotoxicity. Prepare patient for surgical procedures: drainage or excision of abscess.

Continued.

Nursing care plan: ABSCESS—cont'd

NURSING DIAGNOSIS	EXPECTED OUTCOMES	NURSING INTERVENTIONS
Knowledge deficit: diagnostic tests, preparation for surgery, therapeutic and preventive measures	Comprehension of diagnostic, therapeutic, and preventive measures	Explain diagnostic tests to patient and family. Reinforce neurosurgeon's explanation of surgical drainage or excision of abscess (See Chapter 14). Explain rationale for nursing procedures: 1. Positioning with head elevated 30 degrees with straight tracheal alignment to facilitate venous drainage from head. 2. Monitoring neurological status every hour till stabilized.
Potential for complications due to altered physiology:		
Increased intracranial pressure (ICP)	No increased ICP	Administer prescribed osmotic diuretics and corticosteroids. Position with head elevated 15 to 30 degrees. Monitor for signs of decrease or increase in ICP. Maintain accurate intake/output records.
Seizures	No seizure activity	Administer prescribed anticonvulsants (hydantoin). Institute seizure precautions: padded side rails in up position.
Potential for joint contractures and impaired mobility due to loss of muscle tone	No contractures Normal muscle tone	Institute active and passive range-of-motion exercise every 4 hours. Position in correct alignment to prevent abnormal joint adduction or abduction. Apply foot board or high-top tennis shoes to prevent foot drop. Consult with physical therapist.
Impaired skin integrity	Skin integrity	Massage pressure points. Change position every 2 hours. Provide diet with adequate protein and vitamins B and C. Provide kinetic or Roto bed, water or air mattress.

Spinal cord abscess Spinal cord abscesses most frequently affect the anterior cord (motor). Hence, the signs and symptoms of motor rather than sensory deficits predominate.

Etiology. The most common causative organism is *Staphylococcus aureus*. The abscess results from an inward extension of staphylococcal skin infection or osteomyelitis.

Pathophysiology. See Pathophysiology of abscess. The major difference between brain and spinal cord abscesses is the small circumference of the spinal cord, which causes the signs and symptoms to evolve more rapidly.

Nursing assessments

Subjective assessment data

History of boil on back
Localized pain at site of the abscess, which is aggravated by movement
Pain radiating to legs
Spasms of back muscles
Leg weakness
Numbness/tingling in feet and legs
Decreased urination with overflow incontenence
Gastrointestional upsets

Objective assessment data

Fever with increased pulse rate
Pustular lesions on back
Back muscle tenseness
Positive Kernig's or Brudzinski's sign
Hypotonia of leg muscles
Oliguria
Paraparesis progressing to spastic paraplegia within 24 to 72 hours
Sensory impairment in feet and legs
Plantar extension
Initially exaggerated tendon reflexes. In paraplegic state decreased tendon reflexes.
Diagnostic tests:

- CBC: increased segmented neutrophils
- CSF:
  - Color yellow or cloudy
  - Increased protein level
  - Normal glucose
- Myelography: area of abscess edematous, impeding flow of CSF (Fig. 7-6)

Interventions. Patient care is identical to that of brain abscess with exception of:

1. Positioning: Patient should be supine with correct bone/joint alignment.
2. Peripheral circulatory adjunct: Prescribed thigh-high antiembolism stockings should be applied.

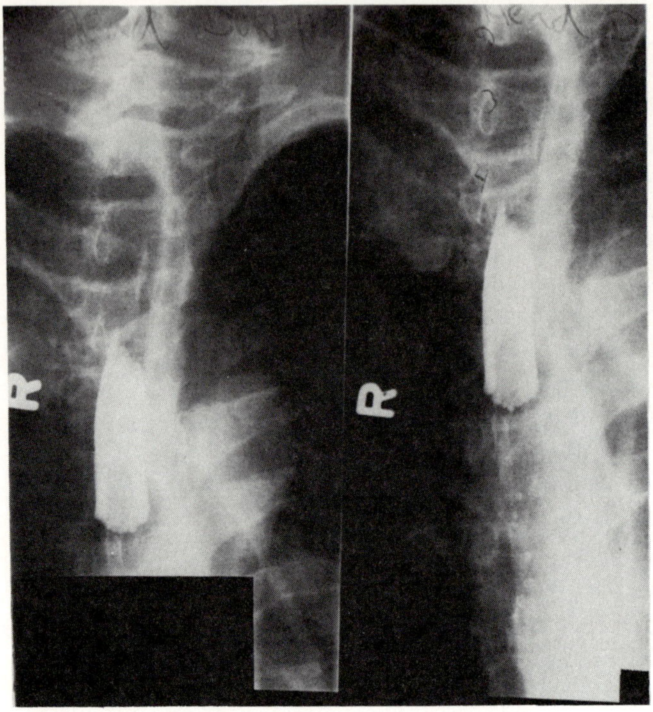

Fig. 7-6 Myelogram: epidural abscess with complete thoracic block. Brush appearance at T4 suggests epidural block.

Neurosyphilis

Neurosyphilis is quite rare today because of three factors:

Availability of penicillin
Improved diagnostic methods
Increased public awareness of the need for and increased access to treatment for primary syphilis

However, there are some patients who have received inadequate or no treatment for primary syphilis. One possible reason given for an increased incidence of neurosyphilis in the future is the acceptance of sexual promiscuity in our culture.

Etiology. Neurosyphilis is caused by the spirochete *Treponema pallidum,* which invades the CNS within 3 to 18 months of the primary inoculation. If the CSF is negative after 2 years, the potential for CNS involvement resulting from the original infection is 1 in 20 (Adams and Victor, 1981).

Pathophysiology. The initial stage of neurosyphilis is characterized by asymptomatic meningitis discovered only by CSF examination. If untreated, a diffuse thickening of

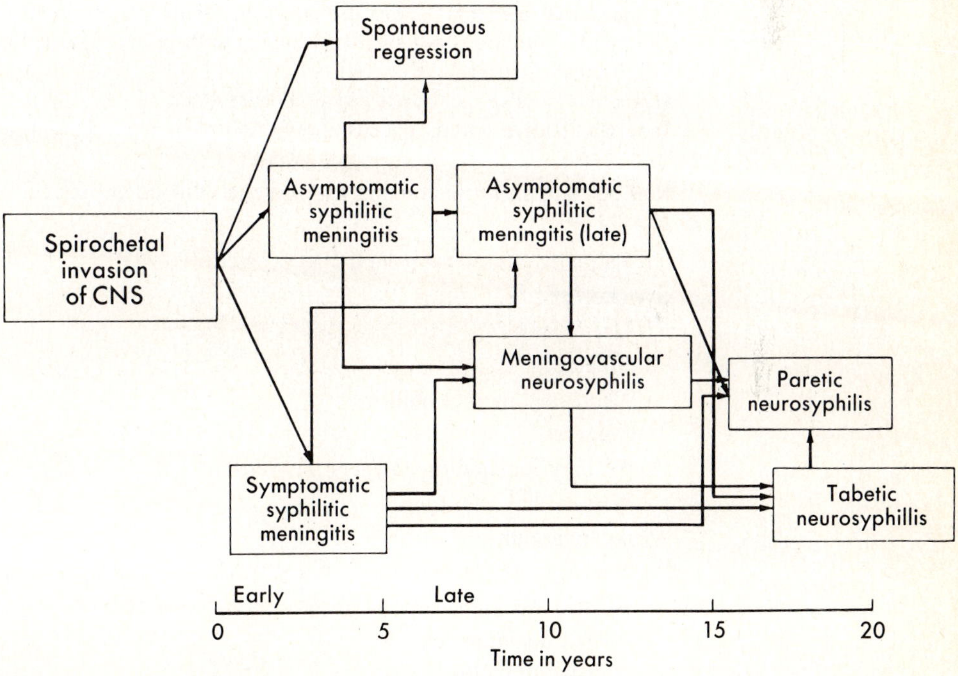

Fig. 7-7 Diagram of the evolution of neurosyphilis. (From Principles of neurology by R. Adams and M. Victor. Copyright © 1981. Used with permission of McGraw-Hill Book Company.)

the meninges occurs causing vascular occlusion, primarily of the frontal and temporal lobes or dorsal nerve roots and posterior columns. Following brain infiltration of the spirochete, perivascular infiltration and glial scarring occur, resulting in atrophy and degeneration of the brain neurons with dilitation of the ventricular system (Merritt, 1979).

Following spirochete infiltration of the dorsal nerve roots, the meninges surrounding the roots thicken and glial scars form, causing the degeneration and atrophy. The spirochete also invades the posterior columns of the spinal cord, usually in the lumbar area, causing degeneration and atrophy of the sensory tracts. Invasion of the spinal cord usually occurs 15 to 20 years after the primary infection (Adams and Victor, 1981). Fig. 7-7 diagrams the evolution of neurosyphilis.

Classification. Neurosyphilis is classified as:

Asymptomatic syphilis meningitis: no or few clinical signs except for Argyll Robertson pupils (small, irregular, unequal pupils that do not dilate to mydriatic agents and that have decreased response to light stimuli. They constrict on accommodation.)

Symptomatic syphilitic meningitis: headache, nuchal rigidity, cranial nerve palsies, decreased mentation, seizures.

Meningovascular: sudden onset of hemiplegia, dysphasia, sensory deficits, visual disturbances, decreased mentation. NOTE: Neurosyphilis should be considered when a young person presents with signs and symptoms similar to those of a transient ischemic attack or cardiovascular accident.

Paretic: progressive mental and physical deterioration.

Tabetic: extensive sensory deficits, Argyll Robertson pupils (Adams and Victor, 1981).

Nursing assessments. Nursing assessments will be delineated according to classification.

Subjective assessment data

- Symptomatic meningitis
  - Headache
  - Stiff neck
  - Decreased mental abilities
  - Seizures
  - Primary inoculation: 2 years previously
  - Nausea and vomiting
- Meningovascular
  - Primary inoculation: 6 to 7 years previously (range: 6 months to 12 years)
  - Muscle weakness and numbness on one side of body (sudden onset)
  - Visual disturbances
  - Speech difficulties
  - Decreased mental abilities
- Paretic
  - Primary inoculation: 15 to 20 years previously

Forgetfulness and memory loss
Speech and writing difficulties
Arm, leg, and facial twitching
Visual disturbances
Convulsions
Behavior changes: irritable, unreasonable plans, inappropriate responses to situations, mood swings, hallucinations

Tabetic
Primary inoculation: 15 to 20 years previously
Leg pains: rapid onset of severe, lancing leg pain (sometimes referred to as "rheumatic pain")
Leg pain increases in cold, damp weather
Severe sudden gastric upsets with stomach pain, nausea, and vomiting lasting several hours to several days
Loss of balance, especially in the dark
Difficulty in walking
Feelings of "walking on cotton balls"
Numbness and tingling feelings around the mouth
Visual disturbances
Urinary dribbling
Loss of libido
Swollen joints especially ankles, knees, hips
Open sores on heels and toes

Objective assessment data

Asymptomatic
Argyll Robertson pupils

Symptomatic
Nuchal rigidity
Decreased extraocular movements
Ptosis
Depressed level of consciousness
No fever
Papilledema and vomiting if ICP increased

Meningovascular
Hemiplegia
Dysphasia or aphasia
Decreased sensation or paresthesias
Decreased extraocular movements
Depressed level of consciousness

Paretic
Slovenly appearance with expressionless facies
Decreased mentation abilities and lack of insight

- Memory loss particularly for recent events
- Disorientation
- Slurred speech, dysphasia
- Intention tremors of eyes, tongue, and fingers
- Increased deep tendon reflexes
- Hypotonic muscles
- Mood/behavior swings
- Unsystemetized delusions, usually paranoid or grandiose in nature
- Bilateral Argyll Robertson pupils
- Decreased visual activity
- Babinski sign present

Tabetic

- Argyll Robertson pupils with ptosis bilaterally
- Vomiting with epigastric pain. Note that there is no abdominal rigidity nor deep tenderness, which differentiates tabetic syphilis from a perforated peptic ulcer
- Ataxia with a positive Romberg sign
- Wide-based station and ''stomping'' gait
- Hypotonic leg muscles
- Smell of urine on clothing and body
- Distended, hypotonic bladder and bowel
- Charcot's joints: swollen, painless, destructive changes in ankle, knee, and hip joint, which restrict movement
- Trophic ulceration on heels and dorsum of toes as a result of decreased sensation in feet, which allows the rubbing of shoes to cause this painless ulceration
- Absent tendon reflexes
- Decreased thermal, tactile, and pain sensation

Diagnostic tests

- Blood: Positive fluorescent treponemal antibody test (FTA). Note that the FTA is more sensitive to seronegative lues than the Veneral Disease Research Laboratory test (VDRL) (Scheinberg, 1977)
- CSF
  - Increased lymphocytes
  - Increased protein: 40-200 mg/100 ml. The globulin component is significantly increased
  - Normal glucose
  - Positive VDRL or fluorescent antibody (FTA)
  - Colloidal gold: First zone curve
- EEG: Slow activity bilaterally over frontal and parietal lobes
- CAT scan: dilation of lateral ventricles

Nursing care plan: **NEUROSYPHILIS**

NURSING DIAGNOSIS	EXPECTED OUTCOMES	NURSING INTERVENTIONS
Inadequate body response to lyse infective organism	FTA: negative VDRL: negative	Administer prescribed penicillin, 10-15 million units over 10- to 20-day period. Monitor FTA or VDRL tests until negative.
Pain, particularly:		
Leg pain in the tabetic patient due to dorsal root involvement	No pain or minimized pain	Administer prescribed carbamazepine (Tegretol) for its antineuralgic effect.
Gastric pain due to hypotonic stomach and intestine	Normal gastric function and fluid/electrolyte balance	Administer prescribed intravenous fluids with electrolyte supplements. Provide foods and fluids according to patient preferences and tolerance. Administer prescribed CNS depressants (phenobarbital or phenothiazines) to control gasatric pain and decrease gastric motility.
Impaired mobility due to deficient position and vibratory senses	Self-locomotion without falls	Maintain light in room (ataxia is more severe in darkness). Provide walking aids (walker or chair placement).
Potential for joint contractures	Increased range of motion Decreased joint destruction	Apply protective joint braces Assist with whirlpool baths and exercises.
Impaired urinary and fecal excretion due to hypotonic bladder/bowel	Normal urinary and fecal elimination	Prepare patients with enlarged prostate glands for surgical transurethral resections. Apply prescribed external catheter and provide perineal hygiene. Establish voiding schedule. Place commode at bedside for fecal evacuation.
Impaired skin integrity due to sensory loss, particularly in extremities	Skin intact	Apply prescribed antibiotic oitments and dressings to trophic foot ulcers. Discourage use of shoes until ulcers are healed, a slow process. Provide warm foot soaks to improve circulation. Establish active/passive range-of-motion exercise program to increase circulation to extremities. Provide diet with adequate protein and vitamins to enhance skin healing.
Self-care deficit ranging from mild to total due to frontal lobe or posterior column and dorsal root degeneration	Can provide self-care within capabilities	Demonstrate and discuss: Hygiene needs, especially foot care. Diet including need for protein and vitamin foods/fluids. Medications: Design a schedule and provide a list of side effects for prescribed medications. Application of joint braces. Safe use of walking aids.
Impaired thought processes due to atrophy of frontal lobe	Presents no danger to self/others	Discuss alternatives available with patient and family Home care Institutionalization

PERIPHERAL/ CRANIAL NERVE INFECTIONS/ INFLAMMATIONS

Herpes zoster

Herpes zoster is a viral infection of the posterior root ganglion primarily of spinal nerves. It causes a painful unilateral vesicular skin eruption along the sensory distribution of the affected nerves. Herpes affects adults, particularly those with debilitating diseases, who have had chicken pox previously. Duration of the infection is 1 to 2 weeks. However 40% to 50% of infected persons suffer postherpetic neuralgia for 1 to 2 years.

Etiology. Herpes virus, the causative agent, is identical to the varicella (chickenpox) virus. The most widely accepted theory is that herpes results from a reactivation of the varicella virus, which has remained dormant in the sensory ganglion following primary chickenpox (Adams and Victor, 1981).

Pathophysiology. The herpes virus causes an inflammatory, hemorrhagic necrosis of the posterior dorsal root ganglion (sensory). The hemorrhagic area is surrounded by lymphocytes that infiltrate the dorsal root ganglia neurons causing degeneration of the gray matter. The inflammatory response spreads along the affected spinal nerves, which results in the characteristic vesicular skin changes within a dermatome area (Fig. 7-8). There is fluid under the epithelium with segmented neutrophils infiltrating the dermis. Occasionally, the cranial neves are affected, most commonly, the ophthalmic branch of the trigeminal nerve (V). The most common areas of involvement in descending order are:

Thoracic
Cervical
Sacral
Gasserian ganglion (Merritt, 1979)

Nursing assessment

Subjective assessment data

Severe pain (burning, stabbing) in a specific dermatome area for 1 to 2 days before observable skin changes
Blisters on skin in the affected area
Muscle weakness in the area of and distal to blisters
Headache
Drowsiness
Difficulty in concentration

Fig. 7-8 Dermatomes indicate areas of body innervated by specific spinal cord segments. Note that spinal cord segments do not correspond with vertebral bodies and that spinous processes correspond with neither. **A,** Segmental innervation of trunk. **B,** Segmental innervation of upper and lower extremities. (From Budassi, S.A., and Barber, J.M.: Emergency nursing: principles and practice, St. Louis, 1981, The C.V. Mosby Co.)

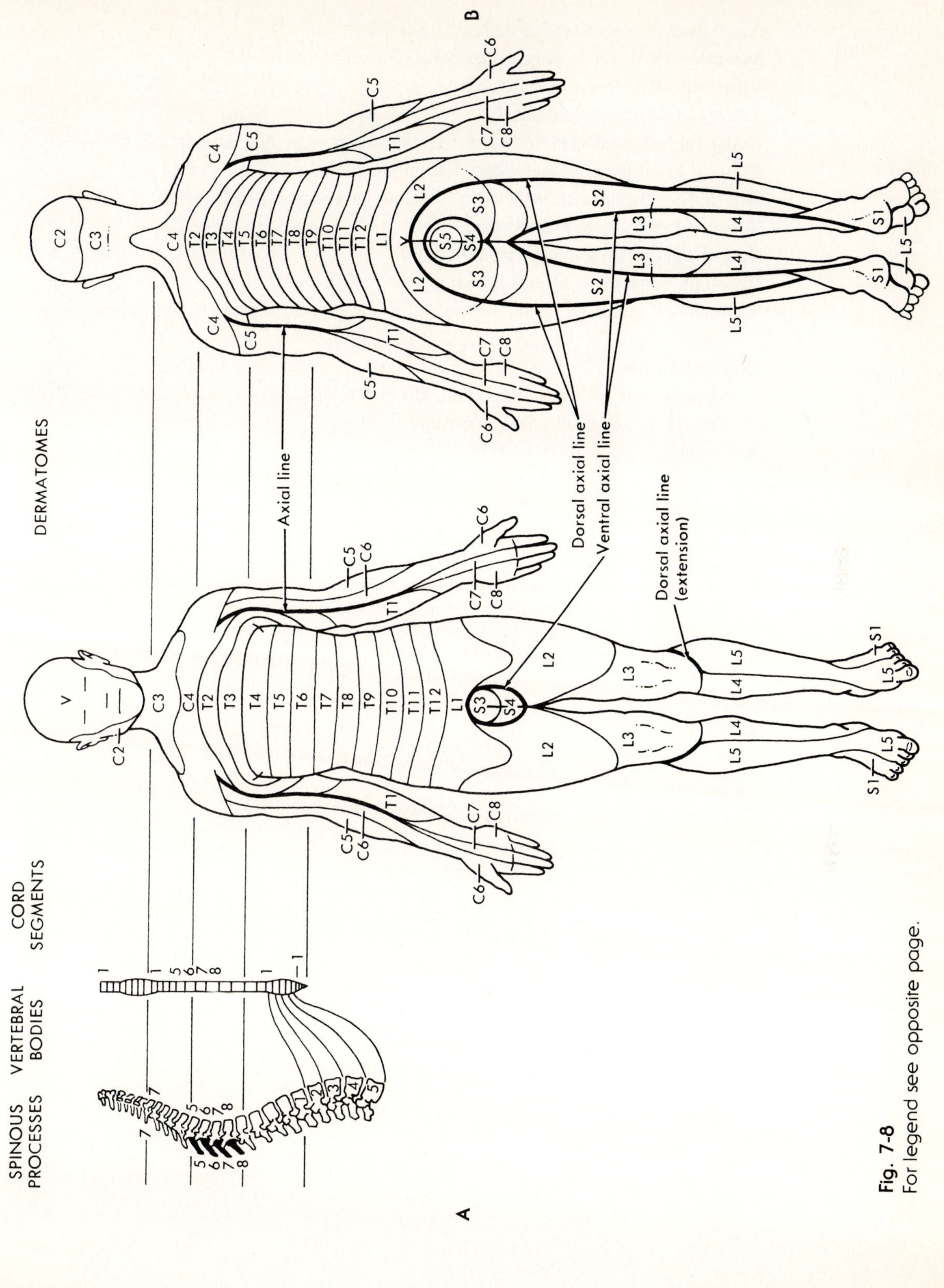

Fig. 7-8
For legend see opposite page.

Facial muscle weakness (facial nerve, VI)
Eye pain and itchiness (trigeminal nerve, V)
Visual disturbances (trigeminal nerve, V)

Objective assessment data

Unilateral reddened skin with vesicular blisters in a specific dermatome.
After 10 to 14 days vesicles scab, leaving an irregular red pigmented scar
Skin hyperesthesia with tenderness to palpation along affected nerve
Regional lymph node enlargement
Nuchal rigidity if meninges are infiltrated
Hypotonic muscles in affected area
Ophthalmic: decreased visual activity, decreased motor eye movement, corneal scarring

Diagnostic tests

Identification of herpes virus with electron microscope
Culture of virus from vesicular fluid

Nursing care plan: **HERPES ZOSTER**

NURSING DIAGNOSIS	EXPECTED OUTCOMES	NURSING INTERVENTIONS
Alteration in comfort: pain	Freedom from or minimized pain	Provide quiet environment. Administer prescribed mild analgesics. NOTE: Acyclover, an analgesic, is in trial presently (Wiederholt, 1982). Apply prescribed topical antiinflammatory and antipruritic agents (calamine, collodian). NOTE: Corticosteroids are not prescribed for immunosuppressed patients (Roelofs, 1982). For severe cases antiviral therapy using vidarabine is prescribed (see Herpes encephalitis).
Potential for infection of vesicles and eyes	No secondary infections and scarring	Maintain skin and eye hygiene. Apply eye patch if patient rubs eyes or has corneal abrasions. Discourage rubbing vesicles on skin. Remove friction-causing clothing. Do not break vesicles. NOTE: Patient and care provider should use gloves when applying ointments to decrease potential for contagion.
Alteration in comfort due to postherpetic neuralgia (40%-50%) of patients)	Minimization or elimination of pain	For ophthalmic herpes apply idoxuridine (IDU) (1%) solution to affected eye every hour. Observe for signs of refractory postherpetic neuralgia: 1. Continuation of sharp, shooting pains. 2. Skin in affected dermatome is sensitive to touch for 1 to 2 years. Administer prescribed carbamazepine (Tegretol) to control pain.

Guillain-Barré syndrome

Synonyms for Guillain-Barré syndrome are (1) GBS, (2) Acute polyradioneuropathy, (3) polyneuritis, (4) Landry-Guillain-Barré-Strohl, and (5) postinfectious polyneuritis. This syndrome is characterized by a rapidly progressing symmetrical ascending flaccid paralysis usually following a viral infection. A history of recent upper respiratory or gastric flu, infectious mononucleosis, or hepatitis is common (Tikkannen, 1982). Recovery is usually complete; however it may take up to 18 months if the degree of involvement has been extensive. Motor recovery typically begins about 10 to 14 days following the onset of symptoms.

Etiology. While the specific etiology is unknown, there are two theories regarding the causation of Guillain-Barré. One theory is that the Guillain-Barré virus infiltrates the spinal and occasionally the cranial nerve roots. Another hypothesis is that the syndrome is a result of an autoimmune response of the body that is precipitated by toxic or infectious agents resulting in segmental demyelination of peripheral or cranial nerves (Tikkanen, 1982).

Pathophysiology. The virus and/or antibodies cause an initial inflammatory response with significant edema, resulting in (1) compression of the nerve roots, (2) segmental demyelination, and (3) wallerian degeneration (Fig. 7-9). Compression of the nerve roots dramatically reduces nerve conduction producing lower extremity paresthesias initially and later in a stocking/glove distribution. Nerve conduction is impeded by the segmental demyelination, resulting in a rapidly ascending flaccid paralysis with sensory loss. When the nerves innervating the intercostal muscles and diaphragm are compressed and demyelinated, potentially fatal respiratory dysfunction occurs. Cranial nerves most commonly affected are VII, IX, X, XI, and XII (Tikkanen, 1982).

Nursing assessments. Because of the rapidly progressing paralysis and the potential for respiratory dysfunction, hourly assessments at a minimum are essential. Care must be taken to minimize the patient's anxiety level by explaining the rationale for repeated assessments and assuring the patient of the proximity of life-support measures (Hickey, 1981).

Subjective assessment data

History of recent respiratory or gastric flu, mononucleosis, hepatitis
Abrupt onset of transient numbness or pins-and-needles feeling in feet, legs, and hands
Leg weakness for 24 to 72 hours progressing to paralysis of legs, trunk, and arms.
Muscle tenderness
Difficulty in walking
Difficulty in swallowing, chewing, breathing
Sagging facial muscles
Drooping eyelids
Constipation
Decreased urinary output
Excessive sweating

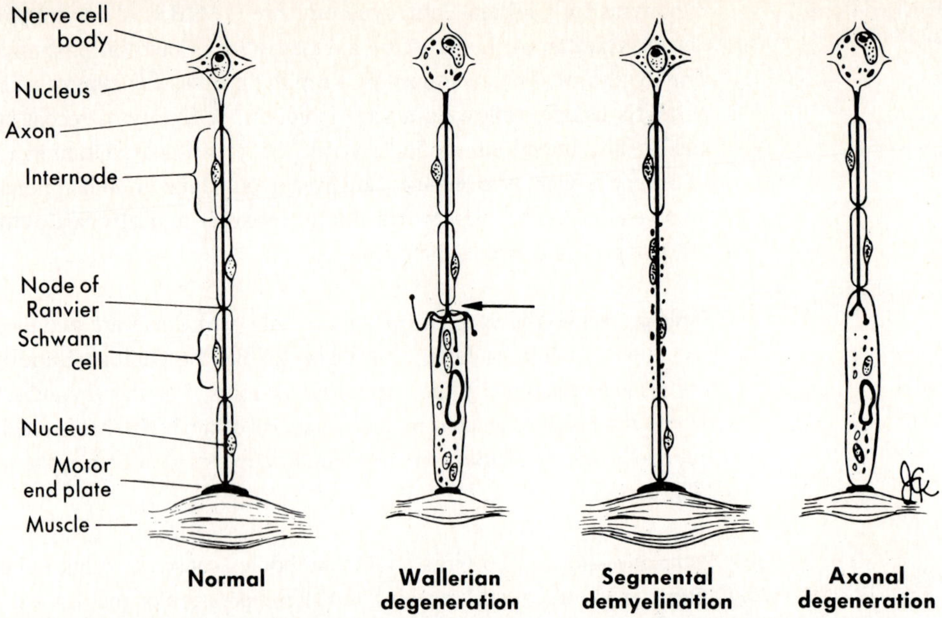

Fig 7-9 Diagram of the basic pathological processes affecting peripheral nerves. In wallerian degeneration, there is degeneration of the axis cylinder and myelin distal to the site of axonal interruption (arrow) and central chromatolysis. In segmental demyelination the axon is spared. In axonal degeneration there is a distal degeneration of myelin and axis cylinder as a result of neuronal disease. Both wallerian and axonal degeneration cause muscle atrophy. (From Principles of neurology by R. Adams and M. Victor. Copyright © 1981. Used with permission of McGraw-Hill Book Company.)

Objective assessment data

Symmetrical ascending flaccid paresis progressing to quadraplegia within 72 hours
Muscles sensitive to pressure
Dyspnea with decreased base lung sounds
Depressed respiratory rate and depth
Absent tendon reflexes
Diminished or absent gag, plantar, and abdominal reflexes
Dysphagia
Decreased facial muscle tone with ptosis
Decreased extraocular movements
Oriented to time, person, and place
Low-grade fever with rapid pulse rate
Widely fluctuating blood pressure with postural hypotension
Oliguria with distended bladder

Papilledema if respirations decreased, with carbon dioxide retention
Diagnostic tests:
- CSF:
  - Slightly increased opening pressure
  - Increased protein: 75-200 mg/dl caused by serum protein leakage into subarachnoid space and the CSF
  - WBC: less than 10/ml
- Electromyography: diffuse slowing and decreased velocity in nerve conduction
- Vital capacity: reduced if respiratory impairment exists. If under 800 cc, ventilatory assistance is required.
- Arterial blood gases indicating need for ventilatory assistance:
  - O_2 decreased.
  - CO_2 increased.
  - pH decreased.

Nursing care plan: **GUILLAIN-BARRÉ SYNDROME**

NURSING DIAGNOSIS	EXPECTED OUTCOMES	NURSING INTERVENTIONS
Potential for ineffective breathing pattern due to paralysis of intercostal muscles/ diaphragm	Adequate ventilation with vital capacity 800-1000 cc	Observe for dyspnea. Ascultate lung sounds. Assess vital capacity. Under 800 cc indicates need for mechanical assistance. Monitor respiratory rate, rhythm and depth, muscles used and excursion. Position in semi-Fowler's with head and thorax elevated to 30 degrees. Keep patient's arms off rib cage as pressure inhibits lung excursion.
Potential for impaired gas exchange due to diminished contractability of bronchi	Maintenance of P_{O_2} at 80-100 mm Hg	Monitor arterial blood gases. Administer physician- or protocol-prescribed oxygen usually at 6 L/min per cannula. Have tracheostomy tray and mechanical ventilatory assistance equipment readily available. Aseptically suction tracheostomy tube according to agency policy. Note that secretions are copious during the first 12 hours, necessitating very frequent suctioning. Suctioning is preceded by one minute of ambu bag or Lardol pocket mask oxygen administration at 25 squeezes/minute (Shea, 1981). Initiate intermittent maximal inspiration technique: maximal inspiration, hold for 20 seconds, exhale slowly.

Continued.

Nursing care plan: **GUILLAIN BARRÉ SYNDROME—cont'd**

NURSING DIAGNOSIS	EXPECTED OUTCOMES	NURSING INTERVENTIONS
Decreased cardiac output secondary to autonomic involvement and immobility	Normal blood pressure and pulse rate	Monitor and record vital signs. Change position and perform passive range-of-motion exercises every 2 hours. Establish and maintain a turning schedule. Apply prescribed antiembolism stockings. Observe for sympathetic nervous system stimulation: facial flushing, diaphoresis, fluctuating blood pressure, and pulse rate.
Impaired physical mobility due to demyelination of nerves	Return of motor/sensory function Maintenance of muscle tone and joint mobility	Administer prescribed antiinflammatory agents: ACTH intravenously if endotracheal tube is in place Oral corticosteroids (prednisone) Provide roto or kinetic bed, water/air mattress. Assess motor/sensory function every 2 hours and record on flow sheet (Fig. 7-10). Initiate passive and active range-of-motion exercises every 4 hours. Assess and record muscle mass and tone. Position in alignment to prevent contractures.
Potential nutritional and fluid deficiencies	Maintenance of positive nitrogen balance, adequate hydration	Check gag reflex before giving food/fluids Provide preferred soft, semi-solid foods. Note that tepid foods and fluids are more easily aspirated than hot or cold ones (Samonds, 1980). Have oral suctioning equipment readily available. If patient is dysphagic: 1. Position patient on side to enhance saliva drainage. 2. Initiate gastric gavage every 6 hours or by continuous drip. NOTE: Because of the paralytic ileus and gastric distention common during the first week, gastric tube placement is recommended (Takkanen, 1982). Monitor for electrolyte imbalances.
Potential for impaired skin integrity	Skin intact	Assess for skin turgor, hydration, and pressure areas. Establish a position-changing schedule. Ensure smooth, dry bed linen. NOTE: Because of sensory loss, skin integrity is often compromised.
Potential for altered elimination	No constipation/impaction Normal urinary output (2-3 L/day)	Maintain accurate output record including feces and emesis and estimate insensible losses through diaphoresis, rapid respirations. Auscultate for bowel sounds. Administer prescribed stool softeners or laxatives. Provide preferred fluids and roughage foods such as peeled apples, prunes, seedless grapes, oranges, plums.

Continued.

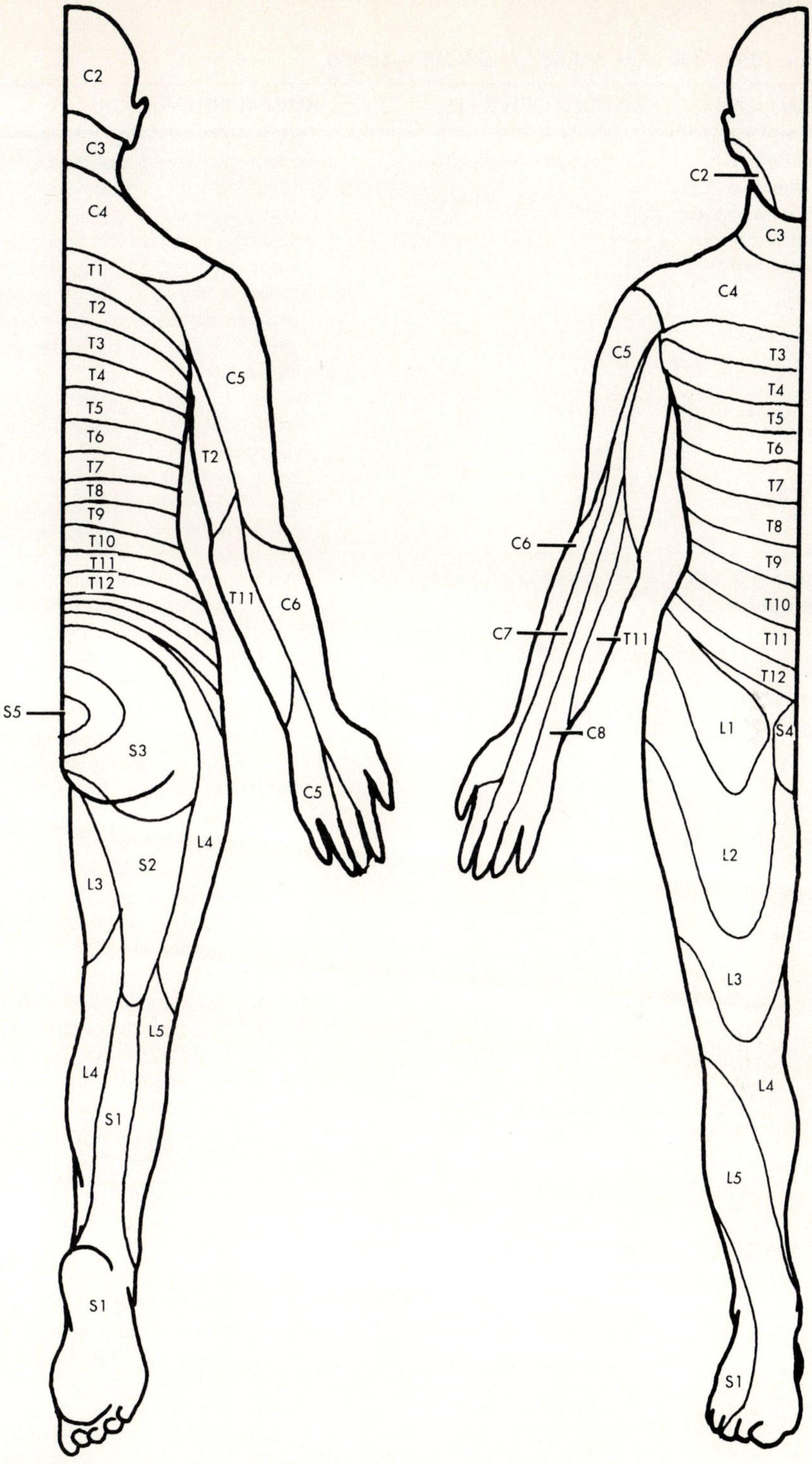

Fig. 7-10 GBS flow sheet (Courtesy Margarethe Cammermeyer, Clinical Nurse Specialist, Veterans Administration Medical Center, San Francisco).

Nursing care plan: GUILLAIN BARRÉ SYNDROME—cont'd

NURSING DIAGNOSIS	EXPECTED OUTCOMES	NURSING INTERVENTIONS
Anxiety (moderate to severe) due to abrupt onset of paralysis and dependence on machines and others	Decreased anxiety level	Explain characteristics of the disease process: gradual return of sensation and motor function in 95% of cases within 2 years. Encourage verbalization and expression of anxiety and depression. Establish a communication method, such as a bell or magic slate, for patients who are aphonic because of paresis of phonation muscles or presence of tracheostomy tube. Ask yes/no type questions. Locate patient close to nursing station. Allow patient to choose the order of care measures. Encourage family and significant others to visit. Explain treatment measures and the disease process to the family to reduce their apprehension.
Knowledge deficit: self or home care measures	Comprehension of typical rehabilitation process	Initiate patient/family teaching program: 1. Explain the disease process: return of function in descending pattern. 2. Demonstrate range-of-motion and muscle-strengthening methods. 3. Discuss community assistance available to assist with home care: social services, psychological consultants, vocational rehabilitation. 4. Discuss the extended rehabilitation process. Up to 2 years is required for nerve regeneration. 5. Demonstrate maximal inspiration technique used to prevent respiratory tract infections/dysfunctions. 6. Demonstrate use of mobility assistance tools: a. Wheelchair, transferring to and using. b. Crutch walking. c. Walker use. 7. Devise medication schedule for prescribed corticosteroids and discuss precautions: a. Low-salt diet to prevent sodium retention. b. Taking corticosteroids with milk/meals to prevent gastric irritation. c. Need for a tapered decreasing dosage before discontinuing use of corticosteroids.

Bell's palsy

Bell's palsy is an isolated paralysis of the facial nerve (VII) without evidence of other neurological abnormalities. The onset of facial paralysis is abrupt and frequently follows exposure to cold. It is most common in the 30- to 60-year age group.

Etiology. Although the specific cause is unknown, the present hypothesis is that Bell's palsy is caused by a virus. Bell's palsy occurs more frequently in the winter, thus supporting the viral theory (Gilroy, 1975).

Pathophysiology. Following exposure to the infective agent, the facial nerve becomes inflammed and edematous at the point of the bony facial canal where the nerve exits the brain. This results in pressure on the nerve itself, causing a rapidly progressive paresis, and paralysis, resulting in degeneration of the facial nerve fiber (Hickey, 1981).

Nursing assessments

Subjective assessment data

Unilateral facial discomfort/pain 24 to 48 hours preceding paralysis
Unilateral sagging of facial muscles
Inability to close eye completely on affected side
Corners of mouth on affected side turn down. There is an inability to smile/frown on one side of face (Fig. 7-11)
Tearing of one eye
Loss of taste
Inability to chew food on affected side
Drooling of liquids from mouth on affected side

Objective assessment data

Unilateral facial paralysis (unable to smile/frown on affected side)
Dysarthria
Dysphagia with food collected in cheek
Halitosis
Lack of normal facial folds
Decreased salivation
Widened palpebral fissure, unilateral

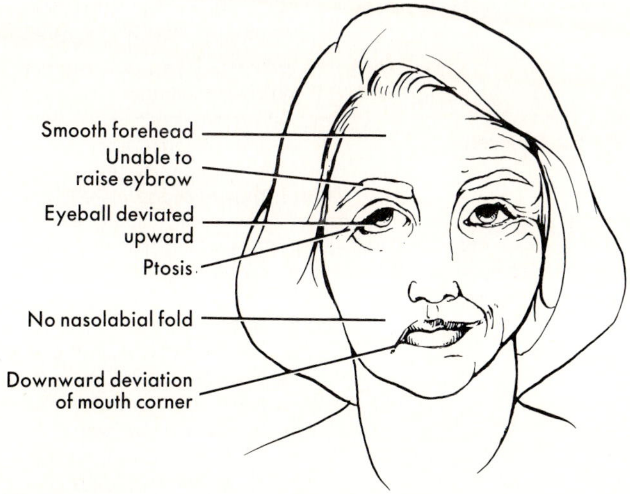

Fig. 7-11 Bell's palsy.

Unilateral tearing with collection of tears in lateral conjunctival sac. NOTE: Tear secretions do not move across eye unless lids are closed
Upward, inward deviation of eyeball
Corneal reflex absent
Nerve stimulation test is positive in spite of facial paralysis

Nursing care plan: **BELL'S PALSY**

NURSING DIAGNOSIS	EXPECTED OUTCOMES	NURSING INTERVENTIONS
Potential fluid/electrolyte imbalance	Normal hydration and electrolyte balance	Provide room temperature fluids. Use catheter to direct fluids toward unaffected side.
Potential for nutritional deficit due to inability to masticate	No weight loss or minimal weight loss	Provide preferred, soft, easily masticated foods to prevent injury to oral mucosa. Monitor skin turgor and weight for hydration and nutritional status. Provide oral hygiene every 2 hours.
Alteration in elimination pattern	Normal bowel evacuation	Maintain accurate intake/output records. Provide fluids stimulating bowel elimination.
Impaired facial mobility	Preservation of facial muscle tone	Initiate facial muscle massage upward from chin. Apply facial sling. Teach active facial muscle exercises in front of mirrow (wrinkle brow, whistling, blowing out cheeks).
Visual sensory deficit due to lack of movement of lacrimal secretions	Return of visual acuity	Provide eye hygiene every 2 hours with artificial tears. Apply goggles/glasses to prevent corneal injury. Butterfly tape eyelid closed.
Inadequate body response to infective agent	Functioning nerve (required time 2 to 10 weeks)	Administer prescribed steroids: ACTH, 40-60 mg IM daily for 2 weeks. Prednisone, 96-128 mg every other day for 10 days. NOTE: Explain need for limitation of salt intake when taking corticosteroids.
Self-esteem disturbance due to altered appearance	Positive self-concept	Encourage verbalization/expression of anxieties due to body-image changes. Explain usual course of Bell's palsy.
Self-care knowledge deficit	Comprehension of home care, possible sequelae, and preventive measures	Institute teaching plan regarding: 1. Scheduling and taking prescribed medications. 2. Application of facial sling. 3. Facial massage methods. 4. Facial-muscle-strengthening exercises. 5. Nutrition: adequate protein and vitamin B food intake; need for easily masticated foods. 6. Potential sequelae: a. Facial tics, which can be controlled by Carbamazepine (Tegretol). b. Crocodile tears (tearing when eating), which subsides usually within 3 months. 7. Eye hygiene and protective methods.

Leprosy (Hansen's disease)

Leprosy is the most common chronic peripheral nerve disease in India, China, Central Africa, South America and the states adjoining the Gulf of Mexico in the United States (Adams and Victor, 1981). The causative agent, the acid-fast bacillus *Mycobacterium leprae* has a predilection for skin and peripheral nerves. Inoculation requires long and intimate contact with a diseased persons's lesions. The incubation period is 3 to 4 years in children and longer for adults. In addition to the skin lesions, the disfigurement associated with leprosy results from the progressive resorption of bones, beginning with the terminal phalanges, and the concomitant shrinkage of the skin.

Etiology. Leprosy is caused by the acid-fast bacillus *Mycobacterium leprae,* which can be isolated from scrapings of the skin lesion.

Pathophysiology. The organism initially invades the skin causing a nonpigmented macule, the center of which is anesthetic. The adjacent superficial nerves are invaded resulting in (1) nodules on the affected nerve; (2) diffuse swelling of the nerve trunks; (3) degeneration of the myelin sheath and the axon; (4) sensory loss in the area supplied by the affected nerve. The disease has a predilection for the coolest body surfaces: ears, dorsum of hand, plantar surface of feet, forearms, and the lateral aspects of the thigh. If treatment of skin lesions is not initiated, the organism infiltrates the adjacent lymph nodes resulting in a symmetrical loss of pain and temperature sense (Adams and Victor, 1981).

Classification. Leprosy is classified as:

Cutaneous: fatal within 10 to 20 years.

Neural: slowly progressive.

Nursing assessment

Subjective assessment data

History of nerve pain preceding sensory or motor loss
Skin sores that do not hurt on hands and/or feet
Decreasing hand and finger strength

Objective assessment data

Nonpigmented macule with anesthetic center on ear, hands, feet, forearm, lateral thigh
Babinski not present
Normal tendon and abdominal reflexes (until late in disease, when they are diminished)
Anhidrosis (lack of sweating) in anesthetic area
Loss of temperature and pain sensation in area of and distal to cutaneous lesion
Prolonged capillary refill time distal to lesion
Trophic ulcerations on knuckles and plantar foot surfaces
Atrophy of thenar (hand and feet) muscles extending to forearm and leg
Hand and feet muscle fibrillations
Claw hand appearance

Diagnostic tests:

Positive Wasserman or Kahn

Mycobacterium leprae bacillus present in lesion scrapings and biopsied nerve tissue

Nursing care plan: LEPROSY (HANSEN'S DISEASE)

NURSING DIAGNOSIS	EXPECTED OUTCOMES	NURSING INTERVENTIONS
Potential for neural infection due to inadequate bacteriocidal treatment	Bacillus not present in skin/nerve tissue	Cleanse skin lesions with hydrogen peroxide solution. Gloves should be worn during cleansing. Administer prescribed sulfone medications: Dapsone 100 mg 6 times/week for life. NOTE: Consult Centers for Disease Control (CDC) for current dosage. Rifampin, 60 mg/day for rapid bacteriocidal activity NOTE: Clofazimine, 100 mg 3 times per week, is used in Japan. Has not as yet been approved by the Food and Drug Administration (Roelofs, 1982). Observe for allergic responses to sulfone: fever, malaise, hepatomegaly, enlarged lymph nodes, ocular palsies, arthritic and neuritic pain. NOTE: Current treatment: 1. Thalidomide, 100-300 mg/day for 2 days 2. Prednisone, 60 mg/day 3. Bed rest 4. Splinting of affected joints
Potential for injury due to impaired sensation or lack of sensation	No injury Skin integrity	Make sure that clean socks and well-fitting shoes are worn when patient is out of bed. Explain need for carefully watching activities involving heat (stoves and bathing, smoking) and potential punctures (knives and pop cans).
Potential for nutritional deficiency due to lack of hand dexterity	Maintenance of muscle mass and tone and positive nitrogen balance	Provide/feed nutritional foods and fluids.
Body-image disturbance due to disfigurement	Toleration of changed appearance	Encourage verbalization of feelings. Cooperatively establish realistic goals. Promote self-care to the extent possible. Use sympathetic approach.
Self-esteem disturbance	Positive self-concept	Focus on abilities not disabilities. Encourage socialization and maintenance of relationships. Provide diversion and recreational activities within the individual's capabilities. Observe and record signs of psychological and physiological depression. Refer to psychologist or spiritual advisor when patient needs exceed nursing competencies.

Nursing care plan: LEPROSY (HANSEN'S DISEASE)—cont'd

NURSING DIAGNOSIS	EXPECTED OUTCOMES	NURSING INTERVENTIONS
Knowledge deficit regarding the disease, treatment, and degree of contagiousness	Comprehension of the disease process and treatment measures	Explain pathophysiology in terms patient understands. Explain the treatment measures and need for long-term medication therapy. Demonstrate skin lesion care. Explain and demonstrate measures to prevent cross contamination: (1) wearing gloves when cleansing skin lesions; (2) wash clothing separately.

Suggested readings

Adams, R., and Victor, M.: Principles of neurology, New York, 1981, McGraw-Hill Book Co.

Budassi, S., and Barber, J.: Emergency nursing: principle and practice, St. Louis, 1981, The C.V. Mosby Co.

Clark, K., and others: Reye's syndrome nursing protocol, J. Natl. Reye's Syndrome Found. **1**(2): 82, 1980.

Conomy, J.: Metabolic disease. In Wiederholt, W., editor: Therapy for neurologic disorders, New York, 1982, John Wiley & Sons, Inc.

Fuerst, R.: Frobisher & Fuerst's Microbiology in health and disease, ed. 15, Philadelphia, 1983, W.B. Saunders Co.

Gilroy, J., and Meyer, J.: Medical neurology, ed. 2, New York, 1975, MacMillan Publishing Co., Inc.

Hickey, J.: The clinical practice of neurological and neurosurgical nursing, Philadelphia, 1981, J.B. Lippincott Co.

Howard, R., and Herbold, N.: Nutrition in clinical care, New York, 1979, McGraw-Hill Book Co.

Merritt, H.H.: A textbook of neurology, ed. 6, Philadelphia, 1979, Lea & Febiger.

NIH Consensus Development Conference Summary, Vol. 4, No. 1, Washington, D.C., 1981, U.S. Government Printing Office.

Richmond, D., and Stair, T.: Reye's syndrome, Ann. Emergency Med. **11**(7):379-383, July 1982.

Rodman, M.: What's new in drugs, RN **45**(3):152, March 1982.

Roelofs, R.: Infectious diseases. In Wiederholt, W., editor: Therapy for neurologic disorders, New York, 1982, John Wiley & Sons, Inc.

Samonds, R.: Guillain-Barré syndrome, Nursing 80 **10**(8):35-41, Aug. 1980.

Scheinberg, P.: Modern practical neurology, New York, 1977, Raven Press.

Shea, J.: Neurologic emergencies, EDNA Scientific Assembly, Toronto, 1981.

Swisher, C., and Williams, A.: Herpes excephalitis: a nursing challenge, J. Neurosurg. Nurs. **13**(1): 34-37, Feb. 1981.

Tikkanen, P.: Landry-Guillain-Barré-Strohl syndrome, J. Neurosurg. Nurs. **14**(2):74-80, April 1982.

Wing, S.: Brain abscess, J. Neurosurg. Nurs. **13**(3): 123-126, June 1981.

CHAPTER 8

Tumors of the brain and spinal cord

The brain and spinal cord may be affected by a variety of tumors. The patient's resulting neurological symptoms and deficits depend upon the tumor's histological type, location, and manner of growth. Early diagnosis of the tumor is imperative to prevent permanent neurological damage. The nurse's role in caring for these patients and their families is very challenging because the patients are faced with many potential physical, psychological, and sociological problems.

BRAIN TUMORS

Etiology

The exact cause of brain tumors is unknown. However, there is strong evidence that several agents may be responsible for specific types of tumors. These agents include heredity, congenital factors, viruses, toxin exposure, and immunological deficits. It has also been suggested that brain tumors may occur secondary to cerebral trauma or an inflammatory disease (Fagan-Dubin, 1979; Larson, 1980, Adams and Maurice, 1977; Merritt, 1979). Metastases to the brain from other areas of the body may also occur. The carcinomas metastasize more frequently to the brain than do the sarcomas. The primary sites of metastatic brain tumors in many patients are the lungs or breasts.

Approximately 2% of all yearly cancer deaths are caused by brain tumors. Figures from the American Cancer Society also show that approximately 12,000 new cases of primary brain and central nervous system tumors are diagnosed each year. Of this total, men are affected slightly more than women.

Pathophysiology

Tumors of the brain may grow in a diffuse manner infiltrating the surrounding tissue without having a definite mass or they may grow in a distinct encapsulated form that causes compression of surrounding tissue, thereby creating local edema. The cell growth may be very slow or rapid. Because of the tumor's effects upon the brain, the patient may experience cerebral edema, increased intracranial pressure (ICP), focal neurological deficits, seizure activity, altered pituitary function, or obstruction of cerebrospinal fluid (CSF) (Harvey, 1980).

Classification

Brain tumors may be classified as being primary (originating within the cranium) versus metastatic (originating outside the cranium), by the degree of malignancy (stages I, benign, to IV, the most malignant), as being intra-axial (originating within the brain substance and affecting the brain by infiltration) versus extra-axial (originating within the skull, meninges, cranial nerves, and pituitary region), or on a histological basis. For the purposes of this manual, a histological classification of primary brain tumors is used.

Gliomas. Gliomas arise from glial cells or connective tissue. These tumors originate in the brain and account for approximately 50% of all brain neoplasms in the adult (Dunphy, 1977). They occur less frequently in children.

Astrocytomas. Astrocytomas grades I and II account for approximately 20% of the gliomas. These tumors grow slowly. In the adult astrocytomas usually occur within the cerebrum as a diffuse form invading the surrounding tissue and they have varying degrees of malignancy. However, in children astrocytomas usually occur within the cerebellum or optic nerve as a benign cyst. The survival rate of children with the cystic form may be indefinite; however, the average survival rate in adults is 4 to 5 years after surgery.

Glioblastomas. Astrocytomas grades III and IV are known as glioblastoma multiforme. Glioblastomas are rapidly growing, infiltrating tumors that account for approximately 50% of the gliomas. In adults glioblastomas occur more frequently in men over the age of 35 years, with the most common sites of tumors being the cerebral hemispheres. In children these tumors rarely occur and the main site usually is the cerebellum. The survival time may range from a few months to a couple of years after surgery.

Ependymomas. Ependymomas grades I to IV account for approximately 10% of all gliomas. These tumors may affect any age group; however, they mainly occur in children, with a greater incidence in males. The main sites are the posterior fossa and the fourth ventricle. The survival rate after surgery may be a few months to years depending upon the degree of malignancy.

Oligodendrogliomas. Oligodendrogliomas grades I to IV account for approximately 5% of all gliomas. These tumors grow very slowly and are calcified. Oligodendrogliomas are rare tumors that usually occur within the frontal lobe of the adult. The average survival rate may be as high as 10 to 15 years depending upon the degree of malignancy.

Medulloblastomas. Medulloblastomas account for approximately 10% of all gliomas. These tumors are invasive and very malignant. Medulloblastomas occur mainly in children under the age of 10 and are more common in males. These neoplasms usually begin in the cerebellum and invade the fourth, third, and lateral ventricles, metastasizing to the subarachnoid space. After surgery, radiation, and chemotherapy the survival rate may be longer than 5 years.

Tumors of supporting structures. Tumors of supporting structures of the nervous system account for approximately 20% of all brain tumors.

Meningiomas. Meningiomas arise from the meninges and grow outside of the brain tissue. Rarely do they invade the cerebral tissue. Meningiomas are very slow growing benign tumors. They mainly occur in adults and are seen more frequently in women. The main sites are the sylvian region, parasagittal area, olfactory grooves, and the sphenoid wing. The survival rate is very good if the entire neoplasm is surgically removed; however, they may reoccur.

Neuromas. Neuromas arise from the nerve cells and grow slowly. These tumors mainly affect the middle-aged adult. Neuromas are encapsulated and usually benign. The most common neuroma affects the acoustic nerve. However, because of the proximity to other nerves the trigeminal and facial nerves may also be involved. If resected early enough, the nerves may be saved and the survival rate is very good.

Developmental tumors. Developmental tumors arise from embryonic cells. They account for approximately 5% of all brain neoplasms. These tumors occur mainly in childhood but may also be found in adults.

Craniopharyngiomas. Craniopharyngiomas are a common form of developmental tumor. They may be cystic and/or solid and tend to grow more rapidly in children. The site of this tumor is in the sella turcica spreading upwards to involve the optic chiasma, pituitary gland, and hypothalamus. Craniopharyngiomas are very difficult to completely excise by surgery.

Pituitary tumors. Pituitary tumors account for approximately 10% of all brain neoplasms. They may affect any age group but occur more frequently in adults. Pituitary tumors are mostly cystic, and as the neoplasms grow they may involve the optic chiasma, cavernous sinus, frontal lobe, hypothalamus, or temporal lobes. There are three tissue types of pituitary neoplasms. *Chromophobic adenoma* is the most common form. These tumors are mainly nonsecretory. Because of the compression of the anterior portion of the pituitary gland, there is a decrease in endocrine activity. *Eosinophilic adenomas* are secretory, causing an excessive amount of growth hormone in the serum. *Basophilic adenomas* are responsible for the excessive secretion of corticotropic, gonadotropic, and thyrotropic hormones. Individuals who have an excessive secretion of these hormones are known as pituitary giants; they usually die in young adulthood.

Metastatic tumors. Metastatic tumors account for approximately 10% of all brain neoplasms and affect all age groups. These tumors arise from malignant cells that originate elsewhere in the body, such as in the lungs, colon, breasts, pancreas, and kidneys. The survival rate is usually poor, possibly a year or two.

When comparing brain tumors in children and adults a major difference can be identified. In children and adolescents approximately two thirds of all tumors are infratentorial, occurring within the cerebellum, fourth ventricle, optic chiasma, and brainstem. In adults brain tumors are chiefly supratentorial.

Nursing assessment

For a more detailed explanation of the signs and symptoms of increased intracranial pressure refer to Chapter 9.

Subjective assessment data

General clinical manifestations (result of increased ICP, obstruction of CSF)
- Headache (note presence, location, severity, onset)
- Nausea/vomiting may or may not occur; vomiting may be projectile and is not related to food ingestion; often associated with headache)
- Dizziness and vertigo
- Mental changes (for example, lethargy, drowsiness, confusion, irritability, apathy, memory failure, inappropriate behavior)
- Seizures (focal or tonic-clonic)

Localized clinical manifestations (result of tumor compression in the specific portion of the brain in which the tumor is located)
- Visual changes (for example, hemianopsia, nystagmus, diplopia, blindness, signs of papilledema)
- Speech changes (for example, aphasia)
- Sensory changes (for example, loss of sensation, pain, sensory hallucinations)
- Motor changes (for example, ataxia, falls, head tilt, weakness, paralysis)
- Bowel/bladder changes (for example, incontinence, urinary retention, constipation)
- Hearing changes (for example, tinnitus, deafness)
- Sexual changes (for example, impotence, delay of secondary sexual characteristics, infertility)

Signs and symptoms of a space-occupying lesion whether it is a tumor, abscess, or hemorrhage are the same. Refer to Table 9-5.

Objective assessment data. Objective data are gathered by conducting a complete neurological examination, which includes an evaluation of the patient's:
- Mental status
- Cranial nerves
- Sensory system
- Cerebellar function
- Motor system
- Vital signs

For a detailed description of the neurological examination, see Chapter 1.

Nursing care plan: **BRAIN TUMORS**

NURSING DIAGNOSIS	EXPECTED OUTCOMES	NURSING INTERVENTIONS
Knowledge deficit: diagnostic procedures	Verbalizes understanding of procedures Verbalizes fears and concerns Cooperates with procedures	Give an explanation appropriate to the patient's and family's level of comprehension and emotional state. Give encouragement and the opportunity to ask questions. Provide psychological support. Make appropriate referrals (such as to a psychiatric nurse). Refer to Chapter 2 for a detailed description of each diagnostic procedure and specific nursing interventions. NOTE: Following a complete history and physical examination conducted by the physician, the following studies may be conducted to confirm the diagnosis: skull x-ray films, computerized axial tomogram (CAT scan), brain scan, electroencephalogram (EEG), echoencephalogram, cerebral angiogram, and chest x-ray films. A lumbar puncture may also be performed; however, it may be contraindicated if there is the possibility of brainstem herniation because of increased ICP. Pneumoencephalograms are infrequently done since the CAT scans have come into general use. Diagnostic procedures for specific tumors include audiometric studies, electronystagmography, caloric tests, and cisternography.
Knowledge deficits: surgery	Verbalizes understanding of surgery Verbalizes fears and concerns	Refer to Chapter 10 for a description of the preoperative and postoperative nursing care for the patient having a craniotomy.
Knowledge deficit: symptomatic medications, potential complications of symptomatic medications, proper administration of symptomatic medications	Cerebral edema is minimal Seizure activity is decreased or under control Early recognition and treatment of untoward effects of symptomatic pharmacotherapy Verbalizes understanding of dosage, administration, and possible untoward effects of drug therapy	Brain tumors create edema in the surrounding tissue. Medications may be administered to decrease the increased ICP. These medications may also be administered postoperatively, with chemotherapy, and during radiation therapy to decrease edema. The more common of these drugs include dexamethasone (Decadron), mannitol, and urea. Nursing interventions are as follows: Monitor intake, output, and electrolytes. Closely monitor blood pressure. Weigh patient daily. Urea is contraindicated in patients with severely impaired renal or hepatic function. Mannitol is contraindicated in patients with severely impaired renal function and with congestive heart failure. Dexamethasone is contraindicated in the presence of active or healed tuberculosis and ocular herpes simplex. Observe for signs of untoward effects of dexamethasone. These may include adrenocortical insufficiency, electrolyte imbalance, and Cushing's syndrome.

Nursing care plan: BRAIN TUMORS—cont'd

NURSING DIAGNOSIS	EXPECTED OUTCOMES	NURSING INTERVENTIONS
Knowledge deficit: symptomatic medications, potential complications of symptomatic medications, proper administration of symptomatic medications—cont'd		Observe for signs of infections since dexamethasone may mask usual symptoms. Refer to a pharmacology text for a detailed description of dosages and administration routes. NOTE: Seizures very often occur preoperatively because of the increased ICP as well as being frequent postoperatively. Many patients are sent home with antiepileptic drugs to prevent further seizures. See Chapter 4 for specific nursing interventions for the major antiepileptic drugs.
Knowledge deficits: potential complications of chemotherapy	Early recognition and treatment of side effects of chemotherapy Verbalizes understanding of dosage, administration, and possible untoward effects of drug therapy	NOTE: Chemotherapy is just one aspect of the approach to control the neoplastic process. Its aim is to attack at the cellular level during one or more phases of the reproductive cycle. The drug of choice and its dosage depend upon the particular tumor, location, and body tolerance. Various combinations of chemotherapeutic drugs may be more effective than their individual components. For a review of different chemotherapeutic drugs, methods of action, usual dosages, routes of administration, untoward effects, and special precautions refer to Table 8-1. Continually assess the patient's degree of acceptance of chemotherapy. Assist the patient in dealing with ambivalent feelings. Continually assess the patient's and family's knowledge and expectations of chemotherapy. NOTE: Chemotherapeutic drugs are very potent and irritating substances. Besides affecting the abnormal neoplastic cells they also cause damage to normal cells. Interventions should be planned according to the major side effects and toxic effects that the patient may encounter. These include nausea and vomiting, alopecia, stomatitis, leukopenia, and thrombocytopenia. Anorexia, nausea, and vomiting (very common: frequently occurs within the first hour after administration; some patients may become nauseated just upon the thought of having to receive chemotherapy): Patient should eat a light meal before chemotherapy. Administer antiemetic before chemotherapy. Seven-up or ice chips may help nausea. Good oral hygiene after vomiting. Small frequent meals may be easier for the patient to handle. Weight should be monitored closely while patient is receiving chemotherapy treatment. Alopecia (common) because the hair follicles proliferate so rapidly that they may be severely damaged):

Continued.

Nursing care plan: **BRAIN TUMORS—cont'd**

NURSING DIAGNOSIS	EXPECTED OUTCOMES	NURSING INTERVENTIONS
Knowledge deficits: potential complications of chemotherapy—cont'd		Use a scalp tourniquet and/or ice packs before, during, and for 15 minutes after administration of alkylating agents. The cuff needs to be 50 mm Hg above the systolic blood pressure. A more useful concept may be the Chemo Cap. Hair loss may still occur. Once the drug is stopped, hair regrows in about 8 weeks. Explore the meaning of the hair loss with the patient to examine body-image changes. Encourage the patient to wear wigs or attractive scarves. Stomatitis (early sign of toxicity): Good oral hygiene. Frequent saline or peroxide mouth rinses. Use of a topical anesthetic mouth rinse. Encourage the patient to eat foods that are bland and served at a mild temperature. Leukopenia (toxic effect that results from myelosuppression): Inform the patient that blood will be drawn frequently (every week and then as long as 2 months after the last dose). The patient may have to be put into protective isolation if the WBC count falls below 2000 mm. Instruct the patient about infection precautions. Instruct the patient about early signs of infections. Thrombocytopenia (toxic effect that results from myelosuppression; the normal clotting time is impaired): Instruct the patient about bleeding precautions and measures to stop bleeding. Signs of bleeding include petechiae formation, nosebleeds, and blood in stool. Meticulous oral hygiene. Use of soft toothbrushes to reduce irritation. The patient should not receive injections. If they are necessary, maintain strict sterile technique and apply sufficient pressure to avoid excessive bleeding. Be prepared to administer platelet transfusions if the platelet count goes below 100,000/mm. Chemotherapy will be withheld if the platelet count is too low. Instruct the patient on the need for frequent blood studies. The platelet count should be checked once a week.

Nursing care plan: BRAIN TUMORS—cont'd

NURSING DIAGNOSIS	EXPECTED OUTCOMES	NURSING INTERVENTIONS
Knowledge deficit: radiation therapy Ineffective family coping	Early recognition and treatment of side effects Verbalizes understanding of radiation therapy	NOTE: Radiation therapy is one aspect of the approach to control the neoplastic process. Its aim is to destroy tumor cells without injury to normal ones. Radiation therapy may or may not precede surgery. If surgery has been performed, the incision site should be healed without the presence of infection before radiation is administered. The dosage used is dependent upon the histological type, location, expected response to radiation, and the patient's tolerance level. Give an explanation appropriate to the patient's and family's level of comprehension and emotional state. Include details of what the patient will experience before therapy (such as preparation of the skin) and during therapy (description of machines and activities of the radiation therapy department). Give encouragement and the opportunity to ask questions. Do not give the patient and family a false hope that the radiation therapy will completely cure the disease. Explain that the patient may experience several side effects from the radiation therapy, which will disappear after treatment is completed. These include fatigue, anorexia, nausea, a skin reaction, alopecia, leukopenia, and thrombocytopenia. Plan nursing interventions appropriately. Fatigue: Plan with the patient a daily activity schedule that has appropriate rest periods. Coordinate with the radiation therapy department and the patient as to what time of day might be best for the therapy. Anorexia and nausea: Refer to nursing interventions mentioned under chemotherapy. Skin reaction (resulting from the loss of the epidermal or epithelial layers of the skin): Do not rub or apply irritating substances such alcohol, tape, or creams to the area. Protect the skin from sunlight. Wash the skin gently with a mild soap and water. Pat dry. Do not remove the dark markings that delineate the irradiation area. Alopecia: Refer to nursing interventions mentioned under chemotherapy. Leukopenia: Refer to nursing interventions mentioned under chemotherapy. Thrombocytopenia: Refer to nursing interventions mentioned under chemotherapy. Assess the patient closely for signs of increased ICP. Radiation may be the cause of increased cerebral edema.

Continued.

Nursing care plan: BRAIN TUMORS—cont'd

NURSING DIAGNOSIS	EXPECTED OUTCOMES	NURSING INTERVENTIONS
Potential occurrences of neurological disturbance	Patient is functioning as independently as possible Patient's dignity and self-esteem are maintained Patient and family have worked through the feelings of anger and guilt	NOTE: The common neurological disturbances resulting from tumors located in the cerebral hemispheres include seizures, aphasia, impaired memory and intellect, visual field defects (such as hemianopsia), hemiparesis, diplopia, dysphagia, paraplegia, and impaired sexual functions. Specific nursing interventions may be found in Chapters 11 and 14 for all of the disturbances listed above except for seizures. Interventions for seizures are found in Chapter 6.
Potential for complication of being bedridden or comatose	Minimal complications have occurred	NOTE: The care of the bedridden or comatose patient centers around proper respiratory care, oral hygiene, nutrition, skin care, bladder and bowel management, and prevention of thrombophlebitis. See Chapter 11 for specific nursing interventions.
Knowledge deficit: self/home care measures and community resources	Patient is functioning as independently as possible Family and patient feel comfortable and are knowledgeable enough to take care of the patient at home if they so desire Appropriate referrals and community resources are utilized for both physical and psychological support	Identify the physical limitations and strengths of the patient. Discuss these limitations and strengths with the patient and family. Include the patient and family in the coordination and delivery of care. Encourage the patient to do as much as possible. Identify appropriate referrals. These may include a (1) nutritionist to discuss ways to maintain nutritional intake and approaches to deal with problems such as stomatitis, diarrhea, and constipation; (2) physical therapist to discuss and demonstrate proper body mechanics and range-of-motion and transfer techniques; (3) occupational therapist to discuss ways of maintaining the patient's activity level and independence; (4) social worker to discuss community resources such as visiting nurses, financial resources, equipment, support groups, and information or other services that can be found by contacting the American Cancer Society. Encourage the patient and family to continue socialization outside the home (such as by maintaining work status if possible, attending church groups or clubs).

Table 8-1 Chemotherapeutic agents*

Drugs	Method of action	Usual dosage	Route administration	Effects	Special precautions
Methotrexate (MTX)	Thought to interfere with DNA synthesis (cell-cycle specific)	12-15 mg once a day for 2-5 days	Does not pass Blood Brain Barrier (BBB), given intrathecally or intraventricularly	Nausea, vomiting, stomatitis, diarrhea, delayed myelosuppression; could be nephrotoxic, hepatoxic	Avoid salicylates (decreases effects), Dilantin, alcoholic beverages, tetracycline and chloramphenicol; may need to administer citrovorum factor to reduce systemic toxicity
Vincristine (Oncovin)	Thought to arrest mitotic division	1.4 mg/m² once weekly	Does not pass BBB; usually given intraveously (push or infusion), rarely by intra-arterial infusion	Very neurotoxic (first sign is constipation),† nausea, vomiting, stomatitis, alopecia, some myelosuppression	Toxicity is dose related; neurotoxicity may be permanent
Vinblastine (Velban)	Thought to interfere with metabolic pathways of amino acids	3.7 mg/m² to start, then slowly increased but not to exceed 18.5 mg/m²; given once weekly (dosage depends on degree of leukopenia)	Does not pass BBB; usually given intravenously (push or infusion), rarely by intra-arterial infusion	Very myelotoxic; also nausea, vomiting, diarrhea, some neurotoxicity	Cumulative toxicity; less active against brain tumors than vincristine
Dacarbazine (DTIC)	Thought to inhibit DNA synthesis (acts as a purine analog)	250 mg/m² per day for 5 days; repeated every 3-4 weeks	Given by intravenous infusion	Nausea, vomiting, anorexia, influenza-like symptoms (fever, malaise, myalgia), alopecia, skin flushing, and myelosuppression	

*From Stewart, C.: Current concepts of chemotherapy for brain tumors, J. Neurosurg. Nurs. **12**(2):99, June 1980.
†Mixed sensory, motor, and anatomic symptoms.

Continued.

Table 8-1 Chemotherapeutic agents—cont'd

Drugs	Method of action	Usual dosage	Route administration	Effects	Special precautions
Nitrosureas BCNU (Carmustine)	Thought to act by inhibiting key enzymatic steps which lead to formation of DNA; thought to act in all stages of cell cycle	200 mg/m^2 in one dose; repeat every 6 weeks	(Lipid soluble) crosses BBB; intravenous infusion	Nausea and vomiting within the first 6 hr after dose; vein discomfort, delayed bone marrow depression	Contact with skin causes brown spots
CCNU (Lomustine)	Thought to act by inhibiting key enzymatic steps which lead to formation of DNA; thought to act in all stages of cell cycle	130 mg/m^2 in one dose; repeated every 6 weeks	Orally	Delayed myelosuppression (4-6 weeks after dose) usually manifest by thrombocytopenia and leukopenia; nausea and vomiting (within first 2 hr of dose), alopecia, anemia, stomatitis, liver toxicity, and skin flushing	

MeCCNU (Semustine)	Thought to act by inhibiting key enzymatic steps which lead to formation of DNA; thought to act in all stages of cell cycles	200 mg/m² in one dose, every 4 weeks	Orally	Delayed myelosuppression (4-6 weeks after dose) usually manifest by thrombocytopenia and leukopenia; nausea and vomiting (within first 2 hr of dose), alopecia, anemia, stomatitis, liver toxicity, and skin flushing	Investigational drug
Procarbazine (Matulane)	Thought to inhibit DNA, RNA, and protein synthesis	50 mg/m² daily for 1 week, then 100 mg/m² until maximum response is obtained or myelosuppression is manifest; 50 mg daily maintenance dose	Moves into CSF rapidly; administered orally	MAO inhibitory actions, myelosuppression, stomatitis, diarrhea, myalgia, lethargy, and skin flushing	Special patient education necessary to avoid tyramine (no cheese, bananas) and ethyl alcohol

SPINAL CORD TUMORS

Etiology

Spinal cord tumors account for about 1% of all cancers. They occur most frequently in the age group from 20 to 60 years and affect both sexes equally. Of the different types of spinal cord tumors approximately 50% occur in the thoracic region, 30% in the cervical region, and 20% in the lumbosacral region (Hickey, 1981). Like the tumors that affect the brain the exact cause of spinal cord tumors is unknown. Refer to the section in brain tumors for possible causative agents.

Pathophysiology

A spinal cord tumor produces pathophysiological changes by compression upon the spinal cord and its nerve roots, by interference with the spinal blood supply, and/or by obstruction of the CSF circulation. The resulting neurological signs and symptoms may develop very rapidly (in hours) or over a long period of time (months to years). This depends upon the neoplasm's rate of growth and its consistency (hard versus soft). Soft, slow-growing neoplasms have a consistency similar to the spinal cord, thus allowing the cord to accommodate for the neoplasm and to adjust its circulation. However, hard, fast-growing neoplasms cause rapid compression of the spinal cord with substantial edema creating rapidly deteriorating neurological deficits. The neurological signs and symptoms the patient is experiencing will also depend upon the location of the neoplasm. Tables 8-2 and 8-3 describe the potential neurological deficits in relationship to the dura and segmented location of the neoplasm.

Classification

Spinal cord tumors may be classified according to the specific locations in which they tend to occur (see Fig. 8-1).

Intradural tumors. Intradural spinal cord tumors arise from the pia arachnoid, denticulate ligament, spinal roots, or inner surface of the dura.

Extramedullary tumors. Extramedullary tumors are located within the dura, but outside the spinal cord. Approximately 40% of spinal tumors are extramedullary (Hickey, 1981). These mainly consist of neurofibromas and meningiomas. Both types of tumors are soft and grow very slowly. Symptoms may manifest themselves over a period of years. Usually these tumors can be removed completely surgically.

Intramedullary tumors. Intramedullary tumors are located under the dura or within the spinal cord itself. Between 5% and 10% of spinal cord tumors are intramedullary. These mainly consist of ependymomas and astrocytomas. Both types of tumors are usually invasive and expansive, making complete surgical removal impossible. They may also be cystic. Ependymomas respond fairly well to radiation.

Extradural tumors. Extradural spinal cord tumors arise in the vertebral bodies, laminae, pedicles, or in epidural tissue. Approximately 55% of spinal cord tumors are extradural. These are mainly metastatic carcinomas, primary sarcomas, and neurofibromas. Both carcinomas and sarcomas are soft and grow very rapidly. Symptoms may develop within a few hours. Postoperative survival may be months to a few years. Some respond fairly well to postoperative radiation.

Table 8-2 Signs and symptoms—tumor relationship to dura*

- **I.** Extradural
  - **A.** Pain: constant or intermittent, dull or dull with sharp overtones localized over the tumor and/or felt along the dermatome(s) involved (radicular pain); worse with bed rest, straining, coughing, sneezing
  - **B.** Weakness: asymmetrical, spastic
  - **C.** Tenderness: spinal processes on palpation
  - **D.** Sensory deficits: segmental, loss of pain, temperature, touch, vibration, girdle sensations
  - **E.** Brown-Séquard syndrome
- **II.** Intradural
  - **A.** Extramedullary
    - **1.** Lateral compression: Brown-Séquard syndrome
    - **2.** Anterior compression: motor deficits
    - **3.** Posterior compression: proprioceptive deficits, paresthesias, ataxia, herpes—dermatome distribution
  - **B.** Intermedullary
    - **1.** Bilateral loss: pain and temperature†
    - **2.** Pain: dull, aching, level of tumor—may be severe
    - **3.** Weakness, atrophy of muscles, fasciculations, loss of tendon reflexes
    - **4.** Analgesia: trunk, legs
    - **5.** Horner's syndrome
    - **6.** Impotence, sphincter disturbances
    - **7.** Symptoms likely to be a combination of the above

*From Taylor, J.W., and Ballenger, S.: Neurological dysfunctions and nursing interventions, New York, 1980, McGraw-Hill Book Co.

†Proprioceptive deficits (position, vibration, touch) occur if tumor is large.

Table 8-3 Signs and symptoms—segmental location of tumor*

I. Foramen magnum
  A. Pain: suboccipital, shoulders (maybe)
  B. Motor and sensory deficits: head, neck, shoulders: weakness, atrophy, quadriparesis
  C. Tumor extension into cranium
    1. Increased intracranial pressure
    2. Vertigo
    3. Dysphagia
    4. Facial sensory loss
    5. Ataxia
    6. Nystagmus
    7. Dysarthria
    8. Tongue atrophy
II. Cervical
  A. Pain: radicular, constant or intermittent; worse with straining, coughing, sneezing. Back of neck, shoulders, arm (midcervical medial arm pain; lower cervical—radial arm pain)
  B. Weakness and atrophy: muscles of above, unilateral or bilateral
  C. Tenderness: spinal processes
  D. Syndromes: Brown-Séquard, Horner's
  E. Quadriparesis, quadriplegia
  F. Sensory deficits: pain, heat, cold, touch, position, vibration, one to two segments below (paresthesias of fingers: midcervical—thumb, index finger; lower cervical—little, ring finger)
  G. Incontinence (late)
  H. Anhidrosis: below level of tumor
III. Thoracic
  A. Pain: radicular, subscapula, shoulder, kidney area
  B. Weakness and atrophy: legs, spasticity and asymmetrical
  C. Tenderness: spinal processes
  D. Brown-Séquard syndrome
  E. Sensory deficits: paresthesias, girdle sensation of abdomen and chest
  F. Reflexes: hyperactive; loss of abdominal reflexes
  G. Anhidrosis: below level of tumor
IV. Lumbosacral
  A. Pain: radicular, back, groin, leg (sciatic nerve distribution)
  B. Weakness and atrophy: hips, legs, spasticity
  C. Tenderness: spinal process
  D. Flaccid paraplegia
  E. Sensory deficits: perineal, genital, anesthesia of sacral dermatomes
  F. Reflexes: loss of cremasteric, knee and ankle jerk; bilateral Babinski's
  G. Sphincter control: decreased (early if lower sacral involved)
  H. Sexual dysfunctions
V. Cauda equina
  A. Pain: back, one or both legs, perineum, bladder, rectum (maybe)
  B. Flaccid paralysis: asymmetrical, atrophy
  C. Sensory loss: radicular
  D. Reflexes: decreased or lost
  E. Sphincter dysfunction
  F. Sexual dysfunctions (if tumor large and impinging on sacral cord)

*From Taylor, J.W., and Ballenger, S.: Neurological dysfunctions and nursing intervention, New York, 1980, McGraw-Hill Book Co.

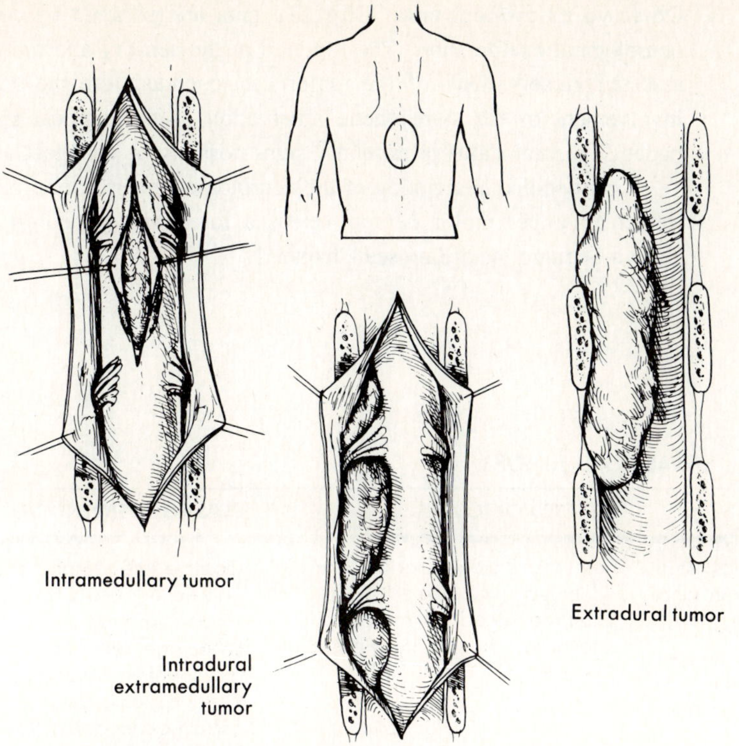

Fig. 8-1 Anatomical location of spinal cord tumors.

Nursing assessment

Subjective assessment data

Pain (most frequent initial symptom). Note:
- Degree (severe, constant or intermittent, minimal, or absent)
- Location (local back or neck, radicular along involved dermatomes)
- Aggravations (sudden movement of spine, bed rest, straining, coughing, or sneezing)

Nonpainful sensory disturbances that begin unilaterally:
- Early (tingling, numbness, coldness)
- Later (loss of touch, vibration, or position sense)
- Hyperesthesia (abnormally increased sensitivity to stimuli)
- Motor disturbances such as ataxia, hypotonia, weakness resulting from involvement of pyramidal or corticospinal tract
- Autonomic disturbances (urgency, difficulty in initiation of urination, loss of bowel control, impotency in males)

Objective assessment data. Objective data are gathered by conducting a complete neurological examination. The function of the sensory and motor systems should be assessed closely. Only if the tumor has extended into the cranium or if there is involvement of the sympathetic innervation of the cervical spinal nerves will the patient's mental status or pupillary signs possibly be changed.

For a detailed description of the neurological examination, abnormal findings that reflect an upper motor neuron versus a lower motor neuron lesion, and also the Brown-Séquard syndrome see Chapter 1.

Nursing care plan: SPINAL CORD TUMORS

NURSING DIAGNOSIS	EXPECTED OUTCOMES	NURSING INTERVENTIONS
Ineffective breathing pattern **Ineffective airway clearance** NOTE: Oxygenation may be impaired due to involvement of the phrenic nerve, ascending spinal cord edema, and paralysis of the intercostal muscles	Respirations are regular and nonlabored Chest movement is symmetrical Arterial blood gases are within normal limits	Observe rate, rhythm, and amplitude of respirators every 1 to 4 hours depending on the location of the tumor. Encourage deep breathing every 2 hours. Monitor arterial blood gases. Check tissue perfusion. Suction as needed. Administer oxygen as needed. Bag ventilate if necessary. Control pain. Reposition every 2 hours.
Alteration in comfort	Pain is controlled with or without narcotics Patient is getting 6 to 8 hours of sleep every night Cord edema is decreased as much as possible Early recognition and treatment of untoward effects of symptomatic pharmacotherapy	Assess patient's degree of pain every 3 to 4 hours. Administer pain and antiinflammatory medications as ordered. Support body position in alignment. Allow rest periods between treatments. Use an alternating pressure mattress. Log-roll patient. Explain all treatments before executing them. Support patient in activities when necessary (such as in walking and bathing). Observe for untoward effects of antiinflammatory agents (dexamethasone). These include adrenocortical insufficiency, electrolyte imbalance, and Cushing's syndrome. Observe for untoward effects of pain medications (meperidine [Demerol]). These include dizziness, nausea and vomiting, decreased blood pressure. Refer to Chapter 11 for additional interventions.

Nursing care plan: SPINAL CORD TUMORS—cont'd

NURSING DIAGNOSIS	EXPECTED OUTCOMES	NURSING INTERVENTIONS
Sensory deficit **Potential for impaired skin integrity** **Impaired physical mobility** **Potential joint contractures**	Tissue perfusion normal Mobility at optimum level	Assess condition of skin every 2 hours. Encourage patient to do activities of daily living (ADLs). Reposition every 1 to 2 hours. Use heel protectors. Keep heels off mattress. Provide footboard. Maintain proper body alignment. Range-of-motion exercise every 2 to 4 hours. Teach proper transfer techniques. Teach patient how to prevent complications from pain and temperature deficits. Test hot water with thermometer. Dress warmly in cold weather. Inspect skin daily. Assess muscle mass, tone, and strength. Refer to Chapter 11 for additional interventions.
Alteration in bowel and bladder elimination patterns **Sexual dysfunction**	Altered elimination program is managed consistent with capabilities Urine output is greater than 2500 ml/24 hours Formed stool every 2 days No urinary or bowel distention No signs of infection Altered perceptions of sexuality and sexual function have been identified and appropriate methods of sexual satisfaction discussed	Bladder: Monitor intake and output closely. Maintain perineal cleanliness. Establish a bladder-control program. Insert an indwelling catheter if necessary. Observe for signs of infection such as cloudy, fecal-smelling urine, perineal itching. Send specimen for culturing if ordered. Offer nonalkalinizing fluids. Bowel: Identify patient's normal bowel habits. Identify the regular time for using toilet. Provide privacy. Encourage a well-balanced diet with adequate fruits and vegetables. Utilize a bowel-retraining program (for example, use a glycerin suppository or mild laxative). Sexuality: Assess the patient's need for information. Make the patient feel comfortable about asking questions. Include the sexual partner in the counseling process. Let the patient's needs, interests, and questions be a guide. Discuss emotional as well as physical aspects of sex. Make appropriate referrals. Refer to Chapter 11 for additional interventions.

Continued.

Nursing care plan: SPINAL CORD TUMORS—cont'd

NURSING DIAGNOSIS	EXPECTED OUTCOMES	NURSING INTERVENTIONS
Knowledge deficit: diagnostic procedures	Verbalizes understanding of procedures Verbalizes fears and concerns Cooperates with procedures	Give an explanation appropriate to the patient's and family's level of comprehension and emotional state. Give encouragement and the opportunity to ask questions. Provide psychological support. Refer to Chapter 2 for a detailed description of each procedure and specific nursing interventions. NOTE: The following diagnostic procedures may be used in diagnosing spinal cord tumors: spinal x-ray films, lumbar puncture, Queckenstedt's sign, myelogram, spinal angiogram, CAT scan, electromyogram.
Knowledge deficit: surgery	Verbalized understanding of surgery Verbalizes fears and concerns	Refer to Chapter 10 for a description of the preoperative and postoperative nursing care for the patient having a laminectomy, which is the main surgical treatment.
Knowledge deficit: chemotherapy and radiation therapy **Potential complications of chemotherapy and radiation therapy**	Refer to brain tumor section	Refer to brain tumor section for general and specific interventions for potential problems. NOTE: The dosage of radiotherapy and chemotherapy used for spinal cord tumors is dependent upon the histological tumor type, location, expected response, and patient's tolerance level. The average dose of radiation is 2000 to 4000 rads administered over 6 to 8 weeks.
Knowledge deficit: self/home care measures and community resources	Refer to brain tumor section	Refer to brain tumor section.

Suggested readings

Adams, R., and Maurice, V.: Principles of neurology, ed. 2, New York, 1981, McGraw-Hill Book Co.

Aminoff, M.J.: Spinal angiomas, London, 1976, Blackwell Scientific Publications, Ltd.

Bergerson, B.S., and Goth, A.: Pharmacology in nursing, ed. 14, St. Louis, 1979, The C.V. Mosby Co.

Damon, J., and Taylor, L.: Brain tumors in children, Nurs. Clin. North Am. **15**(1):99-113, March 1980.

Dunphy, J.E., and Way, L.W.: Current surgical diagnosis and treatment, ed. 3, Los Altos, Calif., 1977, Lange Medical Publications.

Edstrom, S., and Miller, M.W.: Preparing the family to care for the cancer patient at home: a home care course, Cancer Nurs. **4**:49-52, Feb. 1981.

Fagon-Dubin, L.: Causes of cancer, Cancer Nurs. **2**:435-440, 1979.

Gehrke, M.: Identifying brain tumors, J. Neurosurg. Nurs. **12**(2):90-92, June 1980.

Guidetti, B., and Fortuna, A.: Differential diagnosis of intramedullary and extramedullary tumors, In Vinken, P.J., and Brayn, G.W., editors: Handbook of clinical neurology, part I. Tumors of the spine and spinal cord, vol. 19, Amsterdam, 1975, North-Holland Publishing Co.

Harvey, A., and others: The principles and practice of medicine, ed. 20, New York, 1980, Appleton-Century Crofts.

Hausman, K.: Brain tumors in children, J. Neurosurg. Nurs. **10**(1):8-12, March 1978.

Hickey, J.: The clinical practice of neurological and neurosurgical nursing, Philadelphia, 1981, J.B. Lippincott Co.

Larson, E.: The epidemiology of primary brain tumors, J. Neurosurg. Nurs. **12**(3):121-125, Sept. 1980.

Merritt, H.: A textbook in neurology, Philadelphia, 1979, Lea & Febiger.

Sher, J.H., and Ford, D.H.: Primary intracranial neoplasms, New York, 1979, Spectrum Publications.

Stern, W.E.: Localization and diagnosis of spinal cord tumors, Clinical neurosurg. **25:**480-494, 1978.

Steward, C.: Current concepts of chemotherapy for brain tumors, J. Neurosurg. Nurs. **12**(2):97-101, June 1980.

Taylor, J., and Ballenger, S.: Neurological dysfunctions and nursing intervention, New York, 1980, McGraw-Hill Book Co.

Walton, J.N.: Essentials of neurology, ed. 4, Philadelphia, 1975, J.B. Lippincott Co.

Welch, D.: Planning nursing interventions for family members of adult cancer patients, Cancer Nurs. **4:**365-369, Oct. 1981.

Wilson, C., and others: Supportive management of the patient with malignant brain tumor, J.A.M.A. **244:**1249-1251, 1980.

Woods, N.F.: Human sexuality in health and illness, St. Louis, 1979, The C.V. Mosby Co.

CHAPTER 9 Trauma

Since the 1973 implementation of the Emergency Medical Services Act, the number of hospital admissions of trauma victims has increased dramatically (Fincke, 1983). On-site rescue vehicle personnel rapidly assess neurological and physiological deficits, initiate life-saving and immobilization procedures, and transport victims to appropriate agencies. Also, within the past decade vehicular accidents, including cars, motorcycles, and bicycles, which are the primary cause of central nervous system (CNS) trauma, have increased.

Because of the rapidity of events inherent in trauma situations and the potentially devastating outcomes, the patient suffers immediate and sometimes long-term physiological and psychological effects. In severe CNS trauma the patient may exhibit complete or profound loss of neurological and physiological function, making him entirely dependent on health care providers for maintenance of vital and homeostatic functions. Psychologically, the patient's immediate response may be that of denial, disbelief, or anger. Long-term continued dependence on others, financial worries, and the altered self-image resulting from loss of or decreased body function may cause the patient to despair. In the acute postinjury phase, nursing care is directed toward:

Accurate, serial assessment and documentation of vital functions and neurological status.

Implementation of medical or patient care protocols (Table 9-1) to sustain life, protect the patient from further injury, and maintain homeostasis.

Following the acute phase, nursing interventions focus on:

Maintenance and restoration of physiological and psychological functioning.

Prevention of complications.

Facilitating adaptation to trauma-induced limitations (physiological, cognitive, psychosocial).

Including the patient, family, or significant others in the rehabilitation process (Conway-Rutkowski, 1982).

Therapeutic treatment protocols are dependent on the severity of the trauma. For example, conservative treatment, such as immobilization and muscle relaxants, is frequently used for whiplash injuries. In contrast, surgical intervention is necessary for rapidly expanding hematomas. Trauma to the central or peripheral nervous system can result from:

Vehicular accidents: over 150,000 adults per year in the United States.

Falls: increased incidence in infants, children, and the elderly.

Table 9-1 **Standard management protocol for severely head-injured adult patients***

1. Head elevated 30° and in neutral plane
2. Controlled ventilation to maintain $PaO_2 > 70$ mm. Hg. and $PaCO_2$ at 25-30 mm. Hg.
3. Adequate paralysis and sedation
4. Maintain Systemic Systolic Arterial Blood Pressure between 100 and 160 mm. Hg.
5. Maintain normothermia
6. Use prophylactic anticonvulsants
7. Maintain fluid balance with half normal saline

For ICP control

8. Ventricular drainage, if possible
9. Dexamethasone 20 mg. IV q 6 hr.
10. Mannitol 0.25 Gm.-1 Gm./kg. as needed
11. Avoid anesthetics and other drugs that are cerebral dilators

*Reprinted with permission from Bowers, S., and Marshall, L.: Severe head injury: current treatment and research in J. Neurosurg. Nurs. **14**(5):213, Oct. 1982.

Forceful blows: high crime areas and sporting injuries.

Penetrating trauma: more common in war and high crime areas.

Pressure or constriction: traumatic deliveries and occupational injuries, such as from cave-ins, explosions, cutting or roller machinery.

Fractures of bones: vertebral, skull, or extremity fractures.

A major complicating factor, particularly in vehicular accidents and falls, is the presence of concomitant injury to other body systems; for example, the bones protecting the central and peripheral nerve systems, lungs, heart, and abdomen.

Within the CNS, typical healing methods are dependent on the type and location of the trauma. Superficial lacerations heal by gliosis. Lacerations deep in the brain or spinal cord parenchyma cause a consolidation of glia, fibroblasts, and meninges resulting in scar formation. The presence of a foreign body, such as a scalp fragment or bullet, generally results in abscess formation (Adams and Victor, 1980). In this chapter we will discuss trauma to bones, brain, spinal cord, and peripheral nerves.

BONE TRAUMA

Because the CNS is encased by the facial, skull, and vertebral bones, fracture and displacement of these bones frequently results in trauma to the underlying or adjacent nerve tissue.

Skull fracture

The skull bone covering the convexity of the brain is thicker than that in the temporal area. There are four types of skull fractures (Fig. 9-1):

Linear: line fracture
Comminuted: multiple adjacent linear fractures
Depressed: inward displacement of skull bone fragments
Basilar: fracture at base of skull

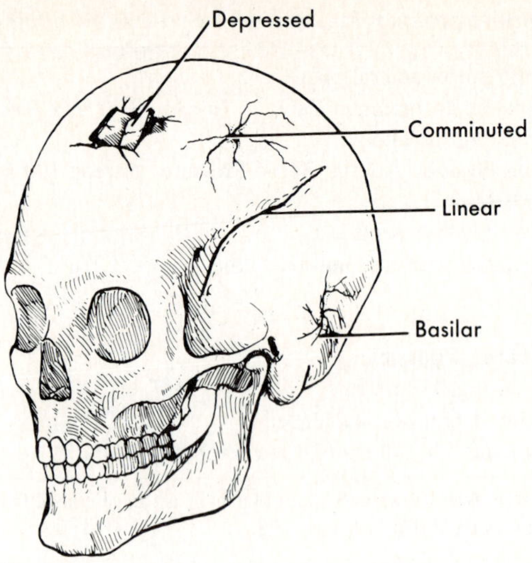

Fig. 9-1 Skull fractures: depressed, comminuted, linear, and basilar.

Linear and depressed skull fractures are visible on x-ray films. Because basilar fractures are not usually visible on x-ray films, astute observation for the typical clinical signs is imperative:

Battle's signs (ecchymosis in the mastoid area); may not occur for 24 to 36 hours after the trauma

Blood behind the tympanic membrane (hemotympanum)

Rhinorrhea or otorrhea; differentiated from other fluids by:

Positive result for glucose when tested with Dextrostix or Tes-Tape

Presence of ''halo'' around bloody fluid collected on a sponge from nose, ear, or head wound; blood migrates to the center and is surrounded by a yellow halo

Raccoon sign: ecchymosis surrounding eyes

Hearing deficit

Severely depressed level of consciousness (LOC)

Unless skull fractures are depressed or are communicating with sinus areas, which increases the potential for infection, conservative management is usually employed. A conservative treatment protocol focusing on observation and prevention includes:

1. Assessing and recording neurological status every 15 minutes to 4 hours depending on the patient's status.
2. Preventing cerebral edema by positioning the patient with the head elevated 30 degrees. Note: Use a 15-degree elevation if otorrhea/rhinorrhea is present.

3. Observing for signs of infection and increased intracranial pressure (ICP).
4. Administering prescribed prophylactic antibiotics and steroids.

In contrast, patients with extensive dural tears, depressed skull fractures, or expanding hematomas require prompt surgical intervention. See Chapter 10.

Vertebral fractures

Because of the mobility of the vertebral column, particularly in the cervical and lumbar areas, and the irregular shape of the vertebral bones, vertebral trauma is relatively common. Trauma to the spinal cord can result from displacement of vertebral fractures. However, *not all* vertebral fractures cause injury to the spinal cord.

Vertebral fractures and their mechanism of injury are classified as (Fig. 9-2):

Simple: usually of the transverse or spinous processes.

Compression (wedge): body of the vertebra is displaced anteriorly usually as a result of hyperflexion.

Dislocated: a disruption of vertebral alignment because of the stretching or tearing of supportive ligaments as a result of either anterior or posterior bone displacement.

Comminuted (burst fracture): the vertebral body is shattered with fragments displaced into the spinal canal and/or cord resulting in neurological deficits (Larrabee, 1977).

The treatment protocol for vertebral fractures includes:

1. Immobilization and stabilization of the fracture with skin or skeletal traction.
2. Administration of prescribed muscle relaxants and analgesics.
3. Assessment and documentation of neurological status every 15 minutes to 2 hours.
4. Observation for signs of spinal cord edema and compression.
5. Maintainence of bone/joint alignment to prevent hip abduction and foot drop during the period of immobilization.
6. Provision of skin care with particular attention to bony prominences.

Extremity fractures

Fractures of long bones in the extremities and in the pelvic girdle can cause stretch, pressure, or sectioning trauma to adjacent nerves. Because of the proximity of nerves and blood vessels to the pelvic and long bones, neurovascular assessment (5 Ps) is imperative when these bones are fractured. The 5 P assessment includes:

Pallor.
Pulses.
Paralysis.
Paresthesias.
Pain (Webb, 1974).

The extent of recovery from bone trauma is dependent upon the:

Severity of the injury.
Amount of edema and hemorrhage.
Location of the insult.
Promptness and accuracy of diagnosis and treatment measures.

A

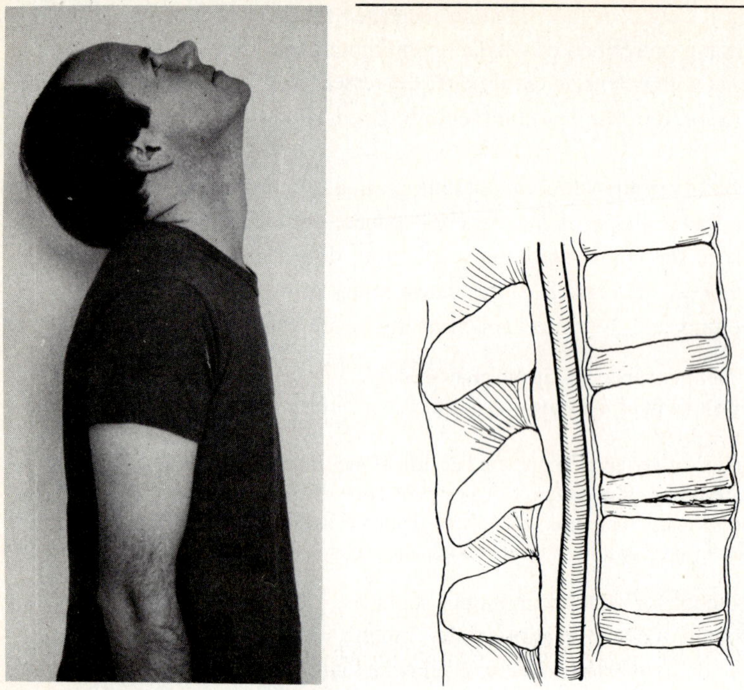

B

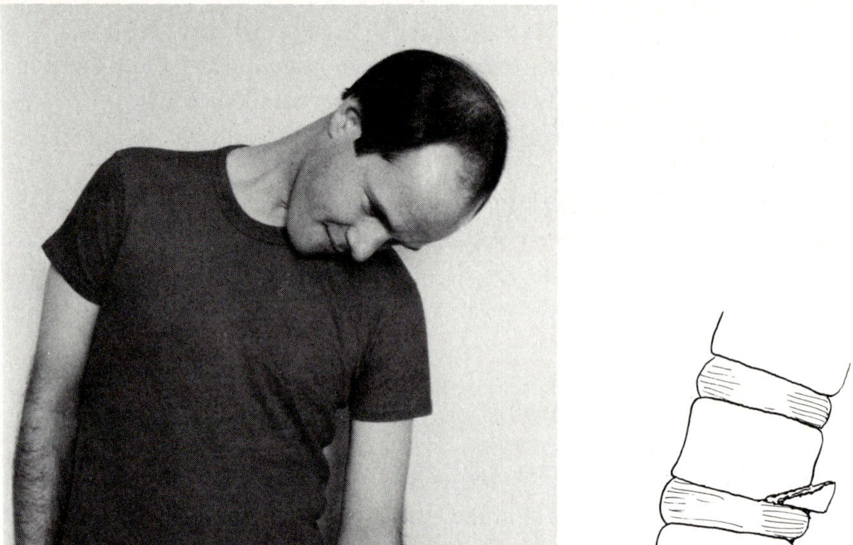

Fig. 9-2 Vertebral fractures. **A,** Disrupted intervertebral disc resulting from hypertension injury. **B,** Wedge fracture resulting from lateral flexion injuries. **C,** Flexion injury resulting in fracture dislocation or wedge fracture with stretching or disruption of intraspinous ligaments.

Continued.

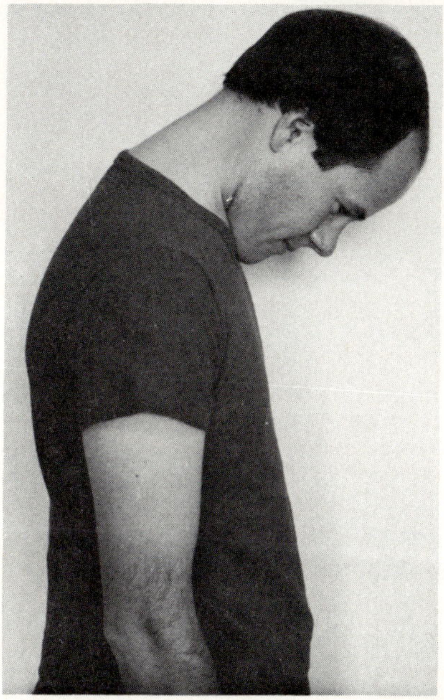

C

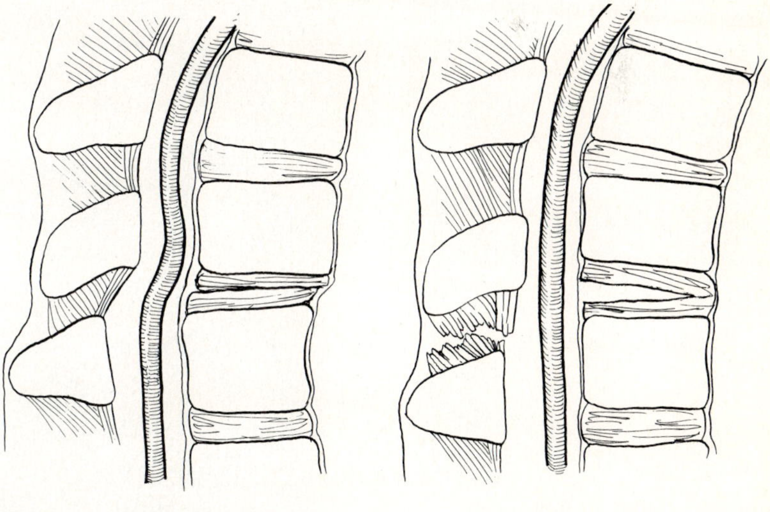

Fig. 9-2
cont'd

Vertebral fractures. **D,** Burst fracture caused by vertical compression as a result of falls form heights or falling objects. Also called comminuted fracture. **E,** Fracture of vertebral body with displacement of body and disc as a result of rotational flexion injury.

D

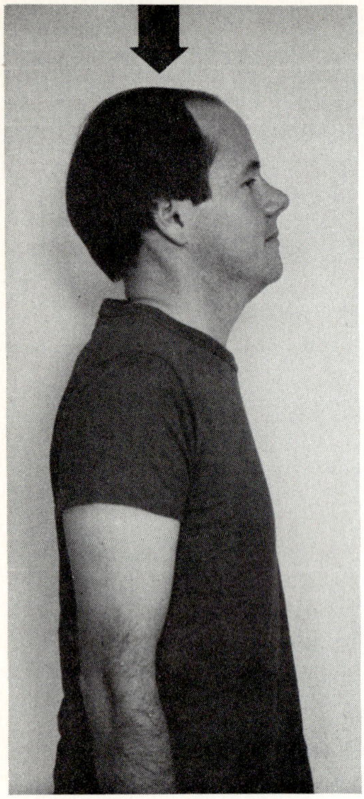

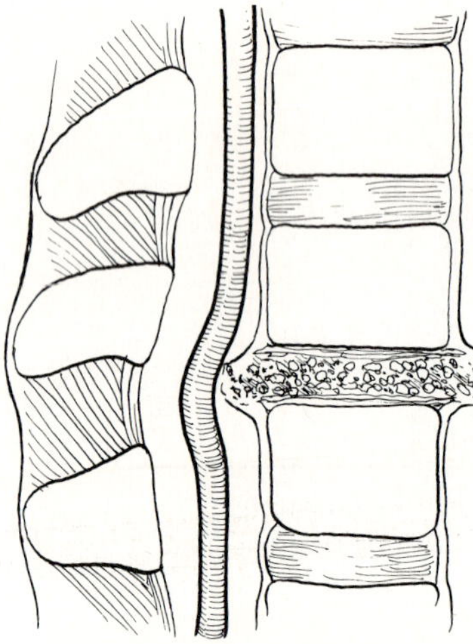

E

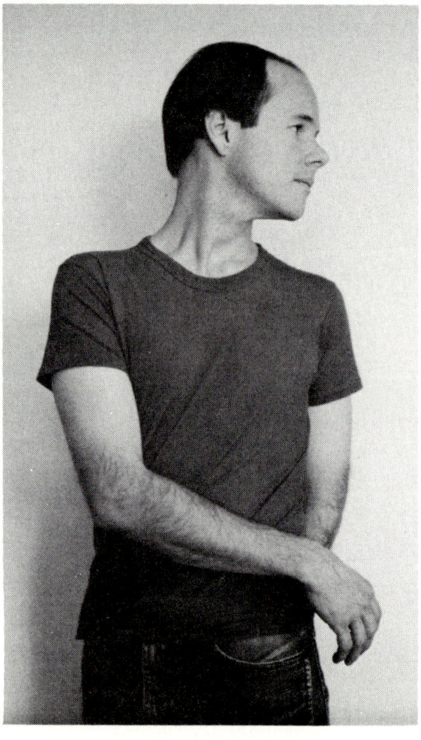

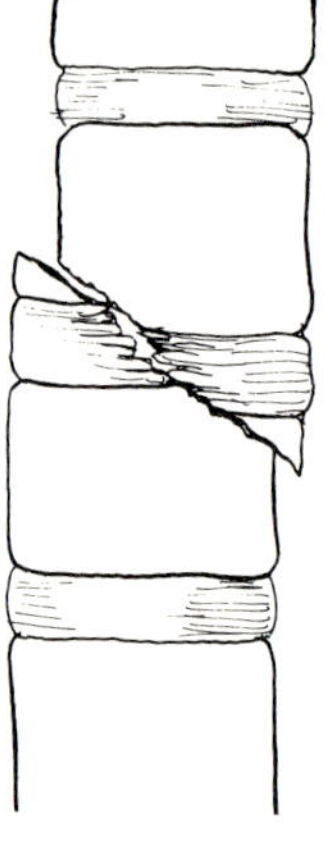

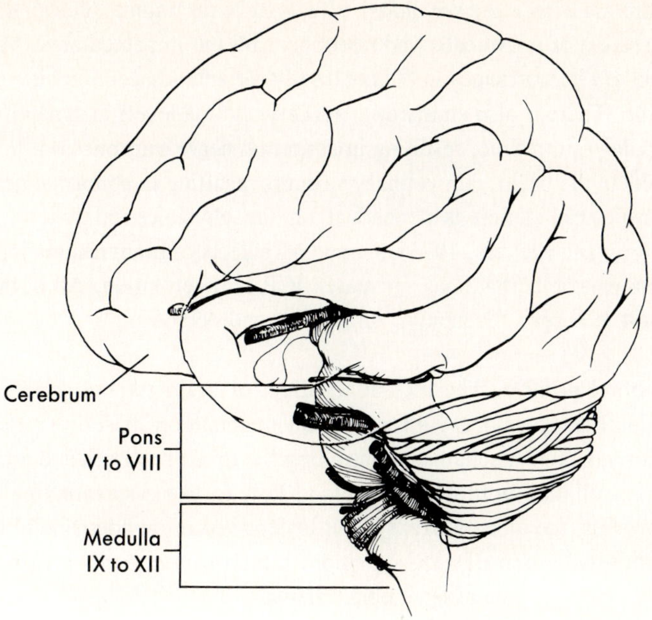

Fig. 9-3 Brain: cerebrum freely movable. Brainstem held stable by cranial nerves.

BRAIN TRAUMA

Anatomically, the brain is protected by the:

Facial soft tissue and bones.

Scalp.

Skull.

Ventricles of the brain and the circulating cerebrospinal fluid (CSF).

Blood.

These structures absorb one quarter to one third of the force of a blow. The cerebrum is soft and movable within the confines of the skull. In contrast, the brainstem is held in place by the cranial nerves (V through XII) that originate in the pons and medulla (Fig. 9-3). Therefore, brainstem movement requires exceptional force, rapidly expanding lesions (hematoma or hemorrhage), or extensive brain edema (Shea, 1981).

Etiology

In descending order of incidence, brain trauma is a result of:

Motor vehicle accidents.

Falls or falling objects.

Blows.

Penetrating injuries.

Traumatic delivery.

Pathophysiology

There are *direct* and *secondary* effects of brain trauma. The *direct* effect is contusion/laceration of nerve cells and fibers beneath the impacted area. Microscopically, small capillary hemorrhages in the contused area and adjacent meninges result in necrosis of tissue. There is also an increase in acetylcholine levels at synapses, which prolongs the depolarization time, resulting in abnormal nerve transmission. Within the injured fiber tracts in the brain, demyelination occurs resulting in abnormal nerve transmission. The neurological deficit is dependent on the physiological function of the injured area (Gilroy and Meyers, 1975). *Secondary* effects of brain trauma include cerebral edema, hemorrhagic hematomas, increased ICP, and herniation. All of these secondary effects result in cerebral ischemia, infarction, and necrosis.

Cerebral edema. The metabolic effect of brain trauma is an increased secretion of antidiuretic hormone with a subsequent retention of sodium and water. Focally, the autoregulatory mechanism controlling the tone of arteries and arterioles fails, resulting in vasodilation with increased blood flow to tissue surrounding the traumatized area. However, the area of *direct* insult is deprived of an adequate blood supply. The result of this is carbon dioxide retention, which causes further vasodilation and acidosis. This, in turn, increases cerebral edema.

The degree of edema correlates with the severity of trauma. As brain volume increases within the confines of the skull and compensatory mechanisms of fluid (CSF and blood) shifts are compromised, the ICP increases. If the pressure is not relieved, signs of herniation develop rapidly (Adams and Victor, 1980).

Hemorrhagic hematomas. Shearing forces in brain trauma may result in laceration or rupture of cerebral blood vessels. The result may be epidural (arterial), subdural (venous), or intracerebral bleeds or subarachnoid hemorrhage. All hematomas act as space-occupying lesions with edematous areas surrounding the hematoma. Physiologically, hematomas:

- Increase the cerebral volume, exerting pressure and causing ischemia and necrosis of brain parenchyma, thereby decreasing neural metabolism.
- Increase ICP by displacing brain parenchyma, thus interferring with normal CSF circulation.
- Can result in supratentorial herniation (Adams and Victor, 1980).

Classification

Head injuries are classified as open or closed.

Open head injury. An open head injury involves an interruption in the integrity of the scalp, skull, and dura. The sequellae of seizure disorders following the acute phase is reported to be 30% (Stevens, 1982). Open head injuries may be:

- Penetrating: a foreign object (bullet, missile) penetrates the skull and dura lodging in brain parenchyma and lacerating blood vessels resulting in (1) localized hemorrhage; (2) edema; (3) open communication with the environment or the presence of a foreign body causing abscesses or other infectious processes.

Compound depressed skull fractures with scalp laceration: bone fragments contuse and lacerate brain parenchyma causing hemorrhage and edema. Open communication with the environment can result in CNS infections.

Basilar skull fractures: may result in displacement and compression of the brainstem.

Closed head injury. Closed head injuries include concussions, contusions, and hemorrhages/hematomas.

Concussion: mild injury, usually a result of hitting the head on a hard object. Neurological impairment is minimal and transient. Complete recovery occurs rapidly.

Contusion: moderate to severe brain injury that involves edema and hemorrhage. There are 2 mechanisms involved in contusions:

Coup: hemorrhage and edema directly under the injured site as a result of acceleration injuries.

Contrecoup: There are two sites of injury, under and directly opposite the site of the trauma, because of acceleration/deceleration or rotational trauma (Fig. 9-4).

Hemorrhage/hematoma: laceration of blood vessels in the epidural, subdural, or intracerebral areas, producing localized bleeds that act as expanding space-occupying lesions causing:

Direct damage with edema, hypoxic tissue, and pressure necrosis.

The secondary effect of increased ICP.

Mechanisms of head injury are illustrated in Fig. 9-5.

Concussion

Concussion is caused by a jostling of brain parenchyma that results in microscopic changes in neurons and nerve fibers. Recovery is usually complete within 48 hours except in cases of multiple concussions where the effects are cumulative, such as with boxers or abused persons.

Nursing assessments

Subjective assessment data

Amnesia for events before and after the trauma
Vomiting without nausea
Pain at site of injury
Dizziness, ''seeing stars''
Irritability
Loss of energy

Objective assessment data

Oriented in three spheres
No pupil abnormalities
No focal neurological deficits
Incomplete history of injury because of transient loss of memory

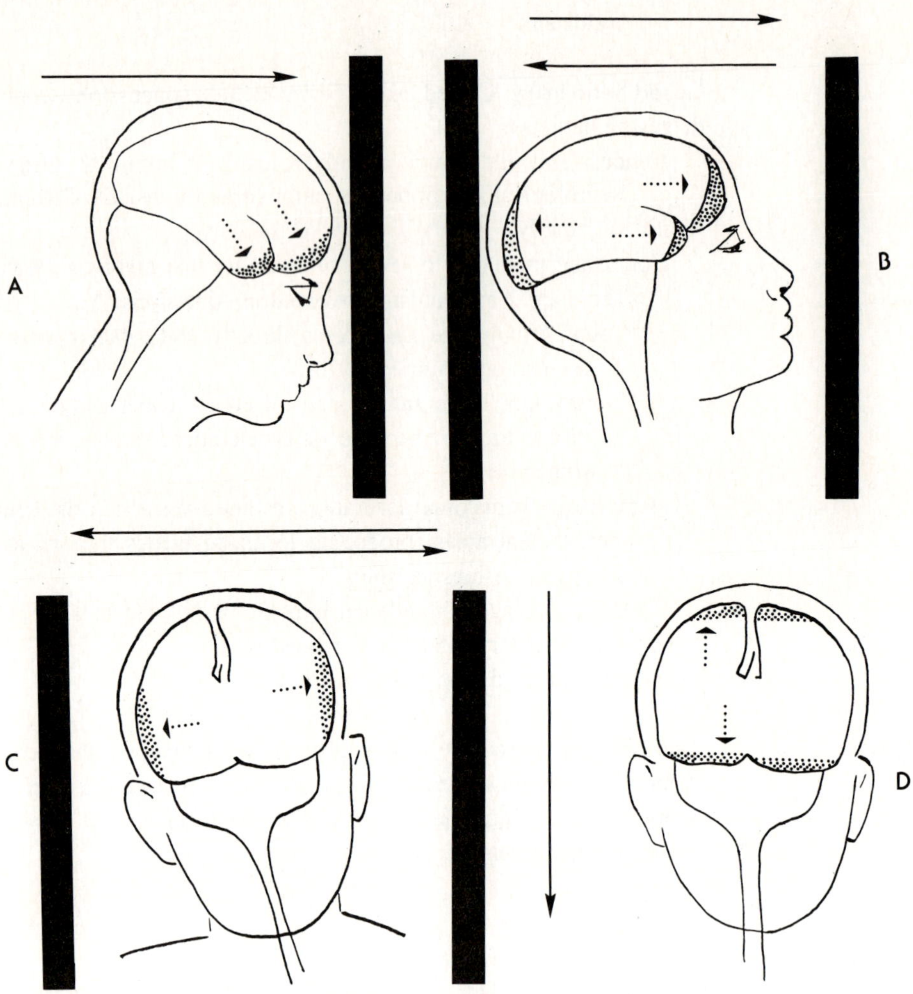

Fig. 9-4 **A,** Coup trauma to frontal lobe. **B,** Contracoup trauma with frontal and occipital lobe trauma because of acceleration/deceleration. **C,** Contracoup trauma to temporal lobes, commonly caused by broadside car accidents. **D,** Contracoup trauma resulting from falls. (Modified from Budassi, S.A., and Barber, J.M.: Emergency nursing: principles and practice, St. Louis, 1981, The C.V. Mosby Co.)

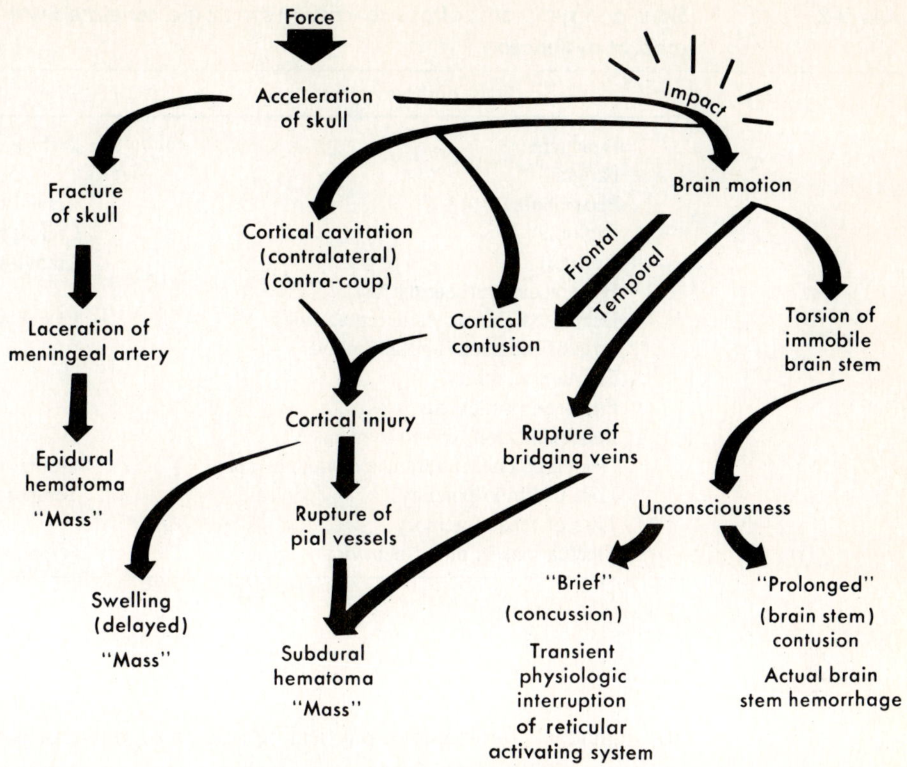

Fig. 9-5 Mechanisms in head injury. (From Warner, C.G.: Emergency care: assessment and intervention, ed. 2, St. Louis, 1983, The C.V. Mosby Co.)

Scalp tenderness at site of injury
Diagnostic tests: skull x-ray film normal

Interventions are focused on observation for signs and symptoms of deterioration indicative of more severe injuries. In cases of multiple concussions patients may experience the postconcussion syndrome.

Postconcussion syndrome

Postconcussion syndrome, a temporary constellation of cognitive, emotional, and personality changes, occurs in a significant number of patients following head injuries. This syndrome can occur up to a year after injury. The signs and symptoms experienced correlate with the area of trauma (Table 9-2).

Before dismissal a plan for home care for both the patient and family should be formulated to prevent or minimize maladjustment at home. Because of memory problems, it is advisable to provide written instructions and the name and phone numbers of persons to call for assistance. The plan of care should address the specific problems of

Table 9-2 Signs and symptoms of postconcussion syndrome correlated with the anatomical area of dysfunction

Signs and symptoms	Area
Headache	Diffuse
Fatigue	
Photophobia	Cranial nerves II and/or III
Diplopia	Cranial nerves III, IV, VI
Vertigo	Cranial nerve VIII
Hyperacoutism/hearing loss	
Decreased abstract thinking abilities	Frontal lobe
Loss of judgment and inhibitions	
Emotional lability	
Focus on past events	
Desocialization, crowd avoidance	
Decreased concentration and attention span	Frontal-limbic
Loss of libido/potency	Temporal-limbic
Loss of recent memory	
Fluctuations in mood/behaviors	Hypothalamus

the individual; for example, physical deficits or cognitive or behavioral dysfunctions (Stevens, 1982). General care measures that should be in the plan include:

1. Demonstration of physical care; for example, exercises, mobility precautions.
2. Discussion regarding environmental modifications, such as toilet seat riser, furniture placement, use of night lights.
3. Ways of structuring daily activities.
4. Reorientation and memory-jogging strategies.
5. Discussion of prescribed medications including their intended action, dosage, route, side effects.
6. Discussion of community referral resources: speech, occupational and physical therapy, community health nursing services, mental health agencies, self-help groups such as Recovery, Inc., and trauma recovery self-help groups.
7. Encouragement of gradual resocialization according to the patient's readiness and fatigue level.
8. Discussion of ways to handle aggressive behavior and the need for time away to maintain the mental health of the care provider (Stevens, 1982).

Contusion

Contusions involve capillary vessel hemorrhage, ischemia, and pressure necrosis of neurons and tracts supplied by the vessels. Secondary effects are relatively common, but vary in intensity related to the severity of trauma and compensation capabilities (see Pathophysiology of brain trauma).

Nursing assessment

Subjective assessment data

History of moderate to severe injury (such as vehicular, fall, sporting accidents)
Altered level of consciousness (LOC)
Weakness or paralysis of limbs
Speech difficulty
Memory loss preceding and following trauma
Headache
Stiff neck
Vision changes

Objective assessment data. Objective signs are related to the traumatized area and severity of trauma.

BRAINSTEM:

Nonresponsive to verbal and painful stimuli
Fever over 102.5° F (may also be caused by dysfunction of the hypothalamus)
Increased pulse and respiratory rate
Profuse perspiration
Pupil alterations:
  Constricted
  Midpoint
  Sluggish or nonresponsive to light stimuli
Vomiting
Hiccoughs
Otorrhea
Battle's sign (ecchymosis in mastoid area)
Flaccid, bilateral paresis or paralysis
Cranial nerve palsies

CEREBRAL HEMISPHERES (FRONTAL, PARIETAL LOBES):

Glascow coma scale: under 7
Depressed LOC
Dysphasia or aphasia (if dominant lobe is contused)
Hemiparesis/paralysis
Decorticate positioning: flexion of arm, wrist, and fingers with inward rotation of hands and shoulders. Legs are extended and internally rotated. (Fig. 4-7)
Rhinorrhea/otorrhea
Seizure activity, focal or generalized
Pupil changes: unilateral dilation with sluggish reaction to light on same side as lesion
Doll's eyes (Fig. 9-6)
Diagnostic tests:
  Skull radiograph: to determine skull fracture
  Echoencephalogram: indicates midline shift
  Brain or CAT scan: identifies location and size of contusion

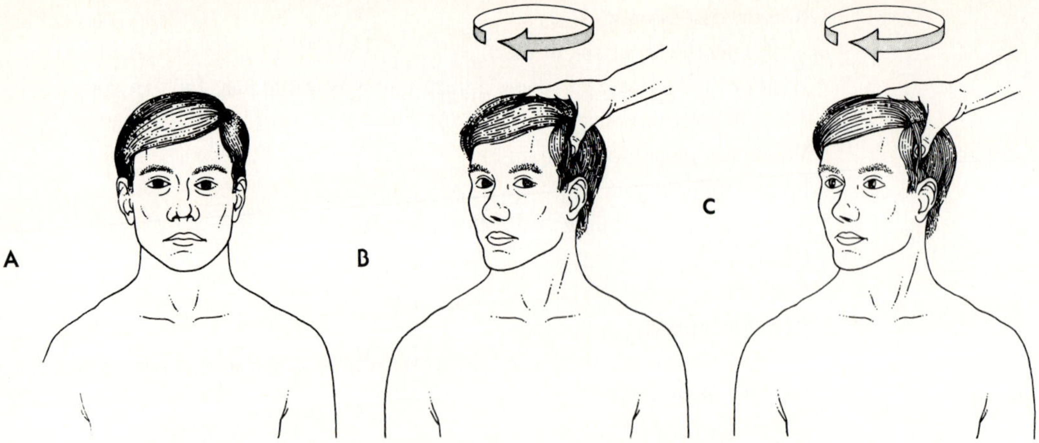

Fig. 9-6 Doll's eye maneuver. **A,** Normal gaze. **B,** Normal reflex: As head is turned to right, eyes rotate to left. **C,** Abnormal or absent reflex. As head is turned to right, eyes stay in midline position. (From Budassi, S.A., and Barber, J.M.: Emergency nursing: principles and practice, St. Louis, 1981, The C.V. Mosby Co.)

Hemorrhage/hematoma

The type and severity of vascular impairment following trauma is dependent on the severity and location of the injury and the source of the bleed. Fig. 9-6 illustrates subdural and epidural hematomas.

Epidural hematomas. Usual sites for epidural hematomas are the temporal lobe or the occiput. This is because of the proximity of arteries to skull in these areas: the basilar artery to the base of the skull and the temporal artery to the thin temporal skull bone. Because of the *arterial* bleeding source, prompt diagnosis and treatment are essential.

Nursing assessment

SUBJECTIVE ASSESSMENT DATA

Blow/penetrating injury to temporal lobe, dural sinuses, or base of skull
Brief loss of consciousness followed by lucid period of minutes to hours (33% of patients), then rapidly progressive depression in LOC
Visual disturbances
Pounding headache
Weakness/paralysis on one side of body
Drowsiness, ataxia, and stiff neck indicative of posterior fossa epidural hematoma

OBJECTIVE ASSESSMENT DATA

Pupil signs: dilated, nonreactive pupil with ptosis of eyelid on same side as hematoma
Depressed LOC with rapid progression to nonresponsive state
Vital signs:
  Blood pressure: increased

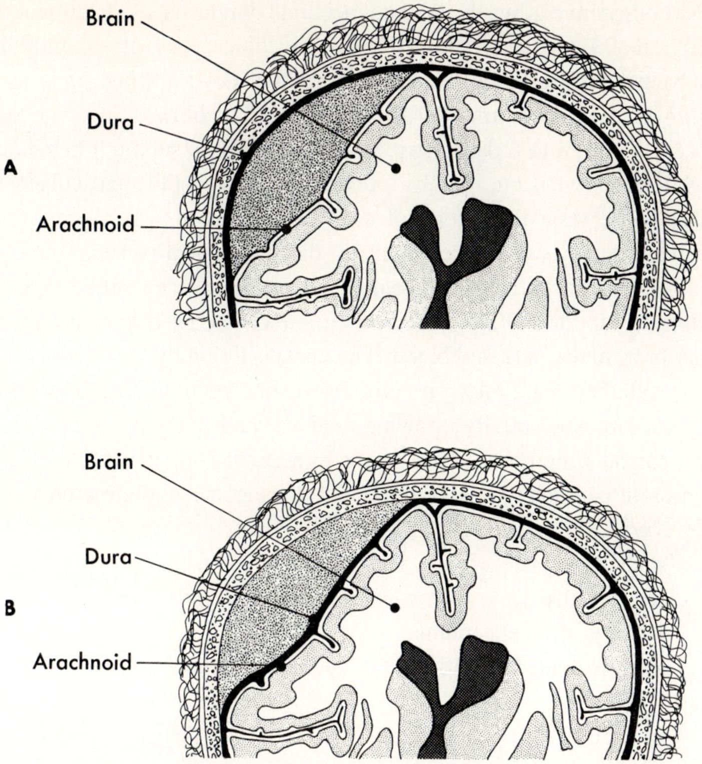

Fig. 9-7 **A,** Subdural and, **B,** epidural hematomas. (From Conway-Rutkowski, B.L.: Carini and Owens' neurological and neurosurgical nursing, ed. 8, St. Louis, 1982, The C.V. Mosby Co.)

Pulse: decreasing rate with arrhythmias
Respirations: decreased rate with irregular patterns
Temperature: normal or slightly elevated

Contralateral hemiparesis/paralysis
Contralateral jacksonian seizure activity
Positive Brudzinski's sign (with posterior fossa hematoma)
Diagnostic tests:
Skull radiograph: fracture of temporal or occipital skull bone; displaced pineal gland
Brain or CAT scan: location and size of hematoma

Subdural hematoma. A subdural hematoma is a collection of venous blood between the dura and arachnoid layer, which results in inward compression and displacement of brain structures (see Fig. 9-7). Unless treated promptly, compression and herniation of the brainstem can result. Without accurate diagnosis and treatment the mortality rate is 60% to 73% (Shea, 1981). There are three types of subdural hematomas: acute, subacute, and chronic. In acute formation deteriorating signs and symptoms occur within 24 to 48 hours after the injury (fall or blow). Subacute subdural hematomas occur within 3 to 5 days after the injury. Chronic subdural hematomas can develop or be detected weeks to months following a blow or fall, particularly in the elderly, who have a decreased elasticity of cerebral vessels and meninges. Subdural hematomas usually occur over the convexity of the frontal and parietal lobes.

In contrast to arterial bleeding, where there is no active mechanism for clotting, chronic subdural hematomas, which are venous in origin, are encapsulated by fibroblasts from the dura and blood. The encapsulation by fibroblasts causes the appearance of a calcified mass on x-ray film. However, when the fibroblasts disintegrate, the clot exerts osmostic activity, drawing fluid to equalize the pressure within the clot to that of the surrounding tissue. This results in an expansion of the clot and increased pressure on brain parenchyma with additional displacement of structures.

Nursing assessment

SUBJECTIVE ASSESSMENT DATA

Acute/subacute

- History of recent trauma
- Variable and fluctuating LOC or loss of consciousness
- Headache
- Irritability
- Weakness of facial muscles
- Weakness of limbs on one side of body
- Visual disturbances
- Infants/children: excessive crying, seizures, restlessness, and irritability

Chronic

- History of past trauma (occasionally forgotten)
- Impaired mental functioning
- Intermittent headache
- Behavioral changes
- Intermittent weakness of limbs on one side of body
- Increasing visual disturbances

OBJECTIVE ASSESSMENT DATA

Acute/subacute

- Fluctuating LOC or nonresponsive
- Contralateral hemiparesis/paralysis
- Babinski sign present
- Pupil signs: unequal, dilated, nonreactive pupil on same side as lesion
- Paresis of extraocular muscles
- Signs of increased ICP (Table 9-5)
- Hyperactive deep tendon reflexes
- Increased ICP readings: over 40 mm Hg or 540 mm H_2O with sustained A waves

- Infants:
  - Bulging fontanels
  - Fever
  - Papilledema
  - Enlarged head size (Fig. 7-3)
- Chronic
  - Depressed, fluctuating LOC
  - Impaired mental function
  - Changing sleep patterns
  - History of alcoholism, epilepsy, taking anticoagulants
  - Mild fever
  - Depressed or fluctuating LOC
  - Increasing ICP readings: 15-40 mm Hg or 200-540 mm H_2O with unsustained B and A waves
- Diagnostic tests
  - EEC: decreased activity over area of hematoma formation
  - CAT or brain scans: location and extent of hematoma, depressed parenchyma, and displacement of brain structures
  - CSF: appearance bloody, pressure elevated, leukocytosis

Intracerebral hemorrhage. Intracerebral hemorrhage usually results from severe blunt trauma, rupture of an existing aneurysm, or uncontrolled hypertension causing vessel rupture. The most common locations are the frontal and temporal lobes. Extensive midbrain and brainstem hemorrhages are usually quickly fatal. The diffuse effects are those of increasing brain volume with increased ICP (Simmons, 1978). Treatment is focused on reducing ICP. See pp. 279 and 280.

Head injury in infants and children

Because of the high activity level and the "exploring" tendency inherent in infants and children, head injuries are relatively common. Falls and bumps are part of growing up. The pathological problems resulting from severe head injury are the same in children as in adults: hematoma formation, acute edema, and transtentorial herniation. The progressive signs and symptoms of herniation include:

Early signs	Rationale
Headache and drowsiness	Tension on dural sinuses
Progressively decreased LOC	Ischemia
Ipsilateral pupil dilation	Compression of cranial nerve III
Contralateral hemiparesis	Compression of cerebral peduncle
Later signs (decompensation)	**Rationale**
Decrease in vital signs	Compression of medulla
Vomiting	Compression of medulla
Continued depression of LOC	Compression of reticular activating system
Bilateral pupil dilation and papilledema	Increased ICP
Decerebrate positioning	Brainstem compression

Aggressive therapy is initiated to decrease cerebral hypertension, thereby decreasing brain volume and the potential for herniation. Therapy includes:

1. Hyperventilation with bag/mask.
2. Administration of mannitol, 0.5-1 g/kg. NOTE: Mannitol is administered only when an expanding lesion is confirmed or when multiple clinical signs of herniation are present; not when unconsciousness is the only sign (Bruce, 1980).
3. Preparation for CAT scan. NOTE: Skull radiographs are not as diagnostically useful in infants and children as in adults. When bradycardia is present 2 to 48 hours after injury, a CAT scan is indicated (Bruce, 1980).

With acute hematoma formation, pediatric neurologists classify the signs and symptoms and the treatment measures by age group:

Signs and symptoms (0 to 1 year)

Commonly associated with child abuse (multiple bruises)
Irritability
Rapid onset of coma following shrill crying
Bulging fontanel
Increasing head circumference
Fixed, dilated pupil
Bradycardia
Seizure activity
Retinal hemorrhages
CAT scan: hematoma formation and shift of midline structures

Treatment protocol (0 to 1 year)

Hyperventilate with bag/mask
Tap fontanel (if retinal hemorrhages are present)
Prepare for surgery

Signs and symptoms (1 to 18 years)

Commonly associated with cerebral laceration resulting from severe trauma
Headache, drowsiness
Depressed LOC progressing to coma
Ipsilateral pupil dilation
Contralateral hemiparesis
Depression of vital signs
CAT scan: hematoma and shift of midline structures

Treatment protocol (1 to 18 years)

Endotracheal intubation and hyperventilation
Mannitol, 0.5-1 g/kg IV. NOTE: Mannitol is used *only* for confirmed expanding lesions, not for loss of consciousness alone.
ICP monitoring
20% of these patients require surgery (Bruce, 1980)

Increased intracranial pressure

Intracranial pressure (ICP) is constantly fluctuating with changes in blood pressure, activity, and altered respiratory patterns. Normally, ICP varies from 80 to 180 mm H_2O or 0 to 10 mm Hg with 15 mm Hg considered the upper limit of normal. When a person stands or exhales, ICP decreases. Table 9-3 delineates factors causing increased ICP (Mitchell and Mauss, 1976). Because of the rigidity of the adult skull, when there is an increase in any of the three intracranial components (brain, blood, CSF), ICP rises. Although fluctuations are normal, prolonged increased ICP results in decreased cerebral blood flow and/or supratentorial or infratentorial herniation. A cerebral blood flow of 30 mm Hg or less causes neural hypoxia and cell death. Herniation results in compression of the vital centers and of the reticular activating system in the brainstem (Hickey, 1981).

Because of the potentially devastating effects of sustained increased ICP, accurate serial nursing assessments are imperative. Many of the clinically observable changes in

Table 9-3 Factors increasing intracranial pressure

Precipitating factors	Caused by	Result
Hypercapnia (Pco_2 over 42 mm Hg)	Shallow respirations Sleep Comatose state Use of sedatives	Vasodilation
Hypoxemia (Po_2 under 50 mm Hg)	Nonpatent airway/endotracheal tube Inadequate ventilation Incorrect suctioning procedures Insufficient oxygen therapy	Vasodilation
Valsalva maneuver	Straining at stool Isometric exercises Turning in bed	Impedes venous flow from brain
Coughing/sneezing	Nonpatent airway Allergic reaction	Impedes venous flow from brain
Positioning	Angular neck flexion Prone/trendelenburg positioning Hip flexion	Impedes venous drainage
REM Sleep	Dreams	Local increase in cerebral activity with increased blood flow
Stress	Patient care measures Anxiety regarding status Family/personal problems Arousal from sleep Unfamiliar environment	Vasodilation

patient status are subtle. Obviously, continuous intracranial monitoring is the most reliable objective sign. However, this procedure is not commonly used outside of specialized hospitals. Therefore, pertinent nursing observation and documentation are essential. Table 9-4 correlates signs and symptoms with three pressure waves identified through intracranial monitoring.

Etiology. Causes of increased ICP are:

Cerebral edema resulting from a traumatic contusion with hematoma formation or after a craniotomy.

Vascular dysfunction because of insufficient cerebral blood flow or a venous obstruction.

Mechanical obstruction from compression or displacement of brain parenchyma or the CSF system.

Excessive CSF production or interferences with CSF absorption (Shea, 1981). Physiological factors precipitating increased ICP are hypercapnea and hypoxemia, both of which cause vasodilation of cerebral vessels.

Table 9-4 Correlation of ICP pressure waves with signs and symptoms with increased ICP

Wave	Signs and symptoms
A (plateau) Pressure: 50-100 mm Hg Time: 5-20 minutes	Decreasing LOC Increased systolic blood pressure with widening pulse pressure Altered respiratory patterns: Cheyne-Stokes respiration, central neurogenic hyperventilation Headache, particularly during position changes Paresis, decorticate or decerebrate positioning Dysphasia Abnormal pupil response Nausea/vomiting
B Pressure: 20-50 mm Hg Time: 0.5-2 min.	Correlates with respiratory changes Drowsiness, increased sleeping Variable, decreased LOC
C (Traube-Hering-Mayer) Pressure: 0-2 mm Hg Time: occurs every 3-8 minutes	Correlates with systemic arterial pressure Not considered clinically significant

Pathophysiology. When the volume of the cranial components increases, the autoregulatory mechanism for the vasculature of the brain is disrupted, thus impeding cerebral blood flow. To compensate for decreased cerebral flow and the subsequent retention of carbon dioxide and hypoxia of cells, the blood vessels dilate to increase cell oxygenation and facilitate removal of cell metabolic waste products. This vasodilation and increased cerebral flow increases the cranial volume resulting in increased ICP. This is called the stage of compensation. When the vasomotor compensatory mechanism fails, arterial and venous vascular collapse ensues, initially in the cerebral cortex, then progressing inward. This is the stage of decompensation (Hickey, 1981).

Nursing assessment. The traditional signs and symptoms of increased ICP correlated with cause are listed in Table 9-5. However, astute observation of the patient for earlier signs and symptoms is necessary. Early signs include:

Restlessness.
Variability in orientation and concentration.
Inability to focus visually (squinting, eye rubbing).
Purposeless movements, such as plucking at clothing or sheets, lip smacking.
Increasing headache, particularly on position changes.
Irregularity of pupils: oval-shaped.
Forced breathing (Mitchell and Mauss, 1976).

Because of the natural fluctuations in ICP, baseline and serial assessments and flow sheet documentation are necessary. Agency protocols state the frequency, commonly every 15 minutes until stable and then gradually prolonging the interval to every 4 hours depending on the patient's status.

Table 9-5 Correlation of signs and symptoms of increased ICP with cause

Signs and symptoms	Causes
Deteriorating LOC	Neural cerebral cortex hypoxia
Ispilateral pupil dilation (on side of lesion) progressing to bilateral dilation	Compression of cranial nerve III
Sluggish/nonreactive pupils	
Decreased extraocular movements	Compression of cranial nerves IV and VI
Increased systolic blood pressure with widening pulse pressure	Ischemia of vasomotor centers
Bradycardia (under 50-60/min) with bounding quality	Cardiac compensation to increase cerebrovascular resistance
Abnormal respiratory patterns	Pattern dependent of level of dysfunction. See Chapter 4, Fig. 4-3.
Decreased motor and sensory function (contralateral to lesion)	Pyramidal and ascending tract dysfunctions
Normal or gradually increasing temperature	Hypothalamic dysfunction
Headache (increased during position changes)	Increased carbon dioxide levels Traction on vessels at base of skull
Papilledema (late signs)	Pressure on optic nerves
Vomiting (projectile, without nausea)	Compression of vomiting centers in medulla

Interventions. Nursing measures are focused on preventing and controlling increased ICP. These interventions include:

1. Ensuring a patent airway by preventing accumulation of oral/pharyngeal secretions. This requires oral swabbing and hygiene or judicious suctioning. However, when ICP is increased, restraint in oral stimulation and suctioning is imperative.
2. Positioning the patient with the head elevated 30 degrees and with nonflexion of the neck to promote venous drainage.
3. Monitoring arterial blood gases to ensure adequate oxygen levels necessary for neural functioning.
4. Providing a cool environment to decrease systemic blood pressure with a subsequent decrease in cerebral blood flow and in metabolic oxygen demand.
5. Assess, document, and compare serial neurological and vital sign data.
6. Space patient care activities to prevent rises in systolic pressure and ICP.
7. Institute an every-2-hour turning schedule and passive range-of-motion (not isometric) exercises. Note that patient participation in these procedures increases ICP significantly.
8. Prevent constipation by providing foods/fluids that stimulate normal elimination.
9. Minimize/eliminate stress situations.

When increased ICP is evident from clinical signs or monitoring equipment, collaborative efforts of the nurse and physician are focused on decreasing cerebral hypertension and/or edema and on treatment of the underlying cause; for example, hematomas, hemorrhage, or infectious processes (Zegeer, 1982). Interventions included in patient care protocols include:

1. Maintenance of an effective airway (see p. 281).
2. Initiation of oxygen therapy with hyperventilation.
3. Administration of prescribed furosemide, mannitol, steroids, and anticonvulsants.
4. Restriction of fluids to 3000 ml for 48 hours.
5. Initiation of hypothermic measures.
6. Institution of ventricular drainage.
7. Initiation of barbituate therapy (Bowers and Marshall, 1982).

Specific information regarding these interventions is included in the nursing care plan on pp. 281 to 288.

Herniation of the brain

Herniation is a shifting of brain parenchyma from one compartment to another through the falx cerebri or tentorium cerebelli. The two most common causes of herniation are cerebral edema and space-occupying lesions. Herniation is classified as supratentorial or infratentorial. Supratentorial herniation involves lateral or downward displacement of cerebrum and midbrain structures. Infratentorial herniation can result in compression of the cérebellum and brainstem or in upward herniation exerting pressure on the midbrain (Merritt, 1979).

Supratentorial herniation. There are three types of supratentorial herniation:

Transtentorial: resulting in downward displacement of the cerebrum, basal ganglia, and midbrain structures.

Uncal: most often caused by temporal lobe expanding lesions resulting in lateral shift and compression/displacement of midline structures.

Cingulate: caused by a unilateral expanding lesions in the cerebrum resulting in displacement of parenchyma to the opposite side. The progressive signs and symptoms of transtentorial (central) and uncal herniation are detailed in Table 9-6. Unless interventions are initiated to decrease the brain edema or to remove the expanding lesion, brainstem herniation with compression of the vital centers in the pons and medulla occurs. Death ensues (Hickey, 1981).

Infratentorial herniation. Because the infratentorial space is small, an expanding lesion results in the rapid appearance of dysfunctional brainstem or cerebellar signs. Brainstem signs include:

Altered respiratory patterns: Cheyne-Stokes respiration, central neurogenic hyperventilation, ataxic, apneustic respirations.

Nonresponsive, comatose state.

Miotic fixed, nonreactive pupils with deviation toward the side of the lesion.

Hemiparesis progressing to hemiplegia.

Ocular and facial paresis.

Decerebrate positioning.

Cerebellar compression signs include:

Incoordination.

Paresthesias particularly in the neck and shoulders.

Stiff, arched neck.

Altered and variable respiratory patterns and pulse rate.

When herniation occurs, rapid neurosurgical intervention is imperative.

Interventions. In acute brain trauma, swift accurate interventions are essential if death and morbid states are to be prevented. As in all trauma, immediate priorities include ensuring:

Airway.

Breathing.

Circulation.

Airway

1. Chin lift or jaw thrust after cervical injury has been ruled out
2. Oral swabbing with tongue blade covered by moistened 4 × 4's
3. Oropharyngeal suctioning
4. Insertion of oral airway
5. Intubation criteria:
   a. Chest does not rise after swabbing/suctioning
   b. Nonresponsive to verbal or painful stimuli
   c. Cyanosis
6. Equipment:
   a. Nasotracheal tube
   b. Esophageal airway (prehospital)

Breathing. Oxygen therapy (100% humidified):

1. If patient can talk, provide nasal oxygen, 4-6 L/min per nasal prongs.
2. If patient is unable to talk, provide hyperventilatory assistance at 18-25 breaths or compressions per minute with pocket mask or Ambu bag. Mechanical ventilation is required (Shea, 1981).

Circulation. In many cases, the patient with brain trauma has multiple injuries and is in hypovolemic shock. When this is the situation:

1. Apply antishock trousers if systolic pressure is below 90 mm Hg (Fig. 9-17). NOTE: After intravenous infusions initiated to sustain blood pressure, follow manufacturer's directions for deflation.
2. Initiate intravenous Ringer's lactate and infuse at a rate to maintain 90 mm Hg systolic pressure. This also permits access for prescribed medications. Because the mortality rate from traumatic hematomas is 60% to 90%, prompt diagnosis and surgical intervention are imperative (Seeling, Becker, and Miller, 1981).

For care of the surgical patient see Chapter 10. For interventions related to hygiene, mobility, skin integrity, and the prevention of joint impairments see Chapter 4.

Table 9-6 Progressive signs and symptoms of central and uncal herniation*†

	Central syndrome				
	Early diencephalon	Later diencephalon	Midbrain—upper pons	Lower pons—upper medulla	Medulla
Pupils	Both small and reactive	⟶	Not equal in size, but each about midpoint and nonreactive	⟶	Dilated and fixed
Extraocular signs	May be normal or slightly roving, then difficulty with upward gaze	Difficulty with upward gaze	And dysconjugate gaze	⟶	⟶
Level of consciousness	Difficulty with concentration and becomes agitated or drowsy; then stuporous	Stuporous; coma	Deep coma	⟶	⟶
Motor	Contralateral hemiparesis to hemiplegia	Plus paratonic rigidity on ipsilateral side which becomes decorticate	Bilateral decerebration	Flaccidity with occasional decerebration	⟶
Sensory	Progressive deterioration	⟶	⟶	⟶	⟶
Babinski sign	No Babinski sign	Bilateral positive Babinski sign	⟶	⟶	⟶
Respirations	Cheyne-Stokes	⟶	And central neurogenic hyperventilation	Shallow	Ataxic, then ceases
Other			Wide variations in temperature (often very high)	Elevated	40.5° C and higher
			Many develop diabetes insipidus		
			Bradycardia	Pulse erratic (fast and then slow)	No vital signs
			Elevated systolic blood pressure	Blood pressure drops	
			Widening of pulse pressure		

	Uncal syndrome				
	Local early signs	Diencephalon—midbrain	Midbrain—upper pons	Lower pons—upper medulla	Medulla
Pupils	Unilateral, dilated pupil; sluggish, nonreactive	Unilateral, dilated, and fixed	Bilateral, dilated, fixed	→	→
Extraocular signs	May have a ptosis; slight weakness → of oculomotor innervated muscles	→ Slight weakness becomes paralysis	→ →	→ →	→ →
Level of consciousness	Little effect on consciousness; may notice restlessness *Once deterioration begins, can proceed to deep coma quickly*	Stupor; coma	Deep coma	→	→
Sensory	Progressive deterioration	→	→	→	→
Motor		With Kernohan's notch, hemiparesis on side of lesion Contralateral hemiparesis to hemiplegia; decerebration	Bilateral decerebration	Flaccidity with occasional decerebration	→
Babinski sign		Bilateral positive	→	No reflexes	→
Respirations		Cheyne-Stokes	Central neurogenic hyperventilation	Shallow	Ataxic, then cease
Other			Bradycardia Elevated systolic blood pressure Widening pulse pressure	Deterioration of vital signs	No vital signs
			Wide variations in temperature; may be grossly elevated	Elevated	40.5° C and higher

*An important point to keep in mind when observing a patient with a possible herniation syndrome is that there is predictable order to the development of signs and symptoms. The neurological deterioration in both central and uncal herniation proceeds in an orderly rostral-caudal scheme; the diencephalon, midbrain, pons, and finally the medulla are affected from the increasing pressure. Signs and symptoms characteristic of each area can be identified. Notice that the last stages of both central and uncal herniation are the same.

†Reprinted with permission from J. Hickey: Clinical practices of neurological and neurosurgical nursing, 1981, Philadelphia, J.B. Lippincott.

Nursing care plan: **BRAIN TRAUMA**

NURSING DIAGNOSIS	EXPECTED OUTCOMES	NURSING INTERVENTIONS
Potential for ineffective airway due to excessive secretions or vomitus	Patent airway	Suction oral pharynx (5 seconds) as necessary, according to agency protocol. NOTE: If rhinorrhea present, no suctioning. Suctioning can increase size of dural tear and risk of infection. Suction endotracheal tube according to agency protocol. NOTE: Hyperventilate before suctioning. Suction for only 15 seconds. Insert nasogastric tube through mouth and connect it to low suction to decompress stomach and prevent vomiting that might: (1) increase ICP; (2) occlude airway.
Potential for impaired gas exchange due to increased ICP, improper positioning, metabolic dysfunctioning, brain herniation NOTE: Carbon dioxide is a potent vasodilator	Po_2: 80-100 mm Hg Pco_2: under 30 mm Hg pH: 7.35-7.45	Position patient in semi-Fowler's position and change position every hour. Maintain tracheal alignment. Monitor serial blood gas analyses. Maintain prescribed oxygen therapy: 100% humidified oxygen at 4-6 liters per minute via Nasal prongs (see Chapter 4 for care of nasal prongs). Endotracheal tube with ventilator. Ventilator should be placed on right side of bed to prevent flexion of the larger left jugular vein (Shea, 1981). Positive end expiratory pressure machine (5 cm). Following acute stage encourage deep breathing and yawning. NOTE: Discourage coughing, which causes increased ICP. Observe for: Dyspnea and altered respiratory rate/pattern (report these to the physician immediately). See Fig. 4-3. Clinical signs of hypercarbia (increased carbon dioxide): Increased pulse, respiratory rate, and blood pressure. Dyspnea. Dizziness and feelings of "full head." Heart palpitations. Muscle twitchings. Convulsions. Progressive disorientation to nonresponsive state. NOTE: Rapidly decreasing carbon dioxide levels may cause ventricular fibrillation. Clinical signs of respiratory acidosis: Dyspnea at rest. Pallor or cyanosis. Tachycardia with dysrhythmias. Hyperkalemia.

Nursing care plan: **BRAIN TRAUMA—cont'd**

NURSING DIAGNOSIS	EXPECTED OUTCOMES	NURSING INTERVENTIONS
Potential for impaired tissue perfusion due to concomitant trauma	Blood pressure: 90 mm Hg systolic Capillary refill: 2 seconds	Regulate prescribed intravenous infusion to maintain 90 mm Hg systolic. Monitor blood pressure, pulses, skin color, and capillary refill.
Potential for cerebral edema with subsequent increased ICP due to cerebral hypertension or cellular edema	ICP: 0-10 mm Hg 80-180 mm H_2O	Position with head elevated 15-30 degrees and with neck straight. Monitor ICP readings (see Chapter 2). Ensure that ICP lines are functioning, that tubing is aligned, and that the ports are closed to prevent infections. NOTE: Some agencies have reported fewer infections with no changing of lines or routine flushing (Jones and Cayard, 1982). Maintain intravenous infusion rate to maintain 90 mm Hg systolic pressure NOTE: Fluid limitations following blood pressure stabilization are: 1000-1500 ml for 24 hours. 2000-3000 ml for 48 hours. Use of a microdrip infusion set increases the accuracy of slow infusion rates. Administer prescribed medications and document: Diuretics (if ICP is over 20 mm Hg): Furosemide (Lasix), 0.5 mg/kg IV (single dose). Mannitol, 0.25 g/kg IV. Dexamethasone (Decadron), 10 mg IV initial dose, then 4 mg every 4 hours. Dexamethasone is administered with Maalox to prevent gastric irritation when given orally. Maintain accurate intake and output records. Consider insensible water losses from diaphoresis and hyperventilation. Aseptically insert retention catheter and connect it to urometer and closed drainage system. Report output under 30 ml/hour to the physician. Discourage exertive activities such as: Valsalva maneuver: Administer prescribed stool softeners. Muscle contractions: Use a turning sheet for position changes. Ask alert patients to exhale when turning. Coughing: Provide liquids and encourage throat clearing. Schedule activities to allow for rest periods. Prepare patients with hematomas/hemorrhages for surgery for clot evacuation or arterial clamping (see Chapter 10).

Continued.

Nursing care plan: **BRAIN TRAUMA—cont'd**

NURSING DIAGNOSIS	EXPECTED OUTCOMES	NURSING INTERVENTIONS
Potential for cerebral hypoxia ischemia due to seizures, hyperpyrexia, or pain NOTE: These conditions increase the metabolic demand for oxygen	Normal cerebral cellular activity No seizures Body temperature: 97.6-98.6 F No complaints of pain	Administer and document prescribed prophylactic anticonvulsant agents. Initiate prescribed hypothermic measures: Cool environment: Remove covers and clothing. Ice water mattress, sponges, ice bags to axilla and groin. Acetaminophen (Tylenol) as prescribed per rectum for fevers over 101° F. If patient is shivering, administer prescribed chlorpromazine (Thorazine), monitoring for excessive decreases in blood pressure. NOTE: There is a 6% increase in cerebral blood flow for each degree of fever (Zeeger, 1982). Administer prescribed mild analgesics to control pain. NOTE: CNS depressants mask respiratory signs of increasing ICP.
Potential for fluid volume deficits due to fluid restriction or hyponatremia caused by the syndrome of inappropriate antidiuretic hormone secretion (SIADH) resulting in cerebral cellular edema	Blood pressure: 90/50 at minimum, normal skin turgor Balance of intake and output Serum sodium (Na^+): 132-142 mEq/L Urinary specific gravity: 1.001-1.010 Urinary osmolality: Dilute: less than 200 milliosmoles/dl	Infuse prescribed fluids at a rate to maintain 90 mm Hg systolic pressure. Monitor for signs and symptoms of dehydration: Skin turgor; Mucous membranes; Urinary output; Maintain strict intake and output records. Provide oral hygiene every 4 hours when fluids are restricted. Monitor electrolyte laboratory studies for imbalances. Observe for signs and symptoms of hyponatremia: Headache Bounding pulse Disorientation Abdominal cramps Test urinary specific gravity: < 1.001: overhydration > 1.010: dehydration NOTE: Low serum sodium, increased urinary sodium, and specific gravity equates with SIADH (Zeeger, 1982).
Potential for nutritional deficit	Maintenance of optimum weight, muscle mass, and tone	If the gag reflex is present in the oriented patient, provide preferred soft, easily masticated and digested foods. If the patient is comatose or lacks the gag reflex, provide gavage feedings (intermittent or continuous). NOTE: Cimetidine (Tagamet) is sometimes prescribed to inhibit gastric secretions, thereby preventing gastric ulceration.

Nursing care plan: BRAIN TRAUMA—cont'd

NURSING DIAGNOSIS	EXPECTED OUTCOMES	NURSING INTERVENTIONS
Altered urinary and fecal elimination due to immobility, decreased autonomic function, fluid restriction, administration of anti-inflammatory agents NOTE: Dexamethasone is ulcerogenic	Normal urinary output (minimum of 30 ml/hour) No fecal impaction or constipation No blood in stool	Assess for abdominal distention. Auscultate bowel sounds. Assess for bladder/colon distention. Maintain accurate output record (urinary and fecal). Note amount, color, odor, and consistency of feces. Provide the patient's preferred methods of promoting fecal elimination, such as prune juice, fruit nectar, peeled fresh fruit, warm water. Test cloudy urine with dipstick. Hemoccult test stools for occult blood. Note: Hemoccult is a more sensitive test than Benzidine (Guiac).
Personal identity confusion due to trauma and/or short term memory loss	Oriented to time, person, place	Address the patient by a familiar name (nickname, title). Converse with the patient while providing care; reorient patient to time, person, and place. Encourage family/significant others to talk with the patient (using a low vocal pitch and speaking slowly). Explain to the family that hearing is a sustained perception and that while there may be no verbal response, the patient may hear. Apply sensory aides (glasses, hearing aids) on the patient. Show the patient pictures of his family or familiar objects. Place a calendar and clock within eye range. Include the family in care provision, such as range-of-motion exercises, massage, hair care, makeup, and shaving.
Spiritual distress due to fear of death, unresolved problems, potential long-term effects of trauma	Spiritual needs met	Communicate availability of spiritual advisors. Call preferred rabbi, priest, or minister. Advise the patient of and turn on televised religious services of patient's preference. Keep religious articles, such as a rosary, prayer book, medals, crucifix, within reach or visual range of patient.
Disturbance in body image due to ICP monitoring equipment, hair shaving before a craniotomy	Positive body image	When the patient has intracranial monitoring equipment in place or has had a craniotomy, remove mirrors. Explain the usual occurrence of the quick return of hair, usually within 6 weeks. Encourage verbalization of fears regarding altered body image. Discuss physical appearance aids: such as wigs, caps, scarves.

Continued.

Nursing care plan: **BRAIN TRAUMA—cont'd**

NURSING DIAGNOSIS	EXPECTED OUTCOMES	NURSING INTERVENTIONS
Knowledge deficit: care measures used in the hospital and home care measures and resources	Understands rationale for procedures used in the hospital Demonstrates physical care measures States situations in which professional or community resources should be contacted	Explain all procedures before their initiation, emphasizing the rationale for actions and the patient's participation. Initiate a patient/family home care teaching plan following an assessment of the learner's physical, mental, and psychological readiness: Motor assessment: hand grasp and plantar flexion/extension. Passive range-of-motion methods. Positioning to prevent deformities. Communication techniques: low vocal pitch, distinct and slow speech. Use of mobility assistance devices: walker, cane. Bed-to-chair and vice versa transfer techniques. Food, fluid, and rest requirements. Discuss psychosocial needs for: Verbalizations of feelings such as fear, anger. Maintenance of some control: Encourage patient participation in determining the order of care measures. Provide written instruction sheets including: Procedures and care measures in sequential steps. Times to be done. Expected results. Listing of occurrences/situations when physician or other health care provider should be notified: Persistent vomiting Seizure activity Paresis/paralysis Persistent high fever or increasing temperature Severe/throbbing headache Double vision, focusing problems, pupil irregularity Name and phone number of whom to call. Inform patient/family of signs of posttraumatic syndrome commonly experienced by brain traumatized patients for several weeks to months and the usual treatment (aspirin). See Postconcussion syndrome (p. 269) in this chapter. Warn patient of lifetime continued sensitivity to CNS depressants including alcoholic beverages. Discuss activities of daily living that cause increases in ICP: Valsalva maneuver. Exercise, aerobic or isometric. Sexual intercourse. Breath holding. Performing multiple activities in rapid succession requires scheduling of exhausting activities at intervals. Inform patient/family of community assistance available such as visiting nurses associations, home health care, rehabilitation centers (speech, mobility), local service organizations that provide mobility or home care equipment, mental health/counseling services. Honestly respond to questions regarding recovery potential and timing.

SPINAL CORD TRAUMA

A high index of suspicion for spinal cord trauma exists with patients who are admitted with brain injury, multiple trauma, or unconscious states caused by vehicular accidents, falls, and sporting accidents. Precise on-site care, careful transport, and accurate initial hospital assessments and interventions are vital to prevention of an increase in the extent of damage and resultant dysfunctions. When cervical cord trauma is suspected, the ABCs for on-site care interventions are altered slightly:

A. Airway
B. Breathing
C. Cervical spine immobilization

Airway. Because hyperextension of the neck is contraindicated, insertion of an esophageal airway, blind nasotracheal intubation, or the use of a fiberoptic bronchoscope over which the endotracheal tube has been placed are recommended.

Breathing. If the breath cannot be felt and the chest is not rising, respiratory resuscitation is obviously essential. When either the endotracheal tube or esophageal airway are in place, oxygen can be administered by Ambu bag, pocket mask, or ventilatory assistance equipment. Oxygen flow at 6 to 10 L/minute is recommended. When the pocket mask or Ambu bag is used, the rate is 18 to 25 compressions/minute. Mouth-to-tube ventilatory resuscitation is another alternative.

Cervical immobilization. Immobilization of the cervical spine is accomplished before extrication and transport. One person is responsible for traction applied to the mandible and occiput during the immobilization procedure. A rigid cervical collar, sand bags, rolled blankets, or cravats are placed at the side of the victim's head. Flexible cervical collars are not effective immobilizers (Shea, 1981). A Velcro strap or adhesive tape is applied over the forehead to immobilize the head thoroughly (Fig. 9-8). Short backboards are used before extrication from automobiles. The patient is log-rolled onto a long backboard. Securing the victim on a long backboard with straps allows for lateral tilting in case of vomiting. It also permits head elevation without hip flexion for patients experiencing dyspnea or for those suspected of concomitant brain trauma.

Etiology

In descending order of incidence, the causes of spinal cord injury are:

- Vehicular accidents: car, cycles, boat.
- Falls from heights greater than the height of the victim or being hit by falling objects.
- Sporting accidents: trampoline, football, diving, gymnastics.
- Direct penetrating injuries: bullets, knife (Adams and Victor, 1981).

These incidents result in:

- Compression.
- Sectioning.
- Hyperflexion, extension, or rotational trauma.

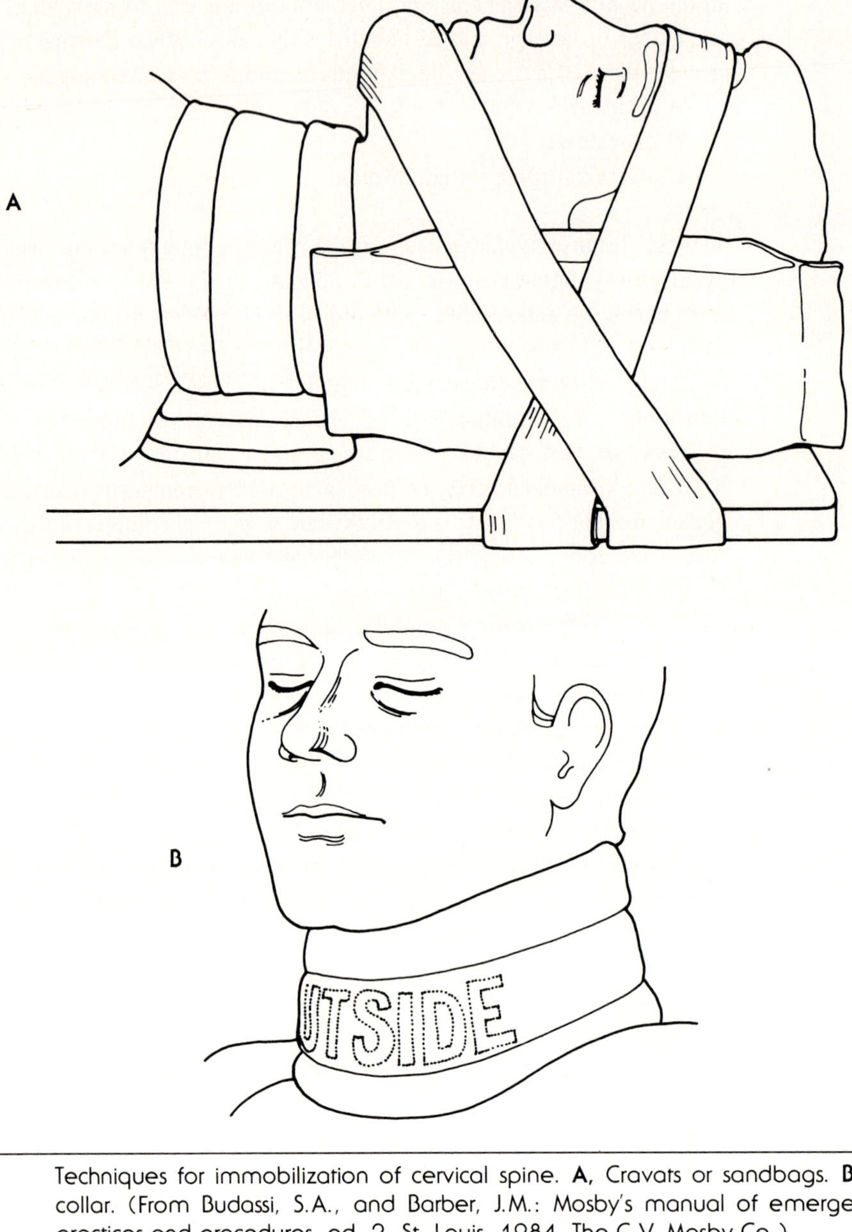

Fig. 9-8 Techniques for immobilization of cervical spine. **A,** Cravats or sandbags. **B,** Cervical collar. (From Budassi, S.A., and Barber, J.M.: Mosby's manual of emergency care: practices and procedures, ed. 2, St. Louis, 1984, The C.V. Mosby Co.)

Pathophysiology

The physiological sequence of events following spinal cord trauma are:

Edema (most significant within 48 hours of the injury).

Microhemorrhage at the trauma site and 1 to 2 segments above and below the lesion.

Compression of neural tissue and the motor and sensory tracts in the spinal cord.

Necrosis of neurons and tracts (Adams and Victor, 1981).

The clinical pathology is related to the extent and level of the edema, compression, and necrosis.

Extent

Transection

COMPLETE TRANSECTION. A complete transection causes a permanent loss of motor and sensory function distal to the transection because of the severance of ascending (sensory) and descending (motor) tracts. (For the location and functions of tracts see Fig. 9-9). Complete transection results in immediate spinal shock. Signs of spinal shock, which may last from several hours to 6 weeks, are listed in Table 9-7.

INCOMPLETE TRANSECTION. An incomplete transection causes a variable loss of motor and/or sensory function on the same side as the sectioning, depending on the tracts involved. With incomplete or complete cervical sectioning, Horner's syndrome occurs. Its symptoms include:

Ipsilateral ptosis of the eyelid and downward rotation of the eyeball.

Miotic pupil.

Ipsilateral facial anhidrosis.

Compression caused by edema or hemorrhage. Compression results in flaccid paralysis with variable sensory losses and sphincter disturbances distal to the compressed area. Because of the proximity to the brainstem and the small size of the cervical vertebrae, compression caused by hemorrhage in the cervical area is the most devastating, usually occurring within 1 to 4 hours after the accident. Clinical signs and symptoms are dependent on the level of the compression:

Cervical. Flaccid quadriplegia with loss of deep tendon reflexes and paresthesias or anesthesia of the trunk and extremities occurs (Fig. 9-10). Pain in the cervical area results from the direct injury or from edema. Autonomic dysfunction causes an absence of perspiration (except in the head, neck, and deltoid areas), decreased blood pressure, priapism (involuntary erection of the penis), and gastric/urinary/fecal retention. If the cervical cord trauma is above C4, respiratory distress or failure occur because phrenic innervation to the diaphragm is lost or diminished.

Thoracic. Compression of the thoracic cord causes high paraplegia involving the legs, trunk, and urinary and rectal sphincters (Fig. 9-11). The paralysis is flaccid initially. After 3 to 4 weeks, mass reflex activity is heightened resulting in spastic paralysis with tremulous, jerking leg movements.

Lumbar. Lumbar cord compression causes a persisting flaccid paraplegia of the legs, bladder, and rectum (Fig. 9-12).

Text continued on p. 297.

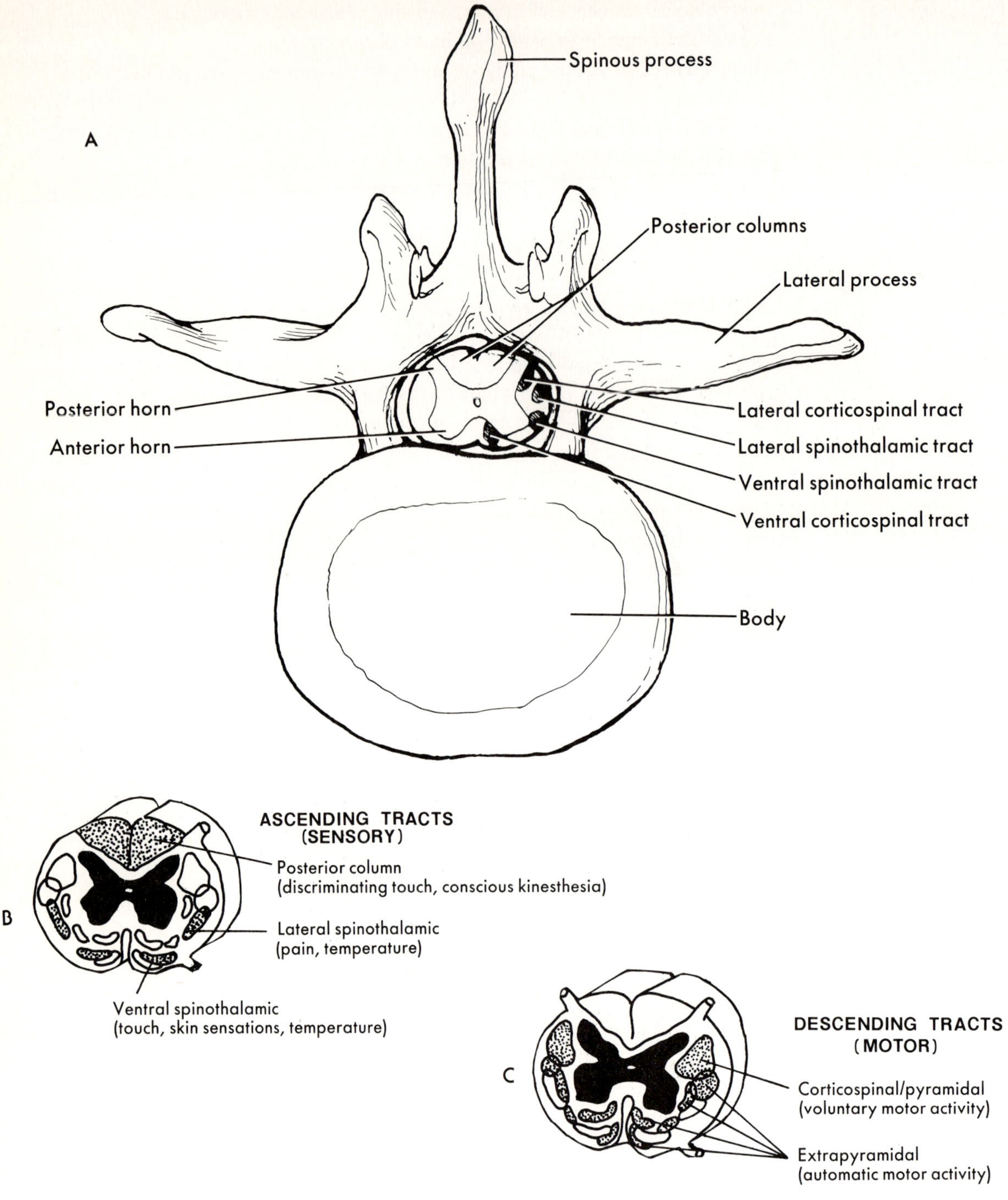

Fig. 9-9 **A,** Spinal cord within vertebra. **B,** Ascending tracts. **C,** Descending tracts.

Table 9-7 Signs of spinal shock

Signs	Rationale
Initial	
Decreased blood pressure (systolic under 80)	Peripheral vasodilation
Decreased pulse rate* (below 60)	
Depressed respiratory rate	Interruption of phrenic nerve
Skin: pink, warm, dry*	Dilation of cutaneous capillaries and sweat gland denervation as a result of inhibition of sympathetic nervous system
Decreased temperature	Inhibition of sympathetic nervous system
Immediate areflexia, flaccid paralysis, and loss of skin sensation below the lesion†	Interruption of ascending and descending tracts
Priapism in males	
24-48 hours after trauma	
Paralytic ileus	Inhibition of parasympathetic nervous system
Urinary retention	Inhibition of parasympathetic nervous system and altered pituitary and adrenal function
7-10 days after trauma	
Stress ulcers	Decreased gastric circulation
Decreased muscle tone/strength	Decreased neural transmission and immobility
Pulmonary/urinary infections	Immobility; urinary retention catheter; lack of respiratory hygiene

*Signs differentiating neurogenic from hypovolemic shock. In hypovolemic shock the pulse rate is increased and the skin is cool and moist.

†Within several weeks affected muscles may become spastic.

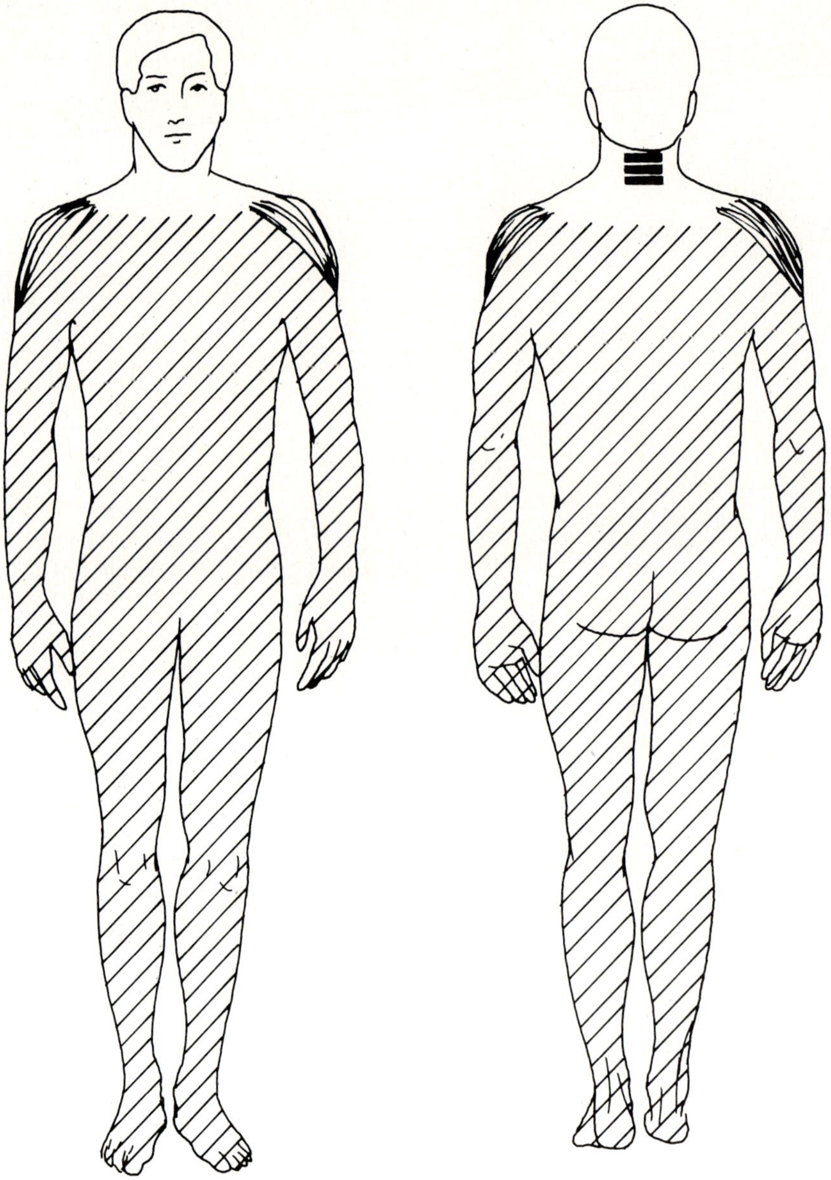

Fig. 9-10 Quadriplegia caused by cervical cord trauma. If cervical injury is at C4, phrenic nerve dysfunction results in respiratory distress.

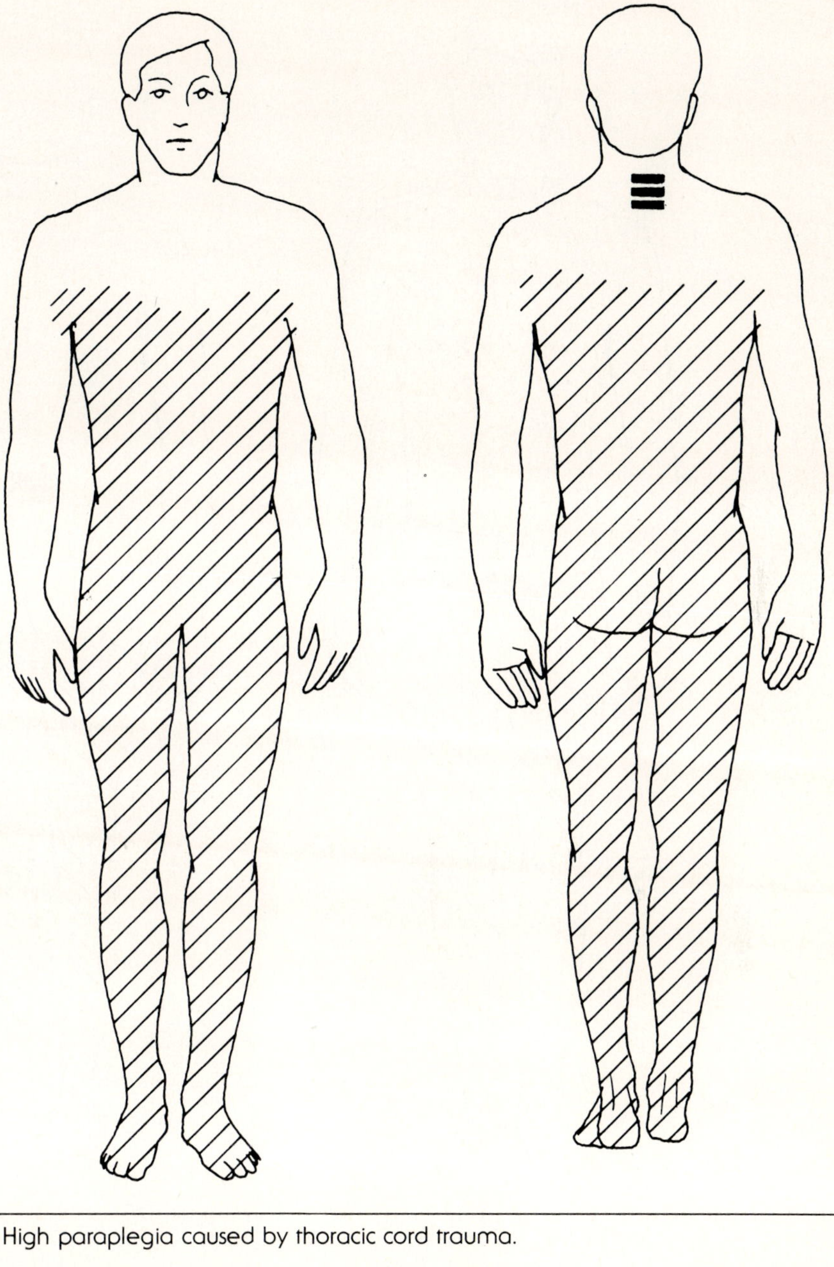

Fig. 9-11 High paraplegia caused by thoracic cord trauma.

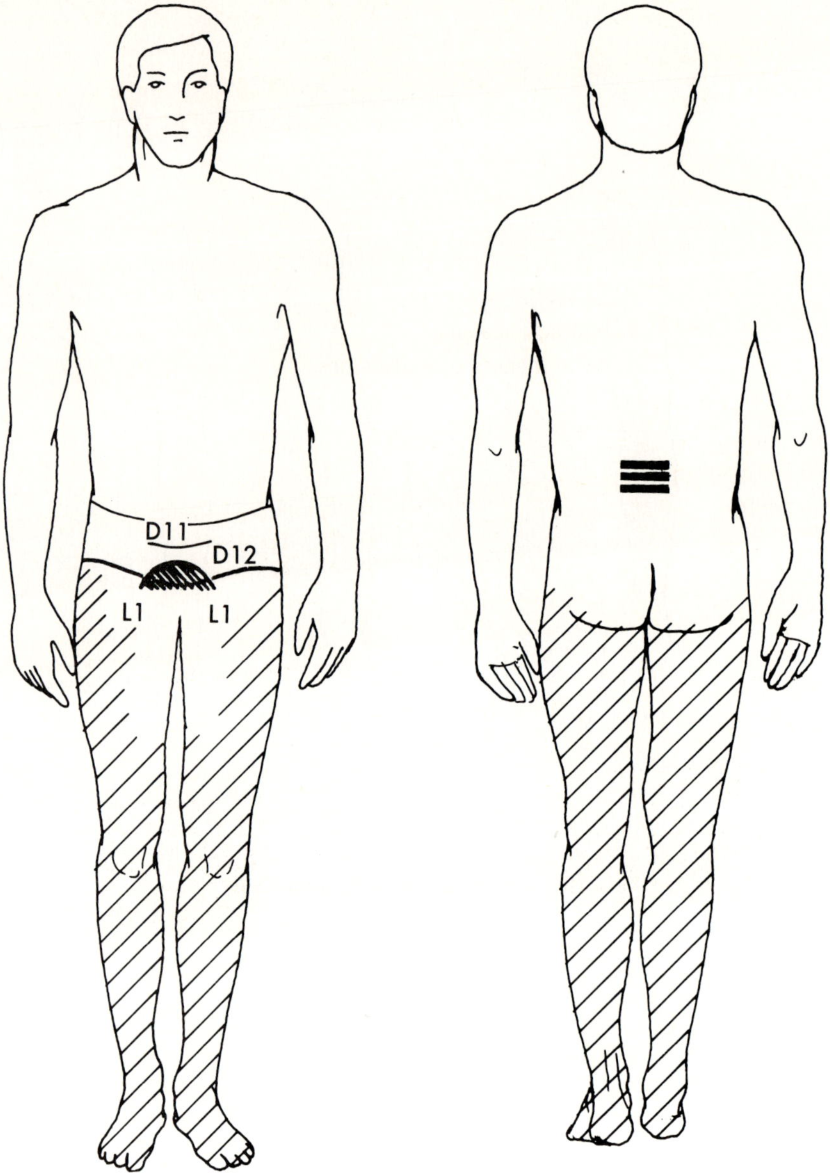

Fig. 9-12 Paraplegia caused by lumbar cord trauma.

Classification

Spinal injuries are classified as:

- Compression.
- Sectioning (complete or hemisectioning).
- Hyperextension, hyperflexion, or rotational trauma (Fig. 9-2).

Nursing assessment

Initial and continuing assessments of the extent of the dysfunction are prerequisite to prompt treatment to prevent further damage to the spinal cord.

Subjective assessment data

History of accident, trauma, fall, injuries involving acceleration/deceleration or rotational movements.

Pain at or above the level of the lesion, sometimes radiating to the extremities in incomplete lesions

Tingling/numbness of extremities

Fever

Lack of perspiration/sweat

Weakness or paralysis of extremities

If the trauma occurred more than 1 week previously, spasticity below the level of the lesion is likely

Difficulty in breathing

Inability to void/defecate or incontinence

Objective assessment data

Flaccid paralysis below the level of the lesion

Pain elicited by movement/pressure

Initial exaggerated tendon reflexes followed by loss of tendon reflexes

Paresthesias or anesthesia distal to lesion

Bladder distention

Bowel distention with sphincter alterations

Rectal examination signs as summarized in Table 9-8

Priapism, indicative of cervical injury

Dyspnea, abdominal breathing

Apnea, indicative of cervical injury above C4

Babinski sign present when sectioning/compression of descending motor (pyramidal) tracts has occurred

Signs of spinal shock (Table 9-7)

Diagnostic tests

- Radiographic. NOTE: It is imperative that the patient remain immobilized on the backboard until x-ray films have been taken and *interpreted* by the physician. Movement must be prohibited if additional spinal cord trauma is to be averted. The nurse or physician should accompany the patient to the x-ray or scan department to protect and support the patient

Table 9-8 **Neurological rectal examination for patient with acute spinal cord injury to determine neurological deficits**

Rectal tone	Rectal sensation	Neurological loss
Present (with bulbocavernosus reflex*)	Absent	Complete
Absent	Absent	Complete
Absent	Present	Incomplete†
Present	Present	Incomplete‡

*Involuntary spinal reflex.
†Chance of greater sensory return.
‡Good recovery is a possibility.

Spinal x-rays: visualization of vertebral fractures and displacements
Myelogram: location of obstruction in CSF flow
Spinal CAT scan: visualization of size and location of lesion

Lumbar puncture with spinal dynamic maneuvers and CSF examination

Lumbar puncture: increased opening pressure

Spinal dynamics procedure: Following the lumbar puncture two maneuvers can be used:

Abdominal straining: Patient is requested to hold breath and strain as if having a bowel movement for 10 seconds. Normal: CSF pressure increases but returns to normal after 30 seconds.

Jugular compression (Queckenstedt's test): Pressure is applied to the jugular veins bilaterally for 10 seconds. Normal: Immediate CSF pressure increase returning to normal within 30 seconds. Abnormal: Slow rise and delayed fall equates with a partial block. No rise after 10 seconds indicates complete obstruction in spinal canal. NOTE: (1) Because of the danger of increased ICP, this test is done infrequently. (2) Before jugular compression, whether done by digit or by a blood pressure cuff, the patient should be warned that facial flushing and warmth and a feeling of a "full head" will be experienced. (3) Spinal dynamics are contraindicated when the patient has a concomitant head injury or increased ICP.

CSF examination: increased protein, bloody CSF
Electrocardiogram: to determine cardiac dysrhythmias or baseline readings
Arterial blood gases: to determine oxygen and pH levels

Interventions

Because of the potentially devastating outcome of spinal cord trauma, regional spinal cord injury (SCI) centers have been designated by many states to provide specialized patient care (MacKechnie, 1982). In some instances, the SCI center develops protocols (Fig. 9-13) to standardize quality care and expedite transfer to the SCI agency. The goal is to sustain vital functions and prevent further injury to the spinal cord.

Table 9-9 Specific dysfunction of spinal neves

Plexus/nerve	Spinal nerve origin	Dysfunctions	Causes
Brachial plexus	C5-T1	External rotation and adduction of arm Impaired arm raising and maintenance Upward, inward fixation of scapula Impaired arm flexion, supination and loss of hand/finger dexterity Sensory deficits: deltoid, triceps, and radial aspect of forearm	Trauma to neck/shoulder girdle Pressure injury
Median nerve	C6	Impaired forearm pronation Loss of thumb/finger opposition and hand dexterity Weak flexion of wrist, hand, and fingers Atrophy of hand and forearm muscles Anhidrosis of hand and forearm Sensory deficits: palm, thumb, index, and middle finger	Shoulder avulsion/dislocation
Ulnar nerve	C8, T1	"Claw hand" (Volkmann's contracture) Atrophy of hand muscles and forearm Loss of hand/finger dexterity Sensory deficits: ring and little finger.	Elbow fracture/dislocation
		Horner's syndrome: ptosis, facial anhidrosis, decreased palpebral fissure, appearance of "sinking eyeball," miosis	Paralysis of cervical sympathetic nerve at C8-T1
Radial nerve	C7, C8	Wrist drop with impaired flexor abilities of elbow, wrist, fingers, and thumb	Pressure from crutches
		Unable to grasp or make fist Impaired forearm supination	Humerus fracture
Femoral nerve	L2-L4	Impaired hip flexion Abduction with external leg rotation Decreased quadriceps muscle tone with atrophy Impaired leg extension Hypoactive patellar reflex Impaired sensation in anterior lateral thigh area	Pressure from pelvic neoplasm or hematoma Pelvis fracture
Sciatic nreve	L4-S3	Lack of knee flexion ability Paresis of lower leg and gluteal muscles Inward rotation of leg Foot drop Thigh pain Sensory deficits: thigh, knee, and lower leg	Fractured pelvis/femur Penetrating trauma Incorrect intramuscular medication administration
Peroneal nerve	S1-S3	Footdroop Inability to evert foot Sensory deficits: instep area and lateral aspect of leg	Leg traction or restraint

INITIAL CARE OF A PATIENT WITH SPINAL CORD INJURY

1. PREPARE EQUIPMENT FOR PATIENT'S ARRIVAL

2. PREVENT FURTHER INJURY TO CORD
   - RECEIVE PATIENT AND MAINTAIN ALIGNMENT ON LONG SPINAL BOARD
   - USE OF SANDBAGS ON EITHER SIDE OF HEAD AND 3" TAPE ON FOREHEAD FOR STABILIZATION IS ESSENTIAL

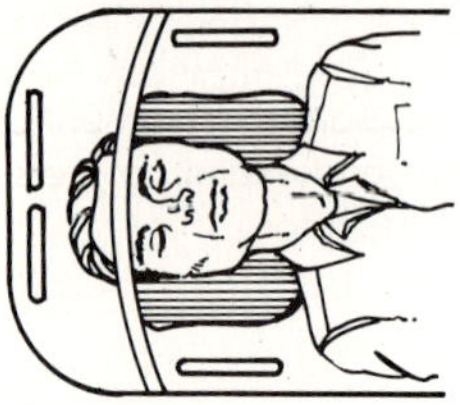

3. TREAT BREATHING DIFFICULTY FIRST
   - MAINTAIN PATENT AIRWAY
   - KEEP HEAD AND NECK IN NEUTRAL POSITION
   - TAPE ORAL AIRWAY IN PLACE AND SUCTION AS NECESSARY
   - O_2 4 L/MIN VIA NASAL CANNULA
   - AMBU-BAG PATIENT AT 12-16 BREATHS/MIN IF RESPIRATORY EFFORT INSUFFICIENT
   - OBTAIN BLOOD FOR BLOOD GASES, TYPE AND CROSS MATCH AND HCT.

4. ESTABLISH CIRCULATION
   - ADMINISTER CPR FOR ABSENT PULSE
   - MONITOR AND RECORD VITAL SIGNS
   - MONITOR CARDIAC PATTERN AND RATE
   - ESTABLISH AND MAINTAIN I.V. WITH LARGE BORE NEEDLE USING D5½ NS AT 100 CC/HR. (UNLESS SUSPECTED HEAD INJURY - RATE K.V.O.)
   - FOR HYPOTENSION ELEVATE FOOT OF LONG SPINE BOARD UNLESS PATIENT HAS SUSPECTED HEAD INJURY (CONTRAINDICATED IN H.I.)

5. REDUCE SPINAL CORD EDEMA
   - GIVE DECADRON 10 MG I.V. PUSH OVER 5 MINUTES AFTER CONTACTING PHYSICIAN (IF NOT ALREADY ADMINISTERED ENROUTE)
   - INSERT SILASTIC FOLEY CATHETER AND START MANNITOL 20% I.V., GIVE IN 500CC OVER 1 HOUR; MAKE SURE SILASTIC CATHETER IS IN PLACE

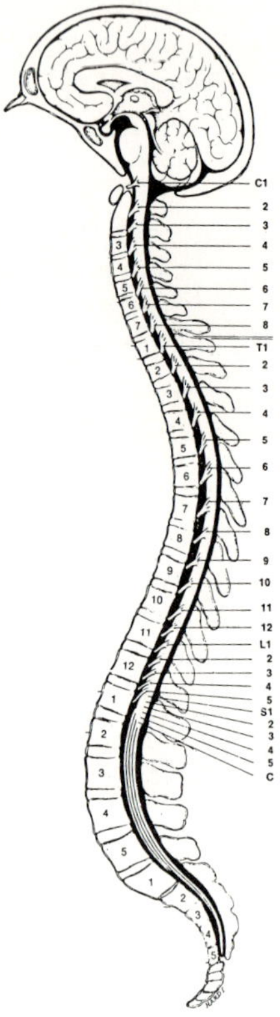

6. TREAT ILEUS
   - INSERT NO. 18 SUMP NASOGASTRIC TUBE

7. PERFORM NEUROLOGICAL ASSESSMENT
   - EVALUATE AND EXAMINE PATIENT FOR LEVEL OF SPINAL CORD INJURY AND OTHER INJURIES
   - DETERMINE LEVEL OF CONSCIOUSNESS
   - EXAMINE PUPILS FOR SIZE, EQUALITY AND REACTION TO LIGHT
   - EXAMINE EXTREMITIES FOR STRENGTH AND RANGE OF MOTION
   - EXAMINE FOR SENSORY IMPAIRMENT
   - MARK THE INITIAL SENSORY DEFICIT LEVEL ON THE PATIENT BY USING A MAGIC MARKER
   - EXAMINE DEEP TENDON REFLEXES

8. OBTAIN APPROPRIATE X-RAYS
   - OBTAIN X-RAYS ACCORDING TO LEVEL OF INJURY
   - SEND ALL X-RAYS WITH PATIENT WHEN TRANSFERRED TO SPINAL CORD CENTER

9. TETANUS PROPHYLAXIS

10. TRANSFER TO SPINAL CORD INJURY CENTER, BAPTIST HOSPITAL, PENSACOLA, FLORIDA

11. EXPEDITE TRANSFER
    - AIR TRANSPORT AVAILABLE VIA LIFE FLIGHT HELICOPTER

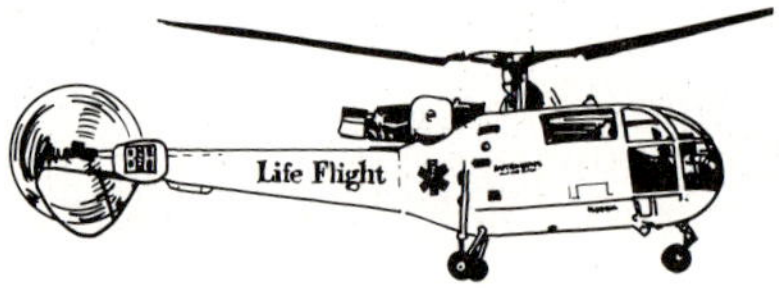

   - A COPY OF THE EMERGENCY ROOM TREATMENT RECORD SHOULD ACCOMPANY THE PATIENT
   - TRANSFERRING PHYSICIAN'S AND ACCEPTING NEUROSURGEON'S NAME SHOULD BE AVAILABLE IF POSSIBLE.

12. CONTACT BAPTIST HOSPITAL SPINAL CORD TREATMENT CENTER BEFORE TRANSFER

BAPTIST HOSPITAL
LIFE FLIGHT
24 Hour Service
CALL: FLA 1-800-342-3222
ALA 1-800-874-1555
LOCAL 434-4555

Fig. 9-13 Initial care of a patient with spinal cord injury. (Courtesy J.N. MacKechnie, Baptist Hospital, Pensacola, Florida.)

Nursing care plan: SPINAL CORD TRAUMA

NURSING DIAGNOSIS	EXPECTED OUTCOMES	NURSING INTERVENTIONS
Ineffective airway clearance	Patent airway	Assess for signs of airway obstruction and hypoxia. If airway is obstructed: Swab/suction oropharyngeal obstruction material. Insert and secure airway: Oropharyngeal. Esophageal obturator. Nasotracheal tube.
Impaired gas exchange	Po_2: 80-100 mm Hg	Provide oxygen therapy: 100% humidified oxygen at 6-10 L/min per bag, mask, cannula until Po_2 is 80. Clean nasal cannula daily with warm water. NOTE: Alcohol disintegrates polyethelene products. Ventilatory assistance equipment used includes: PEEP (positive end expiratory pressure). Mechanical respirator. Following stabilization, maintain scheduled respiratory toilet regime: Deep breathing exercises every 2-4 hours. Position changes every 2 hours. Use of incentive spirometer, blow bottles, maximal sustained inspiration technique. Provide sufficient environmental humidity. Nasal hygiene: warm moist wash cloth to cleanse nares. Monitor: Arterial blood gases. Pulmonary function tests.
Potential for further injury to cord due to patient transfer, position changes, or cord edema	Cord edema decreased Spine immobilized	Maintain immobilization on long backboard until x-rays are interpreted. Administer prescribed steroids: Dexamethasone (Decadron), 10 mg IV push over 5 minutes. In some agencies higher doses are administered. Assess and record initial and serial neurological data. Assessment for concomitant injuries is also necessary. Consistently use log-rolling technique with turning sheet. Assist with application of skeletal traction: Crutchfield tongs. Tippi-Wells tongs (Fig. 9-14). Halo brace (Fig. 9-15). Procedure for application of and care for a patient with a Halo brace are listed in Tables 9-10 and 9-11 (Hummelgard and Martin, 1982) A valuable patient teaching pamphlet entitled "You and your Halo brace" by Janeen Johnson, who wore one, contains practical hints. It is available upon request from Ace Orthopedic Co., Edina, Minn. Position patient on: Bed with firm mattress, bedboards, and flotation mattress. If tongs are applied, position head at bottom of bed. Sryker frame (Fig. 9-16). Rotation bed. See Chapter 11.

Continued.

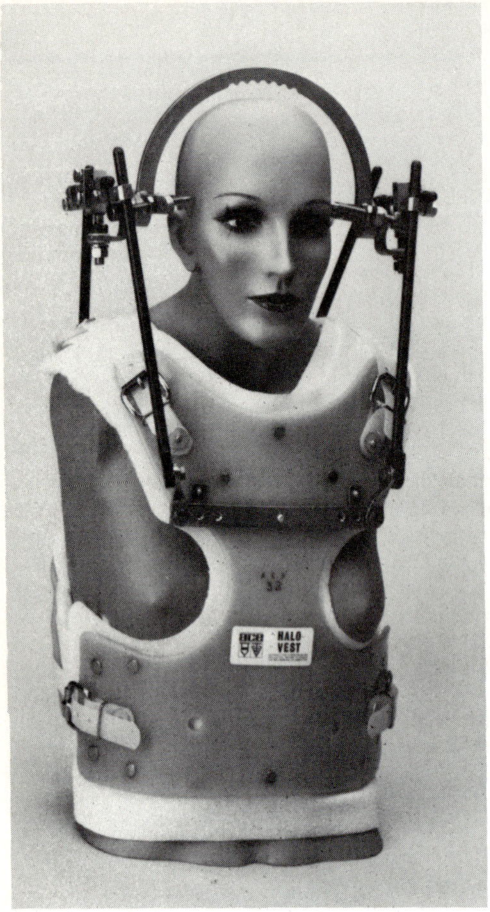

Fig. 9-14

Tippi-Wells tongs. (Courtesy Ace Orthopedic Company, Inc., Edina, Minn.)

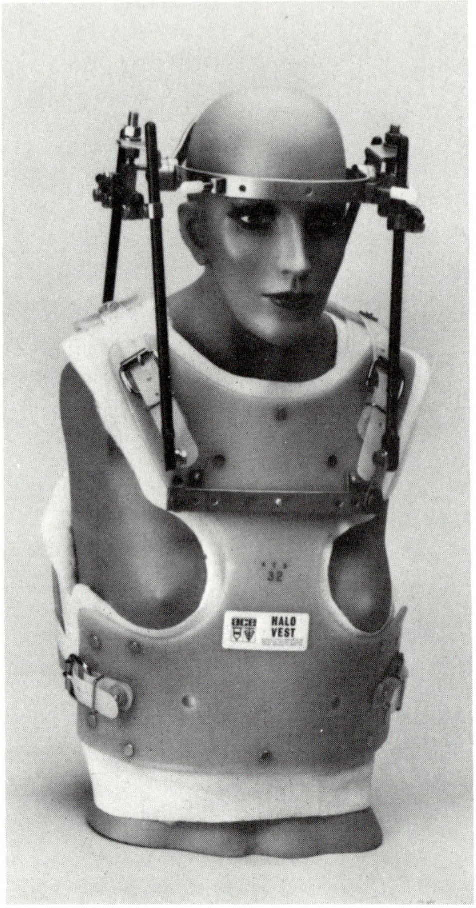

Fig. 9-15

Halo brace. (Courtesy Ace Orthopedic Company, Edina, Minn.)

Table 9-10 Typical sequence for application of halo brace*

Application of the halo ring

1. Measure the patient's head for approximate ring size.
2. Assemble equipment:
   Sterile halos in several sizes.
   Four sterile skull pins and locking plates
   Four sterile positioning pins
   Two torque screwdrivers
   Razor or hair clippers
   Povidone-iodine scrub
   Local anesthetic—1 percent lidocaine
   Sterile syringe and needle
   Sterile gloves
   Positioning board covered with sterile towel (optional)
   Sheepskin-lined vest and superstructure
3. Place the patient in a supine position with the head beyond the edge of the bed or stretcher. The head may be supported by a board placed under the patient's head and back, by an assistant's hands, or both.
4. Shave and trim hair about 5 cm. around each pin site.
   Scrub scalp with povidine-iodine.
5. Position the halo around the head with the raised portion at the back.
6. Place the positioning pins in holes adjacent to those to be used for the skull pins so that the halo is symmetrically around the skull.
7. Infiltrate the 4 pin sites with local anesthetic.
8. Insert all 4 skull pins into holes. Tighten pins by hand, alternating front and back. The patient's eyes should be closed to prevent the skin from puckering around skull pins.
9. When satisfied that skin is not under tension and position is correct, *simultaneously* tighten opposing skull pins with torque screwdrivers to the desired tightness. The suggested maximum is 5-5.5 inch/pounds for adults and 4 inch/pounds for children or adults with osteoporosis. The simultaneous torquing of the screws prevents side to side migration of the halo.
10. Tighten the locking plate on each screw.
11. Remove the positioning pins.

Application of the vest and superstructure

1. Attach the two angled uprights to the posterior vest and the two straight uprights to the anterior vest.
2. Slip the posterior vest under the patient's back so that the shoulder pieces touch the shoulder. (The patient may be log-rolled to one side or lifted to a partial sitting position while alignment is maintained.)
3. Return the patient to the supine position.
4. Attach the threaded uprights (or support bars) to the halo ring and set their position on the posterior upright. Tighten down.
5. Attach linkage assembly to give third point fixation.
6. Place anterior vest on the patient and fasten straps snugly.
7. Attach anterior upright to the posterior upright and tighten down.
8. Verify cervical alignment radiographically.

The skull pins should be retorqued only once. This is done 24-36 hours after application, which allows time for tissue necrosis to occur at the pin site.

*From Hummelgard, A., and Martin, E.: Management of the patient in a halo brace, JNN **14**(3):117, 1982.

Table 9-11 Care of patient with a halo brace

Clean pin sites:
- Swab crusting or drainage away with half-strength peroxide, soap and water, or povidone-iodone. Apply antiinfective ointment.

Time: Initially 3 times daily. More frequently if infected. If infected, administer prescribed systemic antibiotic.

Assess for loose pins or superstructure:
- Pins: Listen for clicking sound.
  - Observe for erythema, skin puckering, or increased drainage at pin sites.
  - Report loosened pins to physician.
- Superstructure: Observe for loosened bolts. NOTE: Superstructure and vest should *never* be used to turn patient.

Assess skin under vest daily for pressure sores. Prevent pressure sores by applying extra padding or by vest trimming by orthotist.

Provide skin care under vest:
- Use a damp washcloth and dry skin thoroughly.
- Ensure a dry sheepskin liner. A cool blow drier can be used.

Change patient's position every 2 to 4 hours.

Remind ambulatory patients of the decreased peripheral vision and the need to adjust their balance because of the extra weight (10 lbs).

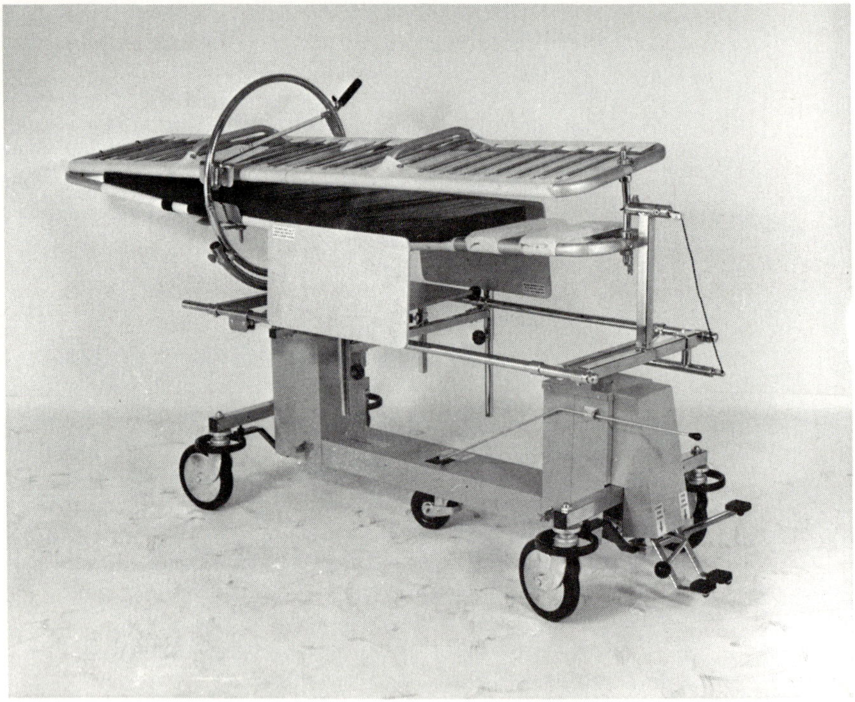

Fig. 9-16 Stryker frame. (Courtesy Stryker Corporation, Kalamazoo, Mich.)

Nursing care plan: SPINAL CORD TRAUMA—cont'd

NURSING DIAGNOSIS	EXPECTED OUTCOMES	NURSING INTERVENTION
Altered tissue perfusion due to impaired circulation caused by immobilization or hypovolemic shock from concomitant injuries	Blood pressure: 90/50 Capillary refill: 2 seconds	Assess circulatory status: Blood pressure. Peripheral pulses. Capillary refill in extremities. Peripheral skin for color, warmth, presence/absence of perspiration. Initiate prescribed intravenous infusion; dextrose in water or half strength saline or Ringer's lactate. Infuse at rate sufficient to maintain 90 mm Hg systolic. Apply antishock trousers per protocol for hypovolemic shock (Fig. 9-17). Manufacturers provide inservice on application if requested. Directions of manufacturer should be followed accurately.

Continued.

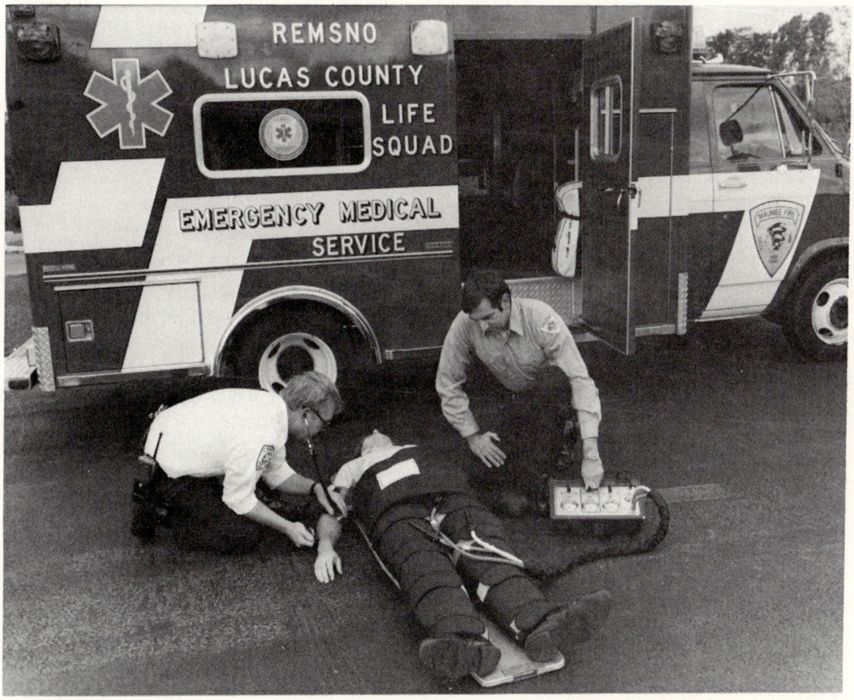

Fig. 9-17 Antishock pants. (Courtesy The Jobst Institute, Inc., Toledo, Ohio.)

NURSING DIAGNOSIS	EXPECTED OUTCOMES	NURSING INTERVENTION
Potential for fluid volume alteration and electrolyte imbalance	Electrolyte balance to ensure normal nerve transmission Adequate hydration to maintain tissue perfusion with balance of intake and output	Assess for signs of dehydration/edema: Skin turgor. Oral mucosa. Lung sounds. Sacral area edema. Peripheral extremities. Body weight. Monitor laboratory tests: Electrolyte studies. Hematocrit. Measure specific gravity of urine. Maintain accurate intake and output records. Following 48 to 72 hours of fluid restriction, encourage fluid intake up to 2500 ml daily.
Potential for autonomic dysreflexia due to stimulation of the sympathetic nervous system. NOTE: Incidence is reported as high as 85% for patients with lesions at T6 and above. Causes summarized in Table 9-12.	Normal autonomic function	Observe for signs and symptoms of dysreflexia: Extreme intermittant blood pressure elevation. Severe throbbing headache particularly behind the eyes. Increased pulse rate, bounding quality, followed by bradycardia with dysrhythmias. Profuse diaphoresis above the level of the lesion. Flushed skin above the level of trauma; pallor below the level of the lesion. Nasal congestion. Visual disturbances. Gooseflesh with piloerection. Nausea; occasionally, complaints of metallic taste. NOTE: Continuing autonomic stimulation can cause: Retinal hemorrhage. Cerebrovascular accident. Seizure activity. Initiate measures to prevent autonomic dysreflexia: Ensure patency of urinary catheter. Cautiously insert catheter, suppositories, and rectal tubes. Keep bed free of sharp objects and wrinkles. Ensure correct placement of urinary drainage bag. Maintain turning schedule. Prevent spastic contractures by using splinting devices and range-of-motion exercises. Initiate physician/protocol procedures to treat dysreflexia: Instillation of lidocaine (Xylocaine) into bladder to reduce excitability. Gently remove fecal impaction. Apply lidocaine or debucaine ointment to rectum to decrease excitability. Administer prescribed adrenergic blockers (phentolamine), vasodilators (dioxide), or ganglionic blockers (guanethidine).
Potential for gastric distention due to spinal-shock-induced interruption of autonomic nervous system	No gastric distress, distention, or vomiting	Insert nasogastric tube and connect it to low intermittent suction.

Table 9-12 Causes of autonomic dysreflexia

Area	Causes
Bladder	Occluded/kinked catheter
	Bladder spasms
	Catheterization
	Irrigation (too fast or cold fluid)
	Drainage bag not lower than bladder level
	Bladder stones or infection
Bowel	Fecal impaction
	Injudicious rectal examination
	Impaction removal
	Suppository/rectal tube insertion
	Enema
	Excessive flatus
Skin	Extremes of heat/cold
	Decubiti
	Lack of position changes
	Catheter pull
	Testicle pressure
	Ingrown toenails
	Infections/rashes/lacerations

Nursing care plan: SPINAL CORD TRAUMA—cont'd

NURSING DIAGNOSIS	EXPECTED OUTCOMES	NURSING INTERVENTIONS
Impairment of urinary elimination due to loss of bladder/sphincter innervation, immobilization, or infection	Normal urinary output No urinary tract infection or stones	Insert retention catheter and connect it to a closed drainage system for 48-72 hours. In some agencies intermittent catheterization has replaced retention catheters to reduce the potential for infection. Monitor and record urinary output. NOTE: Some agencies prefer intermittent catheterization (every 4-8 hours or as needed) until bladder training is initiated. See Chapter 11 for bladder training procedure. Provide acid-ash foods/fluids of patient's preference to maintain urine acidity, thereby decreasing the potential for bladder infections; for example, cranberry, prune, and plum juice, eggs, meat, fish, cereals and bread. Limit milk intake to 8 oz daily to prevent formation of calcium kidney stones (Heaney, 1982). NOTE: Within 24 hours of immobilization, the process of osteoporosis begins. Calcium is drawn from the bones into the blood, resulting in calcium-based kidney stones.

Continued.

Nursing care plan: SPINAL CORD TRAUMA—cont'd

NURSING DIAGNOSIS	EXPECTED OUTCOMES	NURSING INTERVENTION
Potential for nutritional deficit due to immobilization procedures preventing normal sitting position	Adequate nutritional intake to maintain optimum weight Normal muscle mass/tone	Provide high protein/vitamin diet with carbohydrate amount dependent on weight loss/gain. NOTE: Adequate nutrition prevents decubiti formation and preserves muscle mass/tone. Monitor weight weekly. Excessive weight gain should be avoided.
Altered bowel elimination (fecal retention) due to autonomic nervous system dysfunction and immobilization	Normal fecal elimination pattern	Monitor fecal elimination pattern. Auscultate for bowel sounds. Observe for abdominal distention, flatus, and character of stools. Administer prescribed stool softeners/suppositories. Initiate bowel retraining program. See Chapter 11.
Potential for impaired skin integrity	Skin intact	Assess skin for integrity, red areas, rashes. Provide a dry, clean, wrinkle-free bed. Pad and massage bony prominences to prevent skin breakdown. Massage skin with lanolin-based lotion. Initiate an every-2-hour turning or position-change schedule. NOTE: Pressure and dampness on red skin areas cause tissue breakdown in 20 minutes. Initiate range-of-motion exercises of all joints to improve/maintain circulation to skin. Use an alternating pressure mattress. Note that this does not eliminate the need for every-2-hour position changes. Prevent pressure on toes by use of a footboard. When patient is in the supine position, heels should be over the end of the mattress. Position patient on a rotating bed, if available. Following stabilization and callous formation, initiate a mobility program, positioning the patient in a straight-backed chair or wheelchair at least twice daily. NOTE: For wheelchair patients, place a slitted Nerf ball over the arm support edge to prevent finger contractures. Nerf balls are available in toy departments.
Self-care deficit due to immobilization	Clean hair, oral mucosa, teeth, body, and nails	Provide oral hygiene three or more times daily to prevent parotid infections or other oral infections. Assess mouth for lesions and dental caries. Shampoo hair weekly. Soak hands and feet in warm water before trimming nails. Apply lotion to nails to prevent hangnails.

NURSING DIAGNOSIS	EXPECTED OUTCOMES	NURSING INTERVENTIONS
Potential for joint contractures due to immobility, inability to change position by self	No self injury No contractures	Provide a safe environment: Side rails. Restraints if warranted. Removal call light cord and sharp instruments if suicide potential exists. Cautious turning when repositioning. Maintain normal bone/joint alignment to prevent: Contractures—by using splints. Abduction of hip—by using trochanter rolls. Footdrop—by using high-top tennis shoes. Reinforce activities initiated by physical therapist aimed at: Muscle strengthening. Use of mobility-assistance devices. Administer prescribed muscle relaxants to prevent flexion contractures.
Pain	Pain controlled	Assess location and type of pain. Alleviate pain by: Appropriate use of prescribed analgesics. Relaxation techniques. Position changes. Diversionary conversation. Lotion rubs.
Fear regarding present situation and future life due to physiological deficits NOTE: Patient goes through grieving process	Fears alleviated, acceptance of physical limitations Realistic life goals consistent with limitations	Observe for signs and symptoms of psychological depression/anxiety. Initiate referral to psychological counselor if signs of depression/excessive anxiety are observed. Discuss and reinforce realistic potential for rehabilitation (Table 9-13). Encourage verbalization of fears and apprehension. Permit patient to establish time frames for activities following initial dependent stage. Establish and communicate limits related to time and acceptable behaviors. Acquaint patient/family with SCI clubs and groups, such as wheelchair basketball and bowling. Encourage verbalization of feelings regarding the dependence caused by the loss of physical functions and discuss realistic recovery and rehabilitation goals in the motor, sensory, occupational, social, and sexual (Table 9-14) areas. NOTE: Refer to psychological/sexual/occupational counselor if the patient's needs are beyond nursing expertise. Assess patient to determine stage in the grief process: Initial realization of deficit. Denial. Anger/despair. Recognition and cognitive acceptance of the permanence of limitations and potential coping means. NOTE: The progression may involve intermittent regressions to a previous stage.

Continued.

Table 9-13 Rehabilitation potential related to the level of the trauma

Level of trauma	Rehabilitation potential
C4	Upper extremity function only with the use of externally powered devices.
C5	With assistive devices can feed self, some grooming, use a typewriter, push a wheelchair slowly, and help with dressing. Will be dependent for transferring and for bladder and bowel care. Electric wheelchair useful for long distances.
C6	The presence of wrist extension makes grasp and rclease impossible; should be able to dress, handle wheelchair, move efficiently, and transfer with overhead trapeze. May need some assistance with bowel and urinary appliances.
C7-C8	The presence of finger flexors and extensors makes hand activities possible without assistive devices. The presence of triceps makes transfers feasible. Wheelchair independence is possible.
T1	Has normal arm and hand function; therefore, is a high paraplegic. Balance is poor, being mainly dependent upon the latissimus dorsi muscle
T2-T12	Should be fully independent in the wheelchair. Can manage activities of daily living (ADL) including bowel and bladder care.
T12 and below	Possibility of walking with braces and crutches.
L3 and below	May be able to walk with just short leg braces and crutches, depending on strength of the quadriceps.

Table 9-14 Sexual potential for paraplegics and quadraplegics*

Male	Female
Penis: erection	Vaginal wall: secretions inhibited
Fertility: no	Fertility: not affected
During intercourse:	During intercourse:
Scrotum skin: tenses	Clitoris and labia: engorged
Ejaculation: no	Nipples: erect
Vital functions: increases	Breasts: enlarge
Skin color: flushed	Vital functions: increase
	Skin color: flushed

*Potential increases during first year and then stabilizes.

NURSING DIAGNOSIS	EXPECTED OUTCOMES	NURSING INTERVENTION
Potential for ineffective coping	Use of positive coping mechanisms	Assess level of anxiety and patient's coping mechanisms. Encourage communication with other SCI persons to discuss coping approaches. Deal with acting-out behaviors by setting and maintaining behavioral limits. Positively reinforce increasing independent actions (bladder/bowel control, active range-of-motion exercises)
Alterations in socialization	Social and intellectual stimulation to meet self-esteem and belonging needs	Provide intellectual stimulation: books, conversation, school/work materials. Encourage participation in occupational and social/diversional therapy programs. Encourage visits from family and friends.
Spiritual distress	Maintenance of spirituality according to preference	Ask patient if a spiritual counselor is desired. Provide as patient prefers. Provide or read spiritual books or articles at patient's request.
Knowledge deficit: home care	Adequate family/patient knowledge and skill to provide home care	Patient/family teaching; demonstrate and discuss home care measures and procedures: Demonstrate active and passive range-of-motion exercises. Demonstrate hygiene and massage methods to ensure skin integrity. Demonstrate intermittent catheterization procedure; discuss equipment needs and care of retention catheter. Demonstrate and discuss rationale for rectal suppository insertion. Demonstrate transfer techniques: Bed to chair. Chair to bed. Chair to toilet. Discuss means of preventing contractures: Nerf balls over arms of wheelchair. Hydrotherapy including swimming with floats and waist life vests. Positioning changes and alternatives. Application of splints. Discuss nutritional and fluid requirements. Prepare home care equipment list and suggest where available: Toilet seat raisers. Wheelchairs. Adaptive devises for use of typewriter, phone, eating utensils. Over-bed transfer devices. Discuss need for diversion and mental health of home patient and/or care provider: Local volunteers or governmental agencies. Home health care agencies. Counseling services. Physical, occupational, and vocational therapies. Support groups.

PERIPHERAL NERVE TRAUMA

Peripheral nerve trauma can result from (1) crushing injuries; (2) pressure or constriction; (3) penetrating injuries; (4) amputations; (5) fracture of long bones, or (6) from reactions to injections. The nerves most commonly affected are the median ulnar, radial, and sciatic nerves (Merritt, 1979). Return of function is dependent on several factors:

Type of injury such as stretching, pressure, or compression: Relief within 24 hours frequently results in the full return of function.

Degree of degeneration: If the axon and myelin sheath are damaged, degeneration begins within 24 hours of the trauma.

Location: The more proximal to the CNS, the lesser the chance for regeneration of the nerve fiber.

Rapidity and accuracy of diagnosis and treatment: If reanastomosis or homografting of sectioned nerves is accomplished within 6 to 24 hours, the chance for functional return is significantly increased (Merritt, 1979).

Correct care of amputated parts.

The prompt initiation and maintenance of a rehabilitation program.

Etiology

Peripheral nerve dysfunction can result from the following types of trauma:

Crushing injuries: occupational injuries such as cave-ins, power take off or wringer equipment, pinning under motorcycle.

Pressure: ill-fitting or incorrect use of crutches.

Constriction: extensive edema, scar formation, osteoarthritic changes.

Penetrating injuries: gunshot wounds, knife, nails, or pop-can-top injuries.

Amputation: occupational injuries; automobile, cycle, or boat accidents.

Fracture of long or pelvic bones: because of the anatomical proximity of peripheral nerves to long bones and pelvis, fracture displacement can stretch, exert pressure, or section the adjacent peripheral nerve.

Reaction to injections: either physiological reactions to medications or incorrect administration techniques can cause physical laceration of nerves or excessive deposits of medications exerting pressure on nerves (Adams and Victor, 1980).

Pathophysiology

When the axon and the myelin sheath or a peripheral nerve are damaged, degeneration and retraction of the nerve distal to the injury occurs within 24 hours. Unless the axon and protective myelin sheath are reapproximated or surgically reanastomosed, motor and sensory dysfunction distal to the injury occurs. Regeneration is a slow process. Schwann cells of the neurilemma proliferate to form a neural tube for the axon. The axon sends off several shoots that grow towards the distal severed axon (Fig. 9-18). Typically, the regrowth rate is 1 mm per day. Approximation without surgical reanastomosis or grafting can result in variable nerve transmission because of the irregularity of both the axon and the neurilemma (Merritt, 1979).

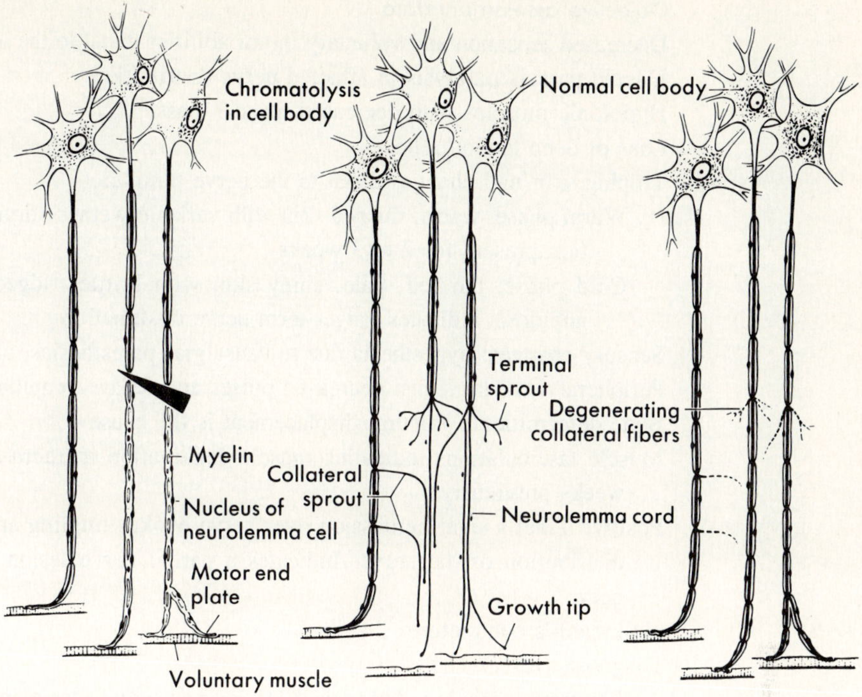

Fig. 9-18 Peripheral nerve degeneration/regeneration process. (From Noback, C., and Demarest, R.: The human nervous system, ed. 2, New York, 1975, McGraw-Hill Book Co. Reproduced with permission.)

Classification

There are two types of peripheral nerve injuries:
- Sectioning injuries
- Pressure trauma

Nursing assessment

Subjective assessment data

History of extremity or pelvic trauma, surgery, use of crutches, painful medication injections

Weakness/paralysis of extremities depending on the location of the trauma

Constant burning sensation distal to the trauma; such as on hands, fingers, and soles of feet. Pain increases with tactile/environmental stimulation

Stabbing pain in affected extremity

History of skin and nail changes in extremities

Objective assessment data

Decreased sensation and voluntary motor abilities distal to the nerve/plexus involved

Flaccid paresis/paralysis in affected nerve distribution

Hypotonic muscles with decreased muscle mass

Loss of deep tendon reflexes

Trophic skin/nail changes distal to the nerve trauma:

- Warm phase: warm, flushed skin with variable wetness/dryness indicates dysfunction present for 2 to 3 weeks
- Cold phase: mottled, pale, shiny skin with brittle, ridged nails, hair loss, and anhidosis indicates longer term nerve dysfunction

Sensory changes: hypesthesia due to causalgia, paresthesias, anesthesia

Peripheral vascular signs: decreased pulses and delayed capillary refill

Bone deformities if fracture/displacement is the cause

Muscle fasciculations indicating muscle denervation if trauma occurred more than 2 weeks previously

Positive Tinel's sign: percussion over nerve evokes tingling and pain along the distal distribution of the nerve. Indicates a partial nerve lesion or regeneration of the nerve

Volkmann's contracture

Diagnostic tests:

- Electromyography: diminished/absent neuromuscular transmission indicative of degeneration or sectioning
- Nerve conduction/velocity studies: diminished/absent strength of nerve transmission
- Muscle biopsy: atrophied/degenerated muscle cells

Interventions

Interventions, whether conservative or surgical, are dependent on the type and extent of trauma. The goals of care are directed toward accurate assessment, maintenance of function, prevention of complications, and rehabilitation (Hickey, 1981).

Nursing care plan: **PERIPHERAL NERVE TRAUMA**

NURSING DIAGNOSIS	EXPECTED OUTCOMES	NURSING INTERVENTIONS
Impaired motor/sensation ability due to compression or sectioning of peripheral nerves	Return of functional motor and sensation abilities	Assess and document degree of function: Motor: presence and degree of paresis/paralysis; tendon reflexes; functional check. Sensory: light touch, pressure, pinch, temperature, paresthesias, or anesthesia. NOTE: Extent of motor testing is dependent on the presence of concomitant injuries. For example, movement of fractures and bones may increase peripheral nerve trauma. Therefore, functional testing is contraindicated. Assess and document: Abnormal motor activity, such as fasciculations, tremors. Alterations in muscle mass and tone. Presence of contractures. For vascular impairments assess: Pulse distal to trauma site. Skin color and temperature: Warm, flushed, and dry correlates with initial autonomic alterations. Mottled, pale, scaly skin with no hair growth and brittle nails with ridges correlates with peripheral nerve injuries that are 2 to 3 weeks old. Immobilize limb in a functional position using: Splints. Skin traction. Casts. Rationale: Immobilization provides rest and decreases the inflammatory response and muscle contractions.
Potential for peripheral vascular impairment distal to dysfunctional nerve due to edema, constricting cast, bandages, or splint	Circulatory sufficiency without venous stasis and dependent edema	Prevent limb edema by: Elevating the limb. Intermittent application of ice bags with absorbent cotton coverings. Assessing for distal vascular and neurological deficiency caused by an excessively tight cast, elastic wrap, splint. Check: Color and temperature of skin. Capillary refill time. Motor and sensation abilities. Provide cast care to maintain integrity of patient's vasculature and skin and the intactness of cast. Assess distal pulses, skin, motor and sensation abilities. Protect skin from breakdown by petaling adhesive over cast edges. Report any drainage or foul odors emitting from the cast to the physician immediately. Protect cast from moisture and pressure to prevent alterations in cast shape.

Continued.

Nursing care plan: **PERIPHERAL NERVE TRAMA—cont'd**

NURSING DIAGNOSIS	EXPECTED OUTCOMES	NURSING INTERVENTIONS
Potential for skin breakdown due to impaired neurological and circulatory status resulting from constriction or sectioning	No skin breakdown	Provide skin care: Examine skin for irritations or sores. Soak nails in warm water, if brittle, and trim straight across. Protect skin against excessively hot or cold temperatures. Assist patient with position changes.
Potential for impaired mobility/dexterity due to ankylosing of unused joints and loss of muscle tone/mass	Normal muscle mass and tone and freely movable joints	Initiate prescribed passive range-of-motion exercises. NOTE: Placing a Nerf ball over the edge of wheelchair arms increases the probability of finger pressure exercises. Assist physical therapist with: Galvanic muscle stimulation procedures to prevent muscle degeneration. Hydrotherapy. Massage affected muscles. Apply prescribed splints/slings. Administer prescribed antiinflammatory and muscle-relaxant agents. Gradually increase activity and exercise.
Self-care deficit due to cast/splint	Increasing independence in ADLs	Assist with ADLs if movement is limited by cast or splint; such as in eating, position changes, ambulation, grooming. Monitor and record weekly weights. Encourage and reinforce efforts towards return to self-care related to extent of abilities. Focus on abilities rather than disabilities. Identify and reinforce beneficial coping mechanisms such as the use of the other hand, competency with self-transfer. Support the rehabilitation program: Physical. Occupational/vocational.

Nursing care plan: **PERIPHERAL NERVE TRAMA—cont'd**

NURSING DIAGNOSIS	EXPECTED OUTCOMES	NURSING INTERVENTIONS
Knowledge deficit: surgical procedure and anticipated results	Understands procedure and anticipated results	Prepare patient for surgical reanastomosis/grafting. Reinforce patient's understanding of the procedure and expected outcomes that were explained by the surgeon in obtaining informed consent. Procedure: Following surgical skin preparation, an incision over the affected nerve is made. Scarred or degenerated tissue is excised. The two nerve segments are approximated. If the nerve is extensively degenerated making approximation impossible, nerve grafts are done. Following skin closure, a flexion cast or splint is applied. Nerve healing and regeneration take approximately 3 weeks. The flexion cast or splint and sutures are then removed. A plastic molded splint with which gradual extension can be accomplished is applied. If the nerve grafting procedure is employed, there is no need for flexion splinting. Nerve healing/regeneration rate: Nerves regenerate at 1 mm per day. Thus the healing process is slow. Prognosis: dependent on the extent and location of the trauma. The more proximate to the CNS, the poorer the prognosis. Expectations regarding common sequelae: Muscle atrophy: begins at time of denervation and progresses until regeneration of the nerve. Joint stiffness resulting from immobilization. Provide postoperative care Immediate care: Assess vital signs. Immobilization and elevation of limb. Make serial observations regarding circulation, edema, skin, motor and sensory function.
Knowledge deficit: self/home care measures and community resources	Understands and demonstrates home care measures. States realistic goals and community resources	Initiate patient/family teaching regarding: Physical needs: Cast care or splint and sling application and care. Hygiene. Muscle/joint exercises. Use of assistive devices (see Chapter 11). Mobility: transfer techniques. Dietary needs: excessive weight gains should be avoided to prevent constriction of cast and need for larger splint. Psychoemotional needs: Discuss and provide list of: Referral resources within community, such as physical/rehabilitation services, vocational rehabilitation agencies. Means of reducing stress caused by physical limitations: Verbal expression in a forthright manner of anxieties. Diversionary activities. Rehabilitation process (see Chapter 11).

Suggested readings

Adams, R., and Victor, M.: Principals of neurology, 1980, McGraw-Hill Book Co.

Bowers, S., and Marshall, L.: Severe head injury: current treatment and research, J. Neurosurg. Nurs. **14**(5):210-218, Oct. 1982.

Cole, T.: Sexuality and the spinal cord injured. In Green, R., editor: Human sexuality: a health practitioner's text, Baltimore, 1975, The Williams & Wilkins Co.

Conway-Rutkowski, B.L.: Carini and Owens' Neurological and neurosurgical nursing, ed. 8, St. Louis, 1982, The C.V. Mosby Co.

Fincke, M.: Changes in the emergency department. In Miller, M.: The nurse manager in the emergency department, St. Louis, 1983, The C.V. Mosby Co.

Gilroy, J., and Meyers, J.: Medical neurology, ed. 2, New York, 1975, Macmillan Publishing Co., Inc.

Hanlon, K.: Description and uses of intracranial pressure monitoring, Heart Lung **5**(2):277-282, 1976.

Heaney, R.: Osteoporosis: the preventable epidemic, Creighton U. Health Science News, pp. 1-2, Nov. 1982.

Hickey, J.: Clinical practice of neurological and neurosurgical nursing, Philadelphia, 1981, J.B. Lippincott.

Hummelgard, A., and Martin, E.: Management of the patient in a halobrace, J. Neurosurg. Nurs. **14**(3):113-118, June 1982.

Johnson, M., and Quinn, J.: The subarachnoid screw, Am. J. Nurs. **77**:448-450, 1977.

Jones, C., and Cayard, C.: Care of ICP monitoring devices: a nursing responsibility, J. Neurosurg. Nurs. **14**(5):255-260, Oct. 1982.

Lanros, N.: Assessment and intervention in emergency nursing, Bowie, Md., 1983, Robert J. Brady Co.

Larrabee, J.: The person with a spinal cord injury: physical care during early recovery, Am. J. Nurs. **77:**1320-1329, 1977.

Lazure, L.: Defusing the dangers of autonomic dysreflexia, Nursing80 **10**(9):52-53, Sept. 1980.

Levin, A.: The use of fiberoptic intracranial pressure monitor in clinical practice, Neurosurgery **1**(3): 266-271, Nov./Dec. 1977.

MacKechnie, J.: Regional spinal cord injury center nursing care: prescription for the present and future, J. Neurosurg. Nurs. **14**(3):133-136, June 1982.

Merritt, H.: A textbook of neurology, ed. 6, Philadelphia, 1979, Lea & Febiger.

Meyd, C.: Acute brain trauma, Am. J. Nurs. **78**(1): 40, 1978.

Mitchell, P., and Mauss, N.: Intracranial pressure: fact and fancy, Nursing76 **••**:53-57, June 1976.

Pepper, G.: The person with spinal cord injury: psychological care, Am. J. Nurs. **77**(8):1330-1335, 1977.

Seeling, J., Becker, D., and Miller, J.: Traumatic acute subdural hematoma: major mortality reduction in comatose patient treated within 4 hours, N. Engl. J. Med. **304:**1511-1518, Mar. 1981.

Shea, J.: Head injuries, EDNA Scientific Assembly, Toronto, Nov. 2, 1981.

Simmons, S.: Evaluating intracerebral bleeds, JEN **4**(5):9-19, Sept/Oct. 1978.

Stevens, M.: Post-concussion syndrome, J. Neurosurg. Nurs. **14**(5):239-244, Oct. 1982.

Webb, K.: Early assessment of orthopedic injuries, Am. J. Nurs. **74**(10):1048-1052, Nov. 1974.

Zegeer, L.: Nursing care of the patient with brain edema, J. Neurosurg. Nurs. **14**(5):268-275, Oct. 1982.

Audiovisual resources

Bruce, D.: Pediatric emergency management of head trauma, New York, 1980, Health Education Programs, Inc.

Patterson, R.: Head trauma, New York, 1976, NCME.

CHAPTER 10 Central nervous system surgery

Surgical intervention is required for a variety of neurological conditions related to trauma and pathophysiology in the brain, cranial nerves, spinal cord and nerve roots, peripheral nerves, and the autonomic nervous system. This chapter will discuss surgery performed for brain tumors (Chapter 8), aneurysms (Chapter 13), spinal cord tumors (Chapter 8), fractured vertebrae, hematomas (Chapter 9), hydrocephalus (Chapter 5), and cranial nerve disorders.

ETIOLOGY AND PATHOPHYSIOLOGY

Diagnosis and assessment of the patient's condition is imperative to the plan of care and treatment. The exact location of tumors, hematomas, and other conditions in the brain and spinal cord needs to be determined before surgery. Tests performed to determine this are the CAT scan, electroencephalogram (EEG), brain scan, spinal and skull X-rays, myelogram, arteriogram, pneumoencephalogram, a complete neurological examination, and visual field evaluations (Chapters 1 and 2).

The physician makes the diagnosis based on clinical findings, patient history, and diagnostic studies and then decides to perform surgery. Intracranial surgery is performed by either a craniotomy or craniectomy, depending on the location of the lesion.

PROCEDURES

Craniotomy

This procedure is performed for supratentorial lesions; that is, for those lesions that are in the area of the brain above the tentorium (fold of the dura mater that separates the cerebral cortex from the cerebellum and brainstem). Craniotomies are performed to remove or correct conditions such as brain tumors, aneurysms and arteriovenous malformations, excision of abscesses, evacuation of hematomas, elevation of depressed skull fractures, tissue biopsies, and temporal lobectomy for seizure control.

Surgically, the cranium is opened via the formation of a bone flap that is attached to muscle tissue. The dura is incised and opened in the direction opposite to the bone flap (see Fig. 10-1, *A*). The closure is done in layers with the closure of the galea being the most important step to promote wound healing.

Craniectomy

A craniectomy is performed by removal of a portion of the skull ranging from burr-hole size to a larger bone segment (Fig. 10-1, *B*). This procedure is performed for infratentorial lesions or for those below the tentorium in the brain. Pathological conditions corrected by craniectomy include those that involve the midbrain, pons, medulla, fourth ventricle, cerebellum, and cerebellar pontine angle (namely, acoustic neuromas and meningiomas). Craniectomies are also performed to aspirate a brain abscess above

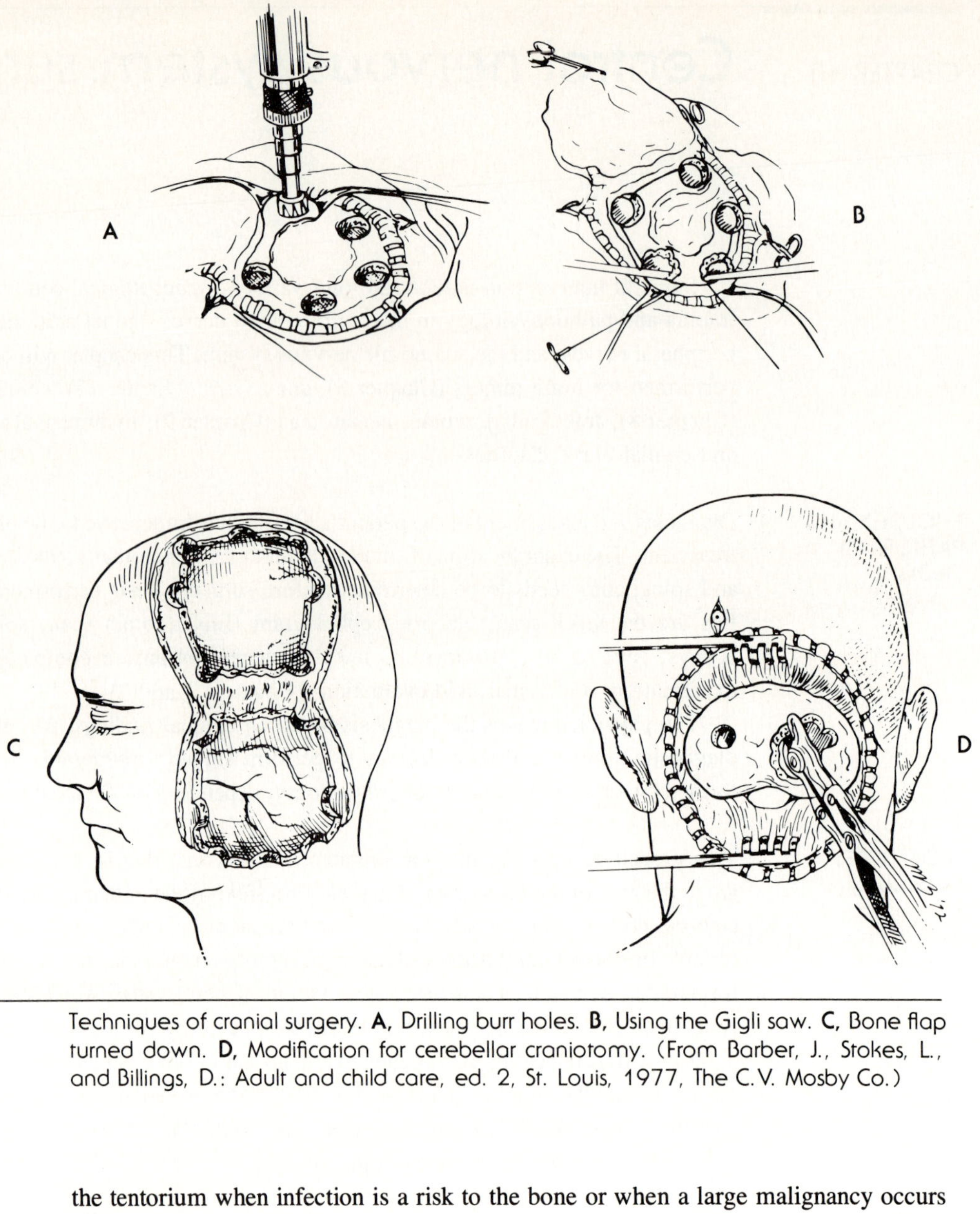

Fig. 10-1 Techniques of cranial surgery. **A,** Drilling burr holes. **B,** Using the Gigli saw. **C,** Bone flap turned down. **D,** Modification for cerebellar craniotomy. (From Barber, J., Stokes, L., and Billings, D.: Adult and child care, ed. 2, St. Louis, 1977, The C.V. Mosby Co.)

the tentorium when infection is a risk to the bone or when a large malignancy occurs and large bone expansion is suspected.

A craniectomy is more complex and takes longer to perform than a craniotomy because there is less accessibility to the operative site. It requires difficult body positioning because of the necessity of avoiding vital areas such as the respiratory and reticular activating systems, and there is a likelihood of increased intracranial pressure (ICP) and compression of additional areas because of displacement from the original pathology. One can expect higher risks and a longer postoperative recovery period for the patient undergoing a craniectomy. Craniectomies are done through a small burr hole to perform a ventriculography, remove a hematoma, perform a biopsy, or to remove pus, cerebrospinal fluid (CSF), or blood. The burr hole is enlarged by gradually chipping away the bone to gain access to the fifth, eighth, ninth, and tenth cranial nerves and to the brainstem and cerebellar portions of the brain.

Carotid endarterectomy

Carotid endarterectomy is the procedure performed to excise atherosclerotic plaques from the common carotid artery. A saphenous vein graft or silicone graft may be sewn into the artery to restore cerebral circulation. This technique is performed to prevent occlusion of the artery or emboli formation from the plaque.

Aneurysms

Aneurysms are repaired by frontotemporal, posterotemporal, or transtentorial craniotomies. Procedures done to repair and to prevent recurrence of bleeding from an aneurysm include placing a metal clip on it to occlude the aneurysm, wrapping a material around it to prevent leaking, ligation, and embolization. Hypotension is maintained during the procedure to decrease blood flow and prevent rupture of the aneurysm. Ligation of the afferent artery may be necessary if an aneurysm cannot be readily clipped. Vascular bypass may be performed to prevent ischemia to a portion of the brain.

Cerebral artery bypass surgery

Cerebral artery bypass surgery is a microvascular technique used to treat patients who have had a stroke or to treat a transient ischemic attack (TIA). Microvascular techniques and instruments enable the surgeon to visualize minute cerebral arteries and to manipulate them in performing a cerebral bypass. One procedure done to achieve this bypass is to anastomase the superficial temporal artery to a branch of the middle cerebral artery to increase blood flow to the frontal and temporal lobes, which include the primary motor and sensory areas for the face, hand, arm, optic radiations, and the dominant hemisphere for speech.

Transphenoidal hypophysectomy

A transphenoidal hypophysectomy is the surgical procedure used for partial or complete removal of the pituitary gland. This procedure is done to remove pituitary tumors, to control the progression of diabetic retinopathy, or to control metastatic carcinoma of the breast or prostate. This procedure is performed through an incision made in the inner aspect of the inner lip and then entering the sella turcica via the floor of the mouth and sphenoid sinus. The dura mater is incised and the tumor or pituitary gland is removed with the use of a microscope. Following removal of the gland, the pieces of bone and cartilage that were removed are packed into the sella turcica or a piece of fascia taken from the anterior thigh is packed into the sella turcica to prevent leakage of CSF. Gel foam soaked in an antibiotic solution is placed in the anterior sella turcica to prevent infection. The nose is packed and a dressing is placed over the base to prevent the packing from slipping out. A nasal airway may be inserted to facilitate breathing. These patients will be mouth breathers after the operation and measures to prevent dry mucous membranes should be implemented.

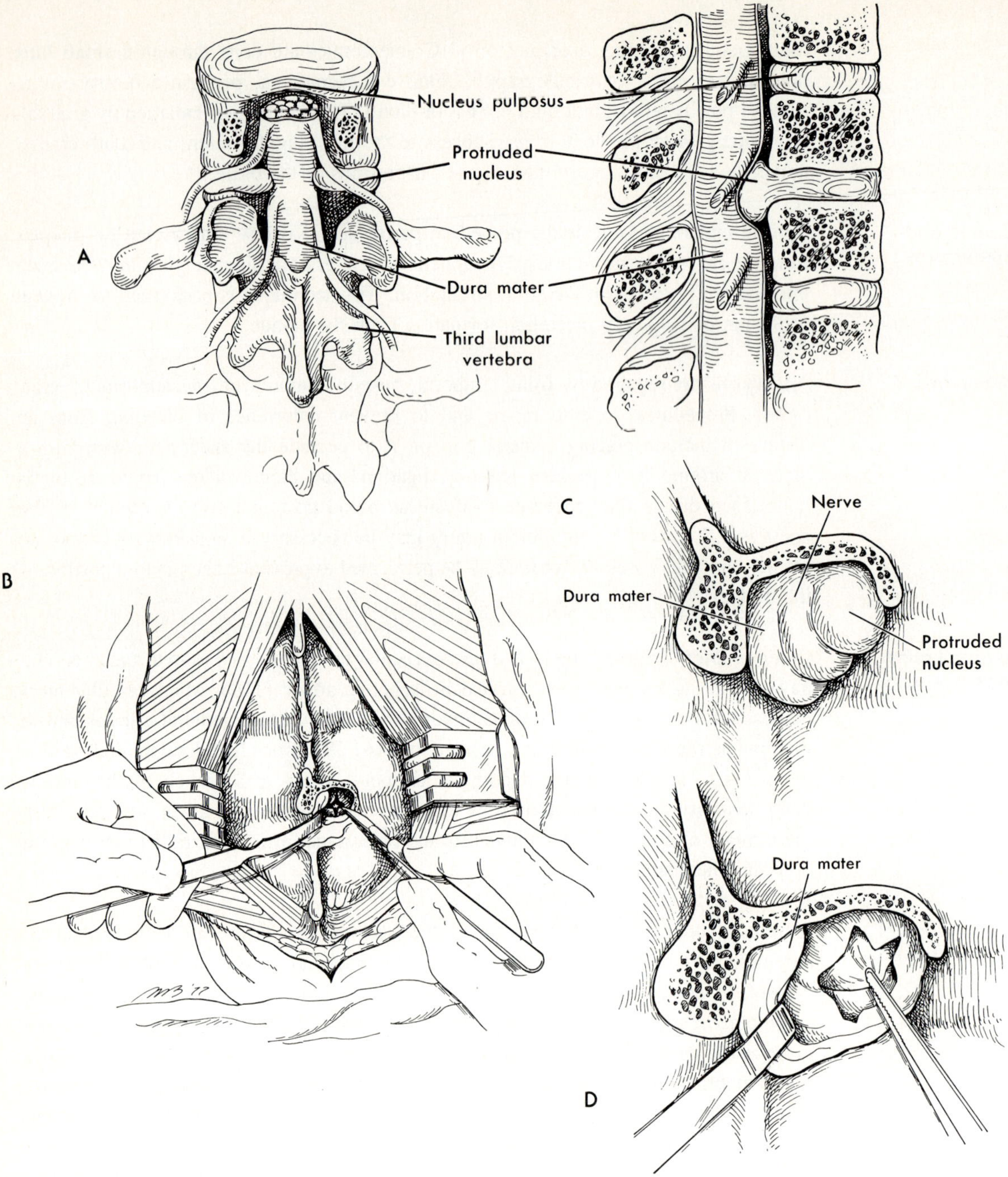

Fig. 10-2 Laminectomy, the surgical procedure performed to remove laminae or portions of them. **A,** Herniation of lumbar intervertebral disc. **B,** Interlaminal removal of herniated disc and removal of part of lamina exposing nucleus pulposus. **C,** Observe relationship of dura mater, nerve, and protruded nucleus. **D,** Removing extruded disc. (From Conway-Rutkowski, B.L.: Carini and Owens' neurological and neurosurgical nursing, ed. 8, St. Louis, 1982, The C.V. Mosby Co.)

Shunts

Several shunt techniques may be used to correct obstructive and nonobstructive (communicating) hydrocephalus including ventriculoureterostomy (Matson), ventriculoperitoneostomy, Choroid plexectomy (Dandy), lumbar subarachnoid ureterostomy (Heile), lumbar subarachnoid peritoneostomy, third ventriculostomy, ventriculocisternostomy, auriculoventriculostomy. Each procedure is different from the others and is performed to continually drain off excess spinal fluid as in obstructive hydrocephalus or to drain off excess CSF to decrease ICP. In all of the procedures a catheter placed into the lateral ventricle drains into the subarachnoid space, into a cistern, or into another body cavity (such as the peritoneum, vena cava, pleura, ureter). A ventriculoatrial shunt is the most common treatment for hydrocephalus. It involves the placement in the ventricle of a catheter with a valve to prevent reflux and the other end is passed through the internal jugular vein into the right atrium, which allows CSF to circulate in the blood stream.

Spinal cord surgery

Tumors of the spinal cord are classified according to their location in relation to the dura (see Fig. 8-1). A *laminectomy* is performed to reach the dura, disc, or cord and is done by making an incision over the involved vertebral area through fascia and muscles to the laminae to remove them or a disc (Fig. 10-2). A *spinal fusion* is performed to stabilize the spine. This may be necessary following removal of a lesion or trauma to the spine. A fusion is performed by removing bone from the involved part and inserting a graft (usually from the iliac crest) or a Harrington rod. A *sympathectomy* is performed for treatment of circulatory disturbances such as Raynaud's disease and other conditions that are pain-producing. The afferent pathways in the sympathetic division of the autonomic nervous system are disrupted as a means for pain control.

NURSING ASSESSMENT

Patient and family education and a thorough assessment of the patient's condition are necessary aspects of the nursing care plan. The surgeon is responsible for explaining the surgical procedure and the reason he or she recommends it to the patient. The risks are critical for neurological procedures since the brain and spinal cord are involved. Some deficits may be permanent and others only temporary. This may cause fears about the loss of function and even death for the patient. The patient needs to understand fully these disabilities and the expected postoperative outcome. Honest information is essential in the preparation of the patient to foster confidence in the surgeon and recommended surgical procedure.

Nurses play an important part in the preoperative care of the patient. Listen to the fears expressed by the patient and the family and provide support by answering questions and reinforcing what the surgeon has said. Patient and family teaching needs to be done about diagnostic tests and the preparation for them as well as about the surgical procedure and postoperative care. This will help alleviate anxiety and fears and give the patient and family a clear understanding of the diagnostic and treatment plan.

The nursing history or data base is beneficial in planning for patient needs as well as assisting in the neurological assessment to help determine the location and diagnosis

Patient name: Date:

Age: Doctor:

Surgical procedure: Allergies:

Surgical permit signed: Yes No

BASELINE PARAMETERS

A. Physical assessment
   1. Neurological status
      a. Visual ability
      b. LOC, orientation
      c. Communication skills
      d. Hearing ability
      e. Neurological assessment to include motor and sensory function
      f. History of neurological symptoms
      g. Handedness (right or left)
   2. Vital signs
      Blood pressure
      Pulse
      Respirations
      Temperature
      Weight
   3. Cardiovascular
   4. Respiratory: Breath sounds
      Auscultation of chest
      Chest x-ray
   5. Hydration
      a. Urine output
   6. Abdomen: bowel sounds, firmness, auscultated

B. Diagnostic test results
   1. Significant findings of CAT, radiographic tests, angiography, scans, EEG, lumbar puncture, ECG
   2. Lab data
      a. CBC: RBC WBC Hb/Hct Diff Plt
      b. Serum electrolytes
      c. Arterial blood gas analysis
      d. Type and cross-matching of blood No. of units
      e. Complete urinalysis
         Urine osmolality
      f. Clotting profile
      g. Cerebrospinal fluid findings
      h. Drug levels (anticonvulsants, antibiotics)

C. General patient information
   1. Anxiety level/fears
   2. Special requests
   3. Medications or other medical-surgical problems

Discuss with the patient and significant others:

A. Physical aspects of the ICU.
   1. Visit ICU and meet staff members.
   2. Location, physical layout, noise level, lack of sleep, lighting, monitors, staffing, visiting rules, approximate duration of stay.

B. Specific nursing care measures and treatment.
   1. Frequent vital signs and neurological checks, I & O, Foley, monitors, respiratory hygiene, (incentive spirometry, postural drainage and percussion when indicated, ventilator, coughing and deep breathing exercises [demonstrate], suctioning), ambulation, large occlusive dressings, tubes (nasogastric, endotracheal, catheters, and drains), shaving of hair, black and swollen eyes, short-term neurological changes, LOC, deficits in motor/sensory functions, visual and hearing deficits (blurred vision, diplopia), vertigo.

Fig. 10-3 Suggested preoperative assessment and teaching guide.

of the pathological condition. The patient or significant other is questioned about the following as subjective and objective assessment data are gathered:

1. Onset, duration, progression, frequency, and specific description of neurological symptoms include alterations in:
   a. Level of consciousness (LOC)
   b. Behavior or personality
   c. Motor function
   d. Sensory function
   e. Balance and coordination
   f. Visual function
   g. Pupils and extraocular movements
   h. Communication skills
2. Seizures should be described by discussing their onset, progression, duration, frequency, type, locality, aura, and incontinence. Also:
   a. Precipitating factors such as emotional upset, environmental stimuli, fever
   b. Variation in seizure activity or episodes if there is multiple seizure activity
   c. Postictal status; injuries sustained, if any
3. Headaches: presence, severity, frequency, duration, precipitating factors, associated other symptoms such as nausea/vomiting, time-related occurrence
4. Cranial nerve dysfunctions
   a. Hearing defects, tinnitus, vertigo
   b. Visual disturbances including diplopia, blurred vision, nystagmus, field defects, papilledema
   c. Smell or taste, swallowing, chewing
   d. Facial numbness, pain, twitching, ability to smile, grimace, wrinkle brow
5. Medications taken for neurological symptoms such as pain medications
6. Previous trauma to head or neuromuscular body parts, previous neurosurgery, or neurological treatment
7. Presence of any other medical or surgical problems and related treatment and medications
8. Patient's reaction to diagnosis, diagnostic studies, treatment, and impending surgery. Explanation of the plan of care and procedures is vital to postoperative care and rehabilitation of the patient
9. Concept of body image: fears of loss of body parts, permanent disability, altered role, altered sexual function, inability to perform activities of daily living (ADL), altered occupation, fear of recurrent pathology, fear of dying

A preoperative checklist can be prepared to facilitate data collection and to serve as a guideline for patient teaching (Fig. 10-3).

POSTOPERATIVE CARE

The postoperative goals of nursing care are (1) prevention of complications and (2) initiation of rehabilitation. Nursing care measures are based on a nursing and medical diagnosis, which is necessary to prevent complications and to produce optimal functioning of the patient.

Nursing care plan: **CENTRAL NERVOUS SYSTEM SURGERY**

NURSING DIAGNOSIS	EXPECTED OUTCOMES	NURSING INTERVENTIONS
Health management deficit: **Development of immediate postoperative complications: hypovolemia, shock, hypostatic pneumonia, pulmonary emboli, thrombophlebitis, abdominal ileus, cardiac tachycardia**	Stable vital signs; absence of complications Maximum neurological function	Loss of large amounts of blood causes a decrease in blood pressure, pulse, respiration, and temperature. Blood volume may need to be replaced by transfusion. Check vital signs according to physician's orders, unit policy, and stability of patient's condition. Vital signs include blood pressure; apical, radial, carotid, and pedal pulses; respirations; temperature; neurological signs especially any sudden change in level of consciousness. Notify the physician immediately of any change in the patient's condition including any signs and symptoms of complications. Observe dressings and drains for large amounts of drainage and report any significant findings. NOTE: Immobility and anesthetic agents lead to a decrease in respiratory, circulatory, and peristaltic functions. Frequently assess breath and bowel sounds and palpate chest and abdomen. Position the patient on the back after spinal surgery to provide pressure on the spine to prevent bleeding.
Increased ICP or hematoma formation		Peak edema occurs within initial 24-hour-postoperative period and it can remain for up to 72 hours. Having the patient's head lower than the rest of the body will increase cerebral edema. Increased circulating blood volume will increase blood flow to the brain resulting in increased ICP. Position the patient on the side with the head of the bed elevated 30 degrees to maintain a patent airway and prevent aspiration. If the patient had a craniectomy, do not place him on the operative side. Avoid hyperflexion or extension of the neck; pillows are not usually allowed. A small pad such as a rolled towel may be placed under the head for support. Monitor fluid and electrolytes. Fluid intake is restricted to 1500-1800 ml/24 hours. A Foley catheter should be in place and urine output and specific gravity should be measured and accurately recorded every hour. If ventricular drains are in place, drain the fluid amount as ordered by the physician. Monitor arterial blood gases at frequent intervals. High levels of carbon dioxide produce cerebral vasodilation, which increases cerebral edema. Administer steroids as ordered to decrease cerebral/spinal cord edema. Decadron, 6-10 mg every 4-6 hours, is the usual immediate postoperative order.

Nursing care plan: CENTRAL NERVOUS SYSTEM SURGERY—cont'd

NURSING DIAGNOSIS	EXPECTED OUTCOMES	NURSING INTERVENTIONS
Increased ICP or hematoma formation—cont'd		Increased ICP or epidural hematoma formation may cause worsening of the neurological deficit. These are assessed by noting changes in neurological status and vital signs. (Refer to Chaper 9 for assessment of increased ICP) Avoid precipitating factors such as hypoxia, hypercapnia, fever, the Valsalva manuever, vomiting. Prevent constipation and ensure that the patient has a bowel movement. Report any sudden incontinence, which may indicate paralysis or other neurological dysfunction. Monitor electrolytes and report any abnormalities. Maintain patient's activity as ordered. If ICP monitoring is done, record pressures (see Fig. 10-4). Normal value: 4-15 mm Hg Prevent kinking of drains to allow adequate drainage. A tight fitting dressing may indicate swelling, a sign of increased ICP or hematoma.

Continued.

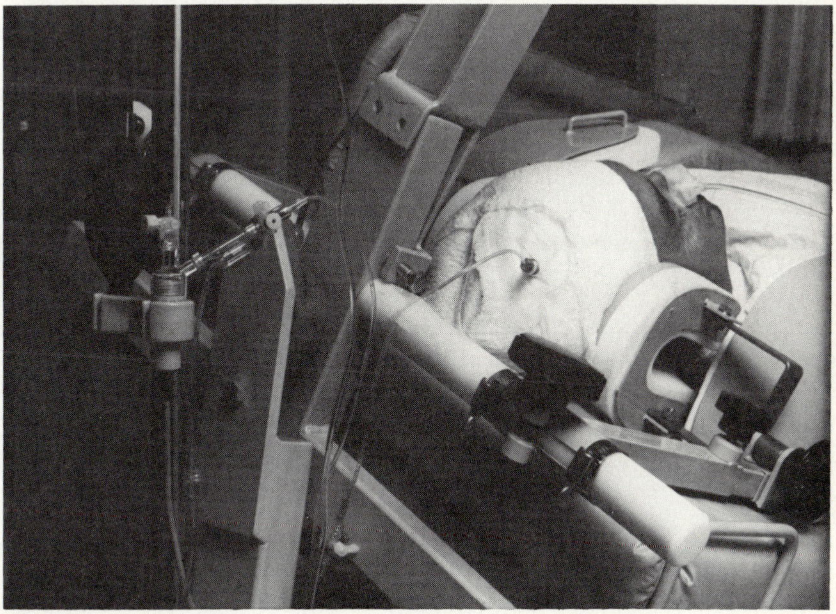

Fig. 10-4 Intracranial screw and pressure monitor. (Courtesy Kinetic Concepts, Inc., San Antonio, Texas.)

Nursing care plan: **CENTRAL NERVOUS SYSTEM SURGERY—cont'd**

NURSING DIAGNOSIS	EXPECTED OUTCOMES	NURSING INTERVENTIONS
Hyperthermia	Normal body temperature; patient is afebrile	NOTE: Increased body temperature increases caloric uptake and decreases oxygen consumption and supply to brain. A rectal probe should be in place continuously to monitor temperature for 24 hours postoperatively. Strip, sponge, and fan patient using tepid alcohol to keep the temperature down and to increase peripheral circulation as a result of vasodilation produced by rubbing. Shivering may be controlled with medications such as chlorpromazine (Thorazine) if a physician prefers it to be used. Administer drugs to control temperature as ordered. A cooling blanket may be ordered to control hyperthermia.
Gastrointestinal bleeding related to central nervous system factors, stress, steroids	Gastric contents have a pH of 7 Absence of blood in stools and gastric contents Patient is free of pain in the gastric region Normal hemoglobin and hematocrit (Men: hemoglobin 14-18 g) hematocrit 38-54 (Women: hemoglobin 12-16 g) hematocrit 36-48	Irritation of the gastric mucosa is caused by an increased production of hydrochloric acid. Antacids may be given orally if the patient has the gag reflex present, is able to swallow and is free of nausea Cimetidine (Tagamet) is administered intravenously if patient cannot tolerate oral medications. Antacids may be given through the nasogastric tube if one is present. Hemoglobin and hematocrit are monitored carefully. Stools and other body excreta may be hematested.
Corneal lacerations	Absence of blindness or corneal ulceration	Provide eye care for the unconscious patient or for the patient with facial paralysis who lacks the ability to blink and lubricate the eye. Blindness can result from dryness and irritation resulting from corneal ulcerations. Apply lubricant or artificial tears to the eyes every 4 hours. Keep the eyes patched with sterile gauze to prevent dryness.
Cranial nerve dysfunctions	Absence of complications rerelated to cranial nerve functions Patient is free of anxiety and accepts altered body image.	Damage to the cranial nerves will interfere with normal neurological function. Deficits may be temporary because of increased ICP following surgery or they may be permanent, depending on the surgical intervention involved.
Oculomotor, trochlear, abducens nerves (nystagmus, ptosis, decreased extraocular movements, diplopia)		Apply alternating eye patch for diplopia. Assess nystagmus. Monitor pupils for size, equality, reactivity, and extraocular movements and observe and report any signs of involvement.

Nursing care plan: CENTRAL NERVOUS SYSTEM SURGERY—cont'd

NURSING DIAGNOSIS	EXPECTED OUTCOMES	NURSING INTERVENTIONS
Trigeminal and facial nerves (loss of facial sensation, loss of corneal reflex)		Protect eye from injury. Record and report any loss of sensation.
Facial nerve (decreased facial muscle strength/expression, facial weakness/paralysis, anxiety related to distorted mouth/altered body image)		Have patient drink with a straw from the unaffected side of the mouth, chew on the unaffected side, and select easily chewed foods. Record asymmetry. Provide good oral hygiene. Remove oral secretions frequently when drooling occurs. Instruct the patient on how to do facial exercises. Provide a means of communication if speech is affected. Encourage ventilation of fears and concerns about appearance to overcome the altered body image.
Acoustic nerve (hearing loss)		Assess hearing loss. Assist with insertion of hearing aid if necessary. Talk to the patient from the unaffected side. Face the patient when speaking to him. Use sign language or gestures if necessary.
Acoustic nerve (disturbance of balance and equilibrium)		Provide safety measures. Assist the patient with ambulation. Remove obstacles. Give support and reassurance. Assist the patient with the use of equipment to encourage independence in activities of daily living (ADL). A physical therapy consultation may be ordered.
Dizziness		Move the patient slowly during position changes. The patient should dangle the legs for a few minutes before standing. Assist the patient with ambulation and other activities.
Glossopharyngeal and vagus nerves (decreased or absent gag, swallowing, cough reflexes; dysphagia; aspiration; nasal, dysarthric speech)		Administer intravenous fluids or give nasogastric feedings. Assess for the presence of the gag reflex and the ability to protect the airway and handle secretions. Suction as needed (prn). Position the patient to prevent obstruction and aspiration. Keep the patient NPO until free of nausea and vomiting and fully alert. Provide frequent oral hygiene. Explain procedures and the need for the intravenous/nasogastric tube. Provide alternative communication methods when speech is impaired.
Hypoglossal nerve (weakness and abnormal movement of tongue)		Assess tongue position and muscle strength. Instruct and supervise the patient in exercises to strengthen the tongue. Give frequent oral hygiene.

Continued.

Nursing care plan: CENTRAL NERVOUS SYSTEM SURGERY—cont'd

NURSING DIAGNOSIS	EXPECTED OUTCOMES	NURSING INTERVENTIONS
Spinal accessory nerve (impaired/absent shoulder shrug and head-turning to the side)		Assess strength and ability to shrug shoulders and turn the head to the side. Assist the patient with ADL. Place objects within the patient's visual field and reach. Assist with exercises to improve the patient's strength.
Seizures	No injuries sustained from seizure activity Control of seizures	Fluid and electrolyte imbalances, hypoxia, fever, and water intoxication are precipitating factors of seizures. Use seizure precautions such as padded siderails, bed height at a low position, a padded tongue blade, anticonvulsants and emergency drugs. Monitor and record seizure activity and notify the physician. Administer drugs to control seizures. Observe for side effects and document the effects of drugs.
Cardiac arrhythmias	Normal sinus rhythm on Electrocardiogram (EKG) monitor Regular heart rate by auscultation and palpation Adequate peripheral circulation observed by skin color, temperature, and palpable pulses.	NOTE: Increased ICP in the brainstem will depress the cardiac center and cause rhythm changes. Ectopic beats or changes in heart rate occur from vagal nerve deficits or irritation. Instruct the patient to avoid vagal stimulation such as with the Valsalva maneuver, coughing, vomiting. Assess the effectiveness of therapy. Administer medications as ordered. Monitor EKG and vital signs. Assess electrolytes.
Hydrocephalus	Absence of headache and signs of increased ICP Bruit auscultated at shunt site Patient is afebrile Absence of infection	An abnormal accumulation of CSF in the cranial cavity may result from a leak of CSF from a ventricle outside the spinal circulation. Increased ICP will result from hydrocephalus. Headache is a classic symptom of a hydrocephalus. Surgery to remove the obstruction may need to be performed (see Ventriculoatrial shunt procedure). Sit the patient up gradually to reduce headache. Assure the patient that the headaches will be relieved when he has adjusted to the shunt. Give instructions about the shunt such as: Avoid participation in sports or strenuous physical activities in which trauma might occur to the shunt because this could obstruct it. Teach the patient/significant others the signs and symptoms of increased ICP, including restlessness, headache, decreased level of consciousness. These should be reported immediately. Teach the signs and symptoms of infection, such as elevated temperature, headache, nuchal rigidity.

Nursing care plan: CENTRAL NERVOUS SYSTEM SURGERY—cont'd

NURSING DIAGNOSIS	EXPECTED OUTCOMES	NURSING INTERVENTIONS
Potential for infection	Patient is afebrile Wound is clean, dry, and not inflamed. Dressings are odor free	There is an increased risk of meningitis if a wound infection develops. Any leak of CSF may increase the chances of infection. Wound rupture leads to saturated spinal dressings and if untreated leads to infection. Foul-smelling cranial dressings unchanged following large amounts of drainage can lead to infection. Note the color and odor of drainage on dressings or from drains, and report any clear or yellow drainage from the incision because this may mean a CSF leak. Reinforce sterile dressings as necessary to prevent contamination Keep the patient's hands away from dressings and sutures. Dressings are generally removed 3 to 5 days postoperatively and the wound is left undressed. Sutures are removed 7 to 10 days after the surgery. Observe dressings and incisional site for redness, tenderness, bulging, separation, drainage, or foul odor. Monitor quality and quantity of drainage emptied from draining device. Monitor temperature as ordered and as needed if temperature is elevated.
Fluid volume deficit	Normal lab serum and urine electrolyte levels Normal values: Calcium (Ca^{++}): 4.5-5.5 mEq/L Chloride (Cl^-): 100-106 mEq/L Potassium (K^+): 3.5-5 mEq/L Sodium (Na^+): 136-145 mEq/L	Decreased sodium and chloride may produce weakness, lethargy, and coma. Low potassium levels may cause confusion and nonresponsiveness. Abnormal serum sodium levels may result from increased aldosterone with increased antidiuretic hormone (ADH) release, which causes sodium retention and decreased sodium levels. Diabetes insipidus may result from increased aldosterone with increased ADH secretion by the posterior pituitary gland following intracranial surgery. The renal tubules stop reabsorbing water. Bowel and bladder function may be lost following spinal cord surgery. Monitor electrolyte levels and report any abnormal results. Electrolyte replacement may be ordered by the physician. Monitor signs and symptoms of dehydration and overhydration: poor skin turgor, peripheral edema, excessive thirst, change in level of consciousness, weight alteration. Observe for frequent urination and high output with low specific gravity of 1.000 or low urine output and high specific gravity. Posterior pituitary hormone, Pitressin (vasopressin tannate), may need to be administered if the diabetes insipidus condition continues past 2 to 3 days. Carefully log-roll spinal surgical patient onto the bed pan. Do not lift patient on while he is lying on his back. Check for deficits in bowel tone.

Continued.

Nursing care plan: **CENTRAL NERVOUS SYSTEM SURGERY—cont'd**

NURSING DIAGNOSIS	EXPECTED OUTCOMES	NURSING INTERVENTIONS
Ineffective airway clearance, breathing pattern, or gas exchange	No pneumonia Normal arterial blood gases Values: (pH: 7.35-7.45) (Po_2: 95-100 mm Hg) (Pco_2: 35-45 mm Hg)	A patent airway is necessary to ensure adequate oxygenation of body tissues and proper respiratory function. Lying the patient on the side with the face dependent facilitates drainage of secretions and vomitus from the airway to prevent aspirations. Body position is dependent on the type of intracranial or intraspinal incision. Supratentorial (craniotomy): Elevate head of the bed 30 degrees to increase venous return and assist breathing. Infratentorial (craniectomy): Keep the patient off his back for up to 48 hours after surgery. Elevate the head of the bed 30 degrees. Spinal cord surgery: Keep the patient in straight body alignment. Log-roll him from side to side maintaining good alignment. Observe for signs of herniation of the brainstem as a result of edema of the medulla oblongata associated with infratentorial operations. Respirations will be depressed. Spinal tumors and/or swelling postoperatively in the upper cervical area can affect muscles necessary for respiration. Measure arterial blood gases at regular intervals. If vomiting occurs, withhold oral feedings; insert a nasogastric tube as appropriate to prevent aspiration. Gently suction the patient's nasopharynx or trachea to clear secretions. Position the patient adequately to prevent the tongue from occluding the airway and to allow adequate lung expansion. A side-lying position with the head in a dependent position (except for spinal surgery and occipital incisions), in a semiprone position, knees flexed when allowed is most suitable. Turn the patient every 2 hours. Encourage the patient to deep breath and cough. Assess breath sounds every hour initially.
Alteration in comfort: pain	Patient is comfortable and painfree.	Analgesics for relief of incisional pain are used with caution to avoid depression of neurological function in the intracranial surgical patient. Morphine sulfate is specifically contraindicated because of its effect on the clinical picture. Codeine is the drug generally prescribed. Patients with spinal surgery may have much pain; narcotics, except morphine, are ordered to relieve it. Assess pain and administer pain medication as ordered. Meperidine (Demerol) and antispasmodics such as diazepam (Valium) may be ordered for spinal surgery. Observe the effects and side effects of medication. Maintain a quiet and peaceful environment. Observe the dressing for tightness and constriction.

NURSING DIAGNOSIS	EXPECTED OUTCOMES	NURSING INTERVENTIONS
Impaired skin integrity Potential joint contractures	Absence of decubitus ulcers and contractures	When the patient is able to eat, give a high-protein, high-caloric diet. A physical therapy consultation may be ordered. Position the patient in good alignment. Turn every 2 hours. Perform range-of-motion exercises to all joints every 4 hours. Keep the skin clean and dry. Stimulate circulation to bony prominences with massage and back rubs. Use an air or foam mattress for long-term care. Use turn sheet to log-roll patients. Do not lift or drag them across the sheets.
Home maintenance management deficit	Patient/family will verbalize fears and concerns Maximum wellness is achieved Patient/family demonstrate techniques of maximal ADL capabilities, safety measures, methods to prevent complications, and can relate signs and symptoms of medical problems	Follow-up care regimen is important to the patient's/family's understanding of the patient's condition. Teaching ADL and a description of medications, diet, safety factors, and activity will provide the patient and family with a thorough understanding of the conditions. Keep the patient/family informed of the patient's condition and progress. Provide emotional support and reassurance. Consult with the physician about the prognosis and potential for optimal recovery. Assist with ADL. Obtain referrals from social service, occupational therapy, physical therapy, communicology, and the dietician as necessary to assist with rehabilitation. Encourage verbalization to allieviate fears. Answer questions honestly. Teach measures to prevent complications, the proper use and maintenance of therapeutic devices and equipment, and skills for maximal independent functioning within capabilities. Assess the level of independence gained to promote as normal a life-style as possible. Describe medications, diet, activity, exercise, and other information related to the patient's progress. Reinforce the physician's teachings about CNS pathology to the patient and the family. Demonstrate safety measures for transfer, ambulation, repositioning, and ADL. Discuss the follow-up plan for care including appointments, specimens, consultations. Key nursing considerations in developing the care plan: Each patient is different and the plan of care must be individualized to meet each patient's needs, depending on the diagnosis, type of surgery performed, and degree of neurological damage. For some patients the prognosis is poor and for others there is total recovery. The nurse must respond accordingly to give the support needed. Good nursing care is the key to the outcome and adaptation of the patient and family to the dilemma that has altered their life-style.

Suggested readings

Conway-Rutkowski, B.L.: Carini and Owens' neurological and neurosurgical nursing, ed. 8, St. Louis, 1982, The C.V. Mosby Co.

Goldfarb, I.W., and Yates, A.P.: Critical care medicine, Pittsburg, 1977, Synapse Publication.

Johanson, B.C., and others: Standards for critical care, St. Louis, 1981, The C.V. Mosby Co.

Jones, D., Dunbar, C.F., and Jirovec, M.M.: Mediolcal-surgical nursing, a conceptual approach, New York, 1978, McGraw-Hill Book Co.

Nursing Skillbook Series, Coping with neurological problems proficiently, Nursing 80 Books, Horshap, Penn., 1980, Intermed Communications, Inc.

Schwartz, S., and others: Principles of surgery, New York, 1979, McGraw-Hill Book Co.

Taylor, J.W., and Ballenger, S.: Neurological dysfunctions and nursing intervention, New York, 1980, McGraw-Hill Book Co.

CHAPTER 11

Rehabilitation of the neurologically impaired individual

Rehabilitation is a part of all areas of nursing practice and is a vital segment of the nursing process. Any change in life-style resulting from illness or injury necessitates the need to adapt and cope in order to maintain homeostasis.

Unfortunately, society is designed for persons to function without physical or emotional limitations. The individual's ability to function in modern culture is based on wellness, work, independence, social justice, and responsibility. When social functioning is interrupted, there is altered ego differentiation. Persons with permanent disabilities find themselves in a minority group when attempting to function in society. The role of rehabilitation nursing is to teach the disabled person to cope positively and to adapt his life-style in order to live and function independently. Rehabilitation is based on attitudes and achievements directed toward the patient and the family in teaching them the coping mechanisms necessary to achieve independence.

The medical profession did not recognize rehabilitation as a part of medicine until World War II. The first rehabilitation medicine service was created in 1946 in New York (Rusk, 1977). Since that time rehabilitation services have slowly been established in other medical settings across the country. In 1973 the Rehabilitation Act became law (Watson, 1977) and it brought a new focus to the vocational rehabilitation of the disabled in the United States. Definitions of handicapped and disabled were defined in legislative bills as early as 1961. A clear definition of severe disability has been difficult for rehabilitators and clients to establish. The prime achievement of all this legislation has been to create a focus on the severely disabled and to recognize a need to create rehabilitation services for them. Provision of vocational rehabilitation programs stemmed from legislation in the 1970s. There has also been recognition of the need for health insurance, case-finding, follow-up care, and the elimination of architectural barriers. Attitudinal changes among employers toward the disabled have also changed. The Comprehensive Rehabilitation Services Amendments law of 1978 has lead to monumental accomplishments in the rehabilitation field in the United States as can be seen today. Funding for research and training of spinal-cord-injured patients was encouraged in the 1980s with an emphasis on methods to allow patients with spinal cord injuries to walk independently. For example, a computerized neuron system is being researched by Dr. Jerrold Petrofsky, of Wright University, Dayton, Ohio.

Rehabilitation is generally associated with patients with neurological problems because these may be permanent and lasting. The actual focus of rehabilitation is applied to the restoration of health and recovery of any individual with a physical or emotional illness. Mobilization is the primary goal of rehabilitation for all diagnostic groups.

Rehabilitation of the neurologically impaired patient involves an intense program coordinated by the nurse with the physician and the physical therapy, social service, occupational therapy, psychology, vocational therapy, recreational therapy, and chaplaincy departments and the family. Qualities to apply in the rehabilitation phase of the nursing process include a strong basic nursing knowledge, compassion, patience, a positive attitude, organization, teaching skills, and the ability to be a strong patient advocate.

CLASSIFICATIONS

The etiologies of disabling diseases are related to the following conditions:

- Spinal cord injuries
  - Quadriplegia
  - Paraplegia
- Cardiovascular diseases
  - Hemiplegia
  - Paresis and weakness
- Trauma/surgery
  - Closed head injuries
  - Craniotomy: tumors, aneurysms
  - Amputees
  - Total laryngectomies
  - Burn victims
- Debilitating and chronic illnesses
  - Arthritis
  - Parkinsonism
  - Cancer
  - Aging and the elderly
  - Infections: poliomyelitis, Guillain-Barré syndrome
  - Toxins: polyneuritis from metal poisonings
  - Congenital deformities: cerebral palsy, spina bifida, Huntington's chorea
  - Degenerative diseases: myasthenia gravis, multiple sclerosis, muscular dystrophy, and atrophy (amytrophic lateral sclerosis)

PATHOPHYSIOLOGY

The causative factors leading to chronic problems that need rehabilitation are discussed in depth throughout this manual. This chapter will focus on the nursing care necessary to prevent the complications of immobilization and to promote independence in activities of daily living (ADL). All body systems are affected by immobilization (Olsen, 1967). A discussion of the complications for each system follows.

Immobility effects

Musculoskeletal system. To maintain the stability and normal metabolism of the musculoskeletal system, it is necessary to provide mechanical stresses through activity to promote strength, endurance, and coordination of the muscles and joints. Muscle pump activity and strength to provide body support are necessary to normal motor function and maintenance of homeostasis among the bones, joints, muscles, and skin. Musculoskeletal complications frequently seen that result from deterioration caused by immobility are osteoporosis, contractures, and decubitus ulcers.

Decalcification of bone results from immobility because there is no strain, which is necessary to the build up of bone, and the destructive process continues until bone calcium levels are depleted. Regardless of the calcium intake, this process occurs and ingested calcium will not be used. Calcium being excreted will be increased in amount by that ingested and be precipated as renal calculi in the urine, deposited in muscles, or deposited in the joints, increasing the complications of immobility. The best method to prevent osteoporosis is to maintain weight-bearing and muscle activity. This can be achieved by the use of tilt tables or other weight-bearing mechanisms, oscillating beds, frequent manual repositioning, standing, ambulation, resistive range-of-motion exercises, and participation in ADLs such as hygiene, eating, and dressing.

Contractures develop because the muscles lack the ability to function within the full range of normal activity either because of damage to innervation from the nervous supply or from prolonged immobilization. Flaccid or spastic paralysis prevents joint flexion and voluntary muscle control. Flaccid paralysis involves the lower motor neuron and causes connective tissue to lose its suppleness and to become hard around body joints. Spastic paralysis involves the upper motor neurons and results from lack of voluntary muscular activity. The joints become tight, shortened, and contracted, which will interfere with their use for walking, bathing, dressing, eating, and other ADLs. Nursing measures to prevent joint contractures must be instituted because this is easier to do than to treat the contractures.

Decubitus ulcers result from the improper circulation and the prolonged pressure on soft tissue caused by decreased muscle activity and immobility. Skin destruction results from three major causes. These are mechanical, physical, and environmental. The longer any of the elements in these categories persist, the more likely it is that skin destruction will result. Nursing intervention is based on the principle that skin destruction is caused by any interference in blood supply or metabolism (Meer, 1981). The categories of causes that lead to skin destruction are:

Mechanical forces

Pressure: Any pressure greater than 55 to 100 mm Hg will cause disruption in blood flow (Meer, 1981). Normal capillary blood pressure ranges from 16 to 33 mm Hg (Van Hook, 1972).

Shear: The capillaries are stretched and elongated when pressure is applied.
Friction: Skin elasticity is lost as a result of shear. When skin skips and drags across surfaces, it tears and burns, causing the capillaries to bleed.

Common body points for shear and pressure include:

- Side of head.
- Occiput.
- Rim of ear.
- Dorsal thoracic area.
- Shoulder.
- Elbow.
- Ischium.
- Sacrum and coccyx.
- Perineum.
- Trochanter.
- Posterior knee.
- Anterior knee.
- Malleolus.
- Heel.

Environmental forces:

Moisture, heat, cold, dryness and prolonged periods in combination with any of the mechanical forces.

Physical conditions:

Emaciation, obesity, anemia, nutritional deficiencies, dehydration, spasm, contractures, coma, incontinence, perspiration, any disease processes that interfere with circulation.

Prevention of decubitus ulcers is the nurses' and patient's responsibility. Techniques to establish a protocol of care to maintain skin integrity include repositioning, maintainence of nutrition, and the use of products to facilitiate these measures.

Manual turning by the nurse provides the patient with some feeling of control over the environment and at the same time allows the nurse an opportunity to gather a total picture of the patient as assessments relating to skin integrity, joint motion, and muscle strength are made. Manual turning is strenuous to the nursing personnel and mechanical devices have been developed as an alternative to provide turning. A patient can be turned more frequently on these devices. The normal sleeping adult has a physiological turning time of every 11.6 minutes (Sullivan, 1981). The concept of the Roto-Rest kinetic bed is based on this principle (Fig. 11-1). Other mechanical beds include the Stryker Turning Frame (see photo in Chapter 9), Stokes-Edgerton bed, and Circo-electric Turning Frame (Fig. 11-2). Foam pads, air and water mattresses, extremity supports, and splints have been developed and are used freely in the prevention of musculoskeletal complications caused by immobilization (Figs. 11-3 to 11-10).

Text continued on p. 345.

A

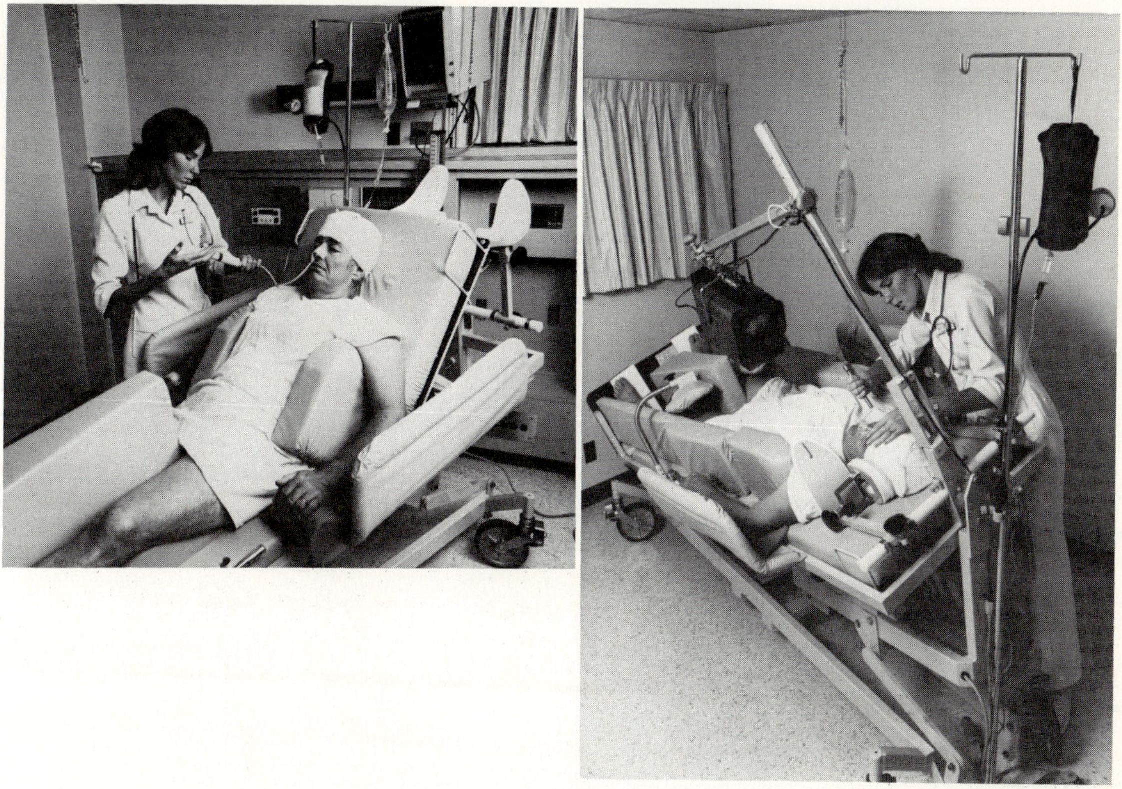

B

Fig. 11-1 **A,** Mark III Roto kinetic bed. It features a sit-up for ease of tube feeding. **B,** Roto kinetic bed to treat immobility. A television is mounted on the table and rotates with it. It is especially useful in supplying audiovisual stimulation to comatose patients. (Courtesy Kinetic Concepts, Inc., San Antonio, Texas.)

A

B

C

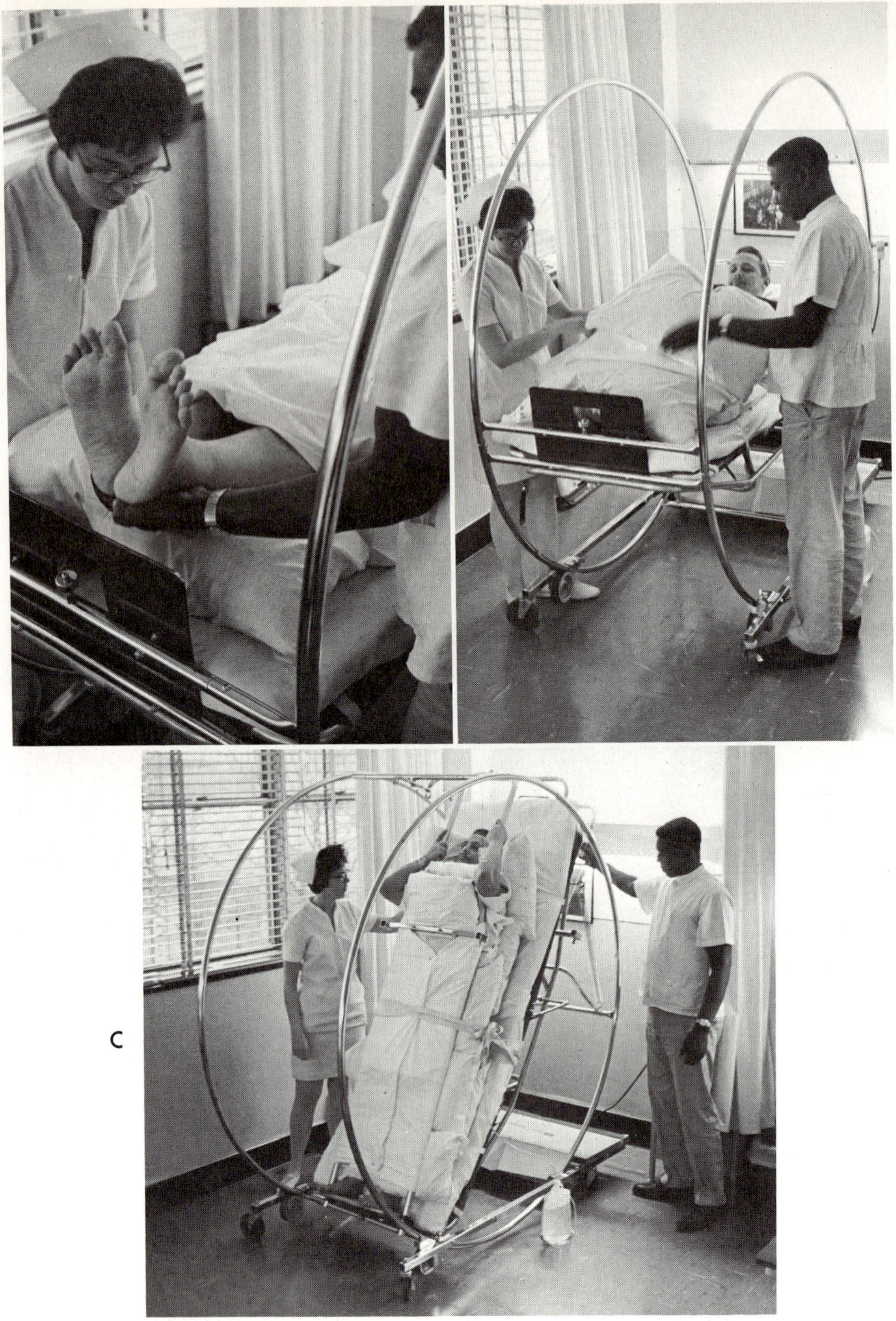

Fig. 11-2 CircOlectric bed. During the turning process the nurse places her hand on the patient's shoulder for reassurance. She observes him for pallor or other signs of vertigo or nausea that can occur the first few times the total body position is changed. (From Rusk, H.A.: Rehabilitation medicine, ed. 4, St. Louis, 1977, The C.V. Mosby Co.)

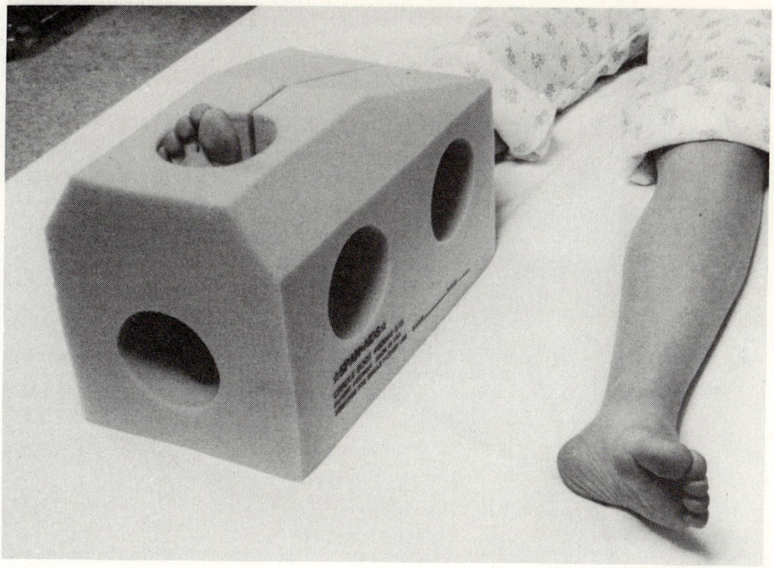

Fig. 11-3 Support to prevent pressure on heels and ankles and to prevent foot drop. (Courtesy Span-America, Inc., Greenville, S.C.)

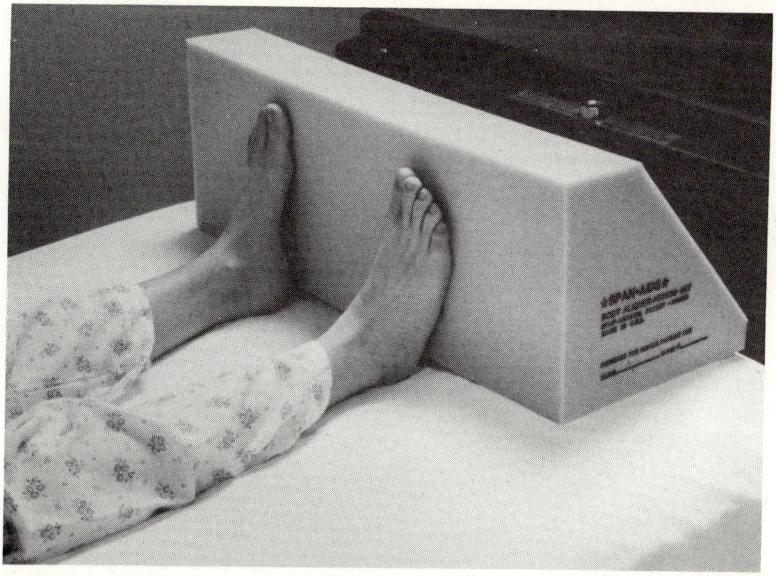

Fig. 11-4 Prevention of foot drop. (Courtesy Span-America, Inc., Greenville, S.C.)

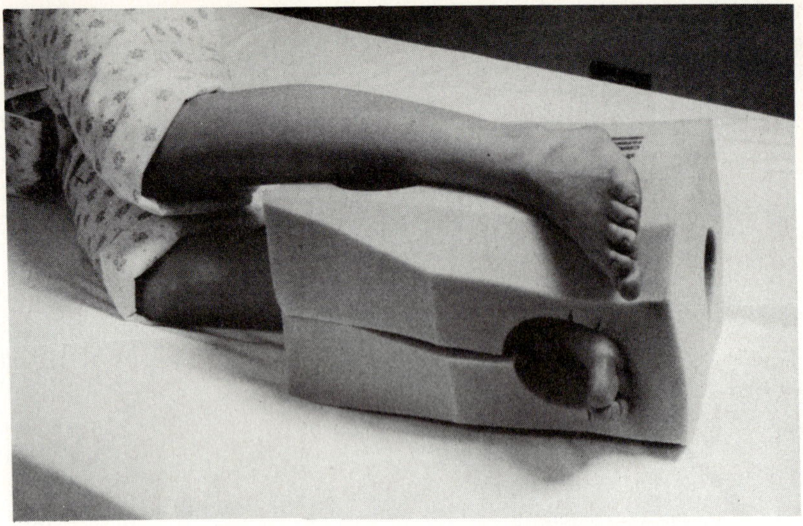

Fig. 11-5 Prevention of pressure on bony prominences of legs and feet. (Courtesy Span-America, Inc., Greenville, S.C.)

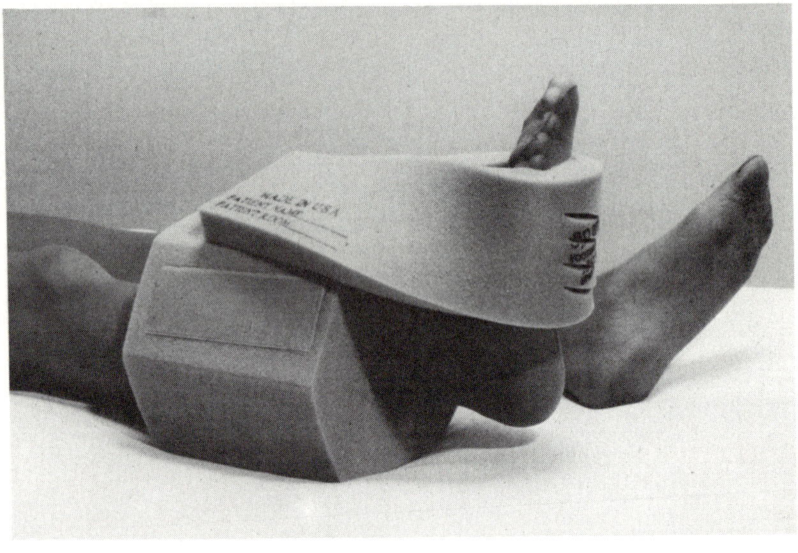

Fig. 11-6 Prevention of heel and ankle pressure and foot drop. (Courtesy Span-America, Inc., Greenville, S.C.)

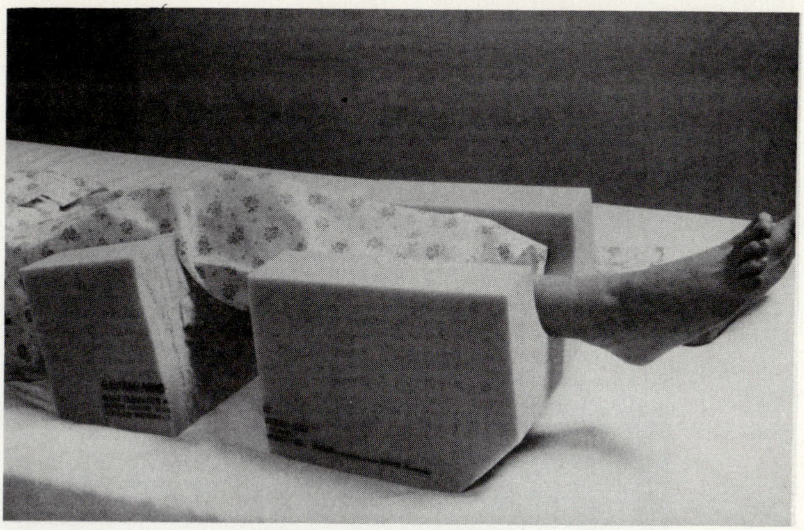

Fig. 11-7 Prevention of pressure at popliteal and heel. (Courtesy Span-America, Inc., Greenville, S.C.)

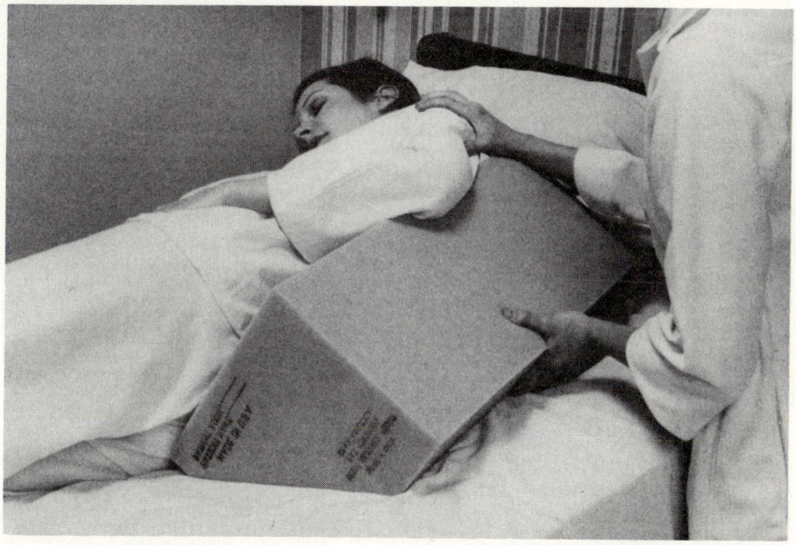

Fig. 11-8 Support to back in side-lying position. (Courtesy Span-America, Inc., Greenville, S.C.)

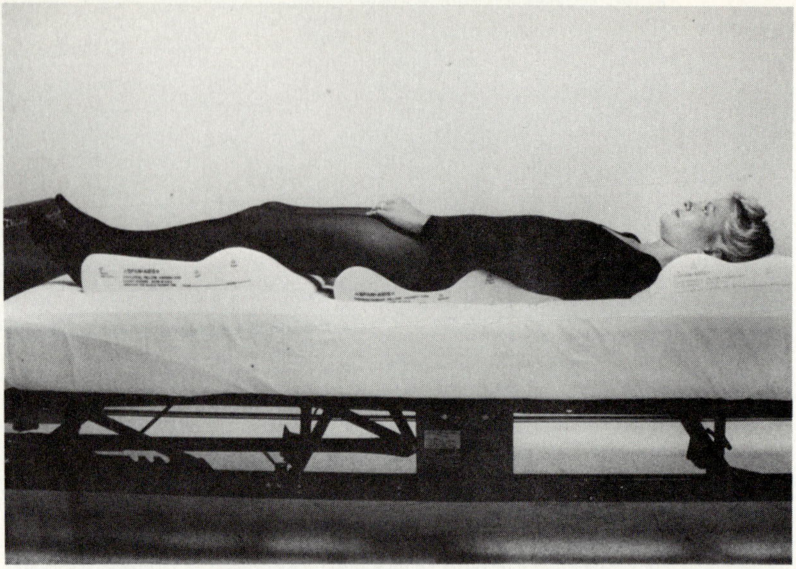

Fig. 11-9 Support to common pressure areas while in back-lying position. (Courtesy Span-America, Inc. Greenville, S.C.)

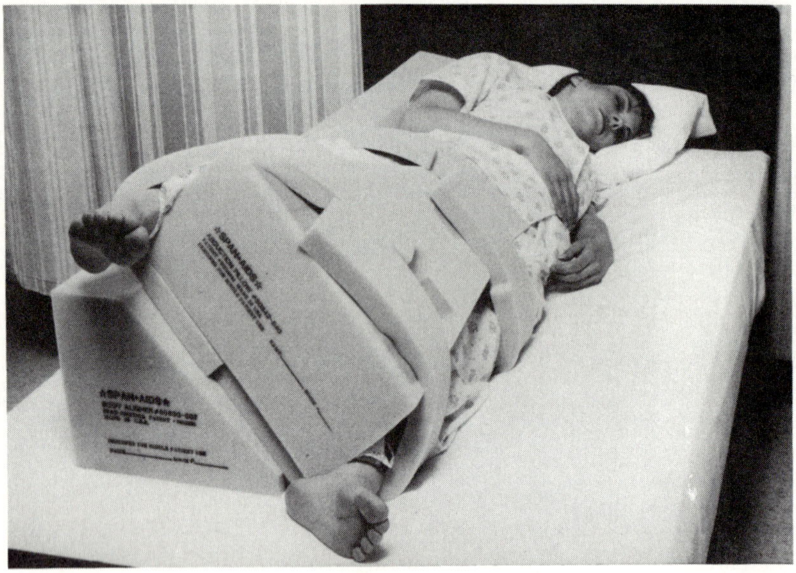

Fig. 11-10 Support of hips in abduction while in side-lying position. (Courtesy Span-America, Inc., Greenville, S.C.)

Cardiovascular system. The three major complications of the cardiovascular system that are caused by immobilization are orthostatic hypotension, increased work load of the heart, and thrombus formation. Orthostatic hypotension is evident when an individual first sits or stands after being supine for a prolonged time; weakness and dizziness occur. This is a result of deterioration of the ability of the autonomic nervous system to equalize blood supply and the loss of the general muscle tone that is necessary to produce the normal pressure on veins that assists venous return to the heart.

The increased work load of the heart is caused by the redistribution of the blood supply while in the recumbent position, and this increases the blood supply to be handled by the heart. Venous stasis, hypercoagulability of the blood, and external venous pressure contribute to thrombus formation in immobilized patients.

Prevention of cardiovascular complications is dependent on nursing interventions such as passive and active exercises, frequent position changes, measures to avoid constipation and fatigue, and the use of antiembolism stockings.

Respiratory system. Respiratory movement is decreased by compression on the thorax when a patient sits too long or lies too long on the back, side, or in a prone position. Any time chest expansion is limited, air exchange in the alveoli is decreased and stasis of secretions occurs. Nursing interventions for preventing such complications include routine assessment of breath sounds; assisting the patient to turn, deep breath, and cough; and postural drainage exercises.

Gastrointestinal system. Anorexia results from prolonged immobility because the nitrogen balance is in a negative state because of immobilization. A protein deficiency develops during immobilization as a result of increased catabolic activity and it causes tissue damage. When patients fail to eat, malnutrition results and body tissues do not receive the normal nutrients necessary for cellular function. An immobilized patient needs adequate nutrients to maintain basal metabolism. This requirement is a minimum of a daily caloric intake of 1000 calories. A high-protein, adequate carbohydrate, and fat diet is required. Small, frequent feedings are more appealing to the anorexic patient. In Ireland immobilized patients are given twenty raw eggs a day with beer to maintain a high-protein diet.

The major complication of immobility of the gastrointestinal tract is impaired bowel elimination. The process of elimination depends upon normal smooth and skeletal muscle activity and visceral reflex patterns. If nerve supply to the external anal sphincter muscle is lacking, the ability to expel formed stool successfully from the rectum is lost. Muscular atrophy, loss of bowel tone, lack of exercise, failure to allow defecation to occur, being unaware of the need to defecate, and the inability to assume the physiological position for defecation lead to constipation, impaction, bowel obstruction, and other complications of bowel elimination. A bowel program must be developed for the patient by the nurse to prevent constipation and other elimination complications.

Table 11-1 Types of neurogenic bladder

Dysfunction	Causes	Characteristics of voiding
Uninhibited neurogenic bladder (NGB)	Brain center conditions such as delayed childhood development, cerebral atherosclerosis, cerebrovascular accident (CVA), brain tumor, brain trauma, demyelination diseases (multiple sclerosis).	Uninhibited contractions that cause delayed voiding and leave the patient with an incontinence. Patient is able to initiate voiding, but cannot stop it.
Reflex NGB	Traumatic transection of the spinal cord	No conscious control of bladder filling or inhibition. Reflex arc is intact and voiding can occur automatically after external cutaneous stimulation.
Autonomous bladder dysfunction	Lesions that involve both motor and sensory components (2, 3, 4) of the sacral spinal cord. Trauma, infection, congenital abnormalities, tumors, radical pelvic surgery, spinal shock following acute spinal cord transection	Reflex arc is lost. There is no motor power to the bladder and perception as well as ability to empty the bladder willfully is lacking.
Motor paralytic bladder	Damage to the anterior horn cells and/or to anterior roots of the S2-S4 cord segments; detrusor muscle has no motor power as a result of this damage. Also caused by medications that affect the peripheral nervous system (atropine, propantheline [Pro-Banthine], chlorpromazine [Thorazine], thioridazine [Mellaril], amitriptyline [Elavil], phenytoin [Dilantin], general anesthesia), pelvic surgery, poliomyelitis, Guillain-Barré syndrome, trauma, tumor, multiple sclerosis.	Patient perceives bladder fullness but cannot initiate voiding.
Sensory paralytic bladder	Lesions of the dorsal horn cells (sensory) or dorsal roots of the sacral cord segments. Diabetes mellitus is the most common cause.	Patient has no perception of bladder fullness, but has the ability to initiate voiding unless overdistention occurs for a prolonged period and the bladder becomes atonic.

Urinary system. Normal urinary function is dependent upon humans being in an erect position and on having an intact nervous supply to the external sphincter, internal sphincter, and detrusor muscle. In the supine position urine remains in the renal pelvis and cannot flow by gravity through the ureters into the bladder. Urinary stasis results as a complication and becomes the cause of calculi formation and the onset of infection. If the reflex action to relax the perineal muscles to enable micturation is lacking, the bladder becomes overdistended. Stress incontinence from an overfilled bladder results, bladder tone is lost because of overstretching, and the sensation of needing to void is no longer present; back pressure and damage to the renal nephrons result.

Bladder function in neurological disorders is related to the location of the trauma and the course of degenerative disease. Bladder, bowel, and sex control are located at S2, S3, S4; if the bladder works, so will the others. There are five types of neurological bladder dysfunctions (see Table 11-1). Nursing care to prevent urinary complications caused by immobilization is based on an understanding of normal micturation, knowledge of the type of neurogenic bladder dysfunction, and an assessment of drug therapy or surgical procedures that may have been performed. Bladder programs are individualized for patients according to the type of bladder dysfunction. Goals of a bladder program are to prevent stasis, prevent distention, and to prevent calculi and infection. A bowel program is discussed on page 367.

Metabolism. The effects of immobilization on metabolic functions have been discussed in the sections on the other complications. To summarize these effects, metabolic processes affected by immobility include protein breakdown and deficiency leading to negative nitrogen balance, development of decubitus ulcers, excretion of electrolytes with accelerated catabolism, demineralization of bone, and formation of urinary stones. Body temperature is also affected by immobilization. Lying in a supine position causes dilatation of the blood vessels and an increase in body temperature. In order to decrease this heat, sweating occurs. Sweating is more profuse in skin folds, such as creases in the neck, axilla, perineum, under the breasts, abdominal folds, and where the arms rest across chest. Bed clothing prevents the loss of heat by conduction and radiation and contributes to the prevention of heat loss. When perspiration is increased, the patient loses potassium, sodium, and chloride, which are essential electrolytes for maintaining metabolic equilibrium. Immobility in combination with physical and psychological stress causes changes in the production of body hormones and in the regulatory function of homeostasis. The reason for this effect is complex and will not be discussed in detail in this manual. Nursing measures to prevent metabolic dysfunction involve the reduction of the effects that cause stress and inhibit the control of body temperatures and preventing all of the other aforementioned dysfunctions.

Psychosocial. Immobility causes disturbances in an individual's ego identify and his self-image as a social being. Following the onset of illness or trauma, the individual goes through a process of adjustment that involves various adaptive behaviors. A person will respond to the situation based on his understanding and ability to learn, his personal drives, self-perception, ability to express self, his ego state, and his flexibility in fulfilling his societal role. In coping with significant physical or emotional dysfunction, an individual must first go through the stages of grief: denial, anger, bargaining, depression, and acceptance (Sire, 1981).

Immobilty reduces sensory stimulation and the ability to relate to one's environment. The American culture centers on wellness, occupation, independence, and social institutions. The role identity of an individual is directly related to family, education, work, religion, sex, and leisure. When this role is disrupted, one's ego differentiation is disturbed and role activities must be adapted to regain optional socioeconomic satisfaction. Nursing care in assisting the patient to adapt in this situation is dependent on compassion and a promotion of independence versus dependence to encourage physical and emotional mobility.

NURSING ASSESSMENT

Patients needing rehabilitation must be evaluated for muscle strength, range of joint motion, ability to function in ADL, and for the home, psychosocial, and vocational situations (Figs. 11-11 to 11-13). In making the initial nursing assessment, the following subjective and objective assessment data must be collected.

History: name, age, sex, marital status, diagnosis, past illnesses, date of admission to the hospital, physician's name, medications, allergies, diet, and appetite.

Physical assessment: bathing (bed, tub, shower, cart, wheelchair), ambulation, assistive devices for ambulation and/or ADL, dressing, communication (type of aphasia, hearing, visual impairments), skin integrity, bladder/bowel function (continency, incontinency), toileting technique, (bedpan, commode, wheelchair bathroom, bathroom, catheterization), muscle tone, analgesia.

Psychosocial: religion, occupation, family role, family members or significant others, education or training, financial (source of income, health insurance), mental status, personality trait pattern and changes that have occurred since the onset of disability, interpersonal relationships, significant coping mechanisms, hobbies and special interests, home environment (physical arrangement, description of living quarters), number of members in household.

Establish goals for the patient and family. Include both short- and long-term objectives.

Develop a discharge plan based on the initial assessment. Include the following: level of independence (supervision, assistive, lifting, or total independence), ambulation method (wheelchair, crutches, other assistive devices such as braces or canes, ambulatory), toilet needs, method of entrance into house (stairs, ramp, other), travel to work (taxi, bus, own car, transfer from wheelchair to car or bus, crossing streets).

The management of immobility is a challenge to all health care professionals. It is the number one goal in the management of acute head injuries, spinal cord injuries, burn victims, multiple system traumas, severe pulmonary disease, comas, and with the aged and debilitated. All body systems are affected by immobilization and a comprehensive plan of care is required to prevent the complications of immobility.

CHART 1

MUSCLE EXAMINATION

Patient's name________________________________ Chart No._________

Date of birth______________________ Name of institution______________________

Date of onset______________________ Attending physician____________________ M. D.

Diagnosis:

	LEFT					RIGHT				
					Examiner's initials					
					Date					
NECK					Flexors					NECK
					Extensors					
TRUNK					Flexor					TRUNK
					Extensors—Thoracic					
					Extensors—Lumbar					
					R. ext. obl. / L. int. obl. } Rotators { L. ext. obl. / R. int. obl.					
					Elevation of pelvis					
HIP					Flexors					HIP
					Extensors					
					Abductor					
					Adductors					
					External rotators					
					Internal rotators					
					Sartorius					
					Tensor fasciae latae					
KNEE					Flexor—Outer hamstring					KNEE
					Flexors—Inner hamstrings					
					Extensors					
ANKLE					Plantar-flexors—Gastroc. & soleus					ANKLE
					Plantar-flexor—Soleus					
FOOT					Invertor—Anterior tibial					FOOT
					Invertor—Posterior tibial					
					Evertor—Peroneus brevis					
					Evertor—Peroneus longus					
TOES (4 lateral)					Flexors—Metatarsophalangeal					TOES (4 lateral)
					Extensors—Metatarsophalangeal					
					Flexor—Proximal interphalangeal					
					Flexor—Distal interphalangeal					
					Abductors					
					Adductors					
HALLUX					Flexor—Metatarsophalangeal					HALLUX
					Flexor—Interphalangeal					
					Extensor—Interphalangeal					

Additional data:

Face____

Speech_______________________________________

Swallowing___________________________________

Diaphragm____________________________________

Intercostals__________________________________

KEY

100%	5	N	Normal	Complete range of motion against gravity with full resistance
75%	4	G	Good*	Complete range of motion against gravity with some resistance
50%	3	F	Fair*	Complete range of motion against gravity
25%	2	P	Poor*	Complete range of motion with gravity eliminated
10%	1	T	Trace	Evidence of slight contractility;no joint motion
0	0	0	Zero	No evidence of contractility
S or SS			Spasm	Spasm or severe spasm
C or CC			Contracture	Contracture or severe contracture

*Muscle spasm or contracture may limit range of motion. A question mark should be placed after the grading of a movement that is incomplete from this cause.

Continued.

Fig. 11-11 Medical assessment for neurologically impaired. (From Rusk, H.A.: Rehabilitation medicine, ed. 4, St. Louis, 1977, The C.V. Mosby Co.)

CHART 1, cont'd

LEFT										RIGHT
					Examiner's initials					
					Date					
SCAPULA					Abductor—Serratus anterior					SCAPULA
					Adductor—Middle trapezius					
					Adductors—Rhomboids					
					Elevators					
					Depressor					
SHOUL-DER					Flexors					SHOUL-DER
					Extensors					
					Abductors					
					Horizontal abductor					
					Horizontal adductor					
					External rotators					
					Internal rotators					
ELBOW					Flexors					ELBOW
					Extensors					
FORE-ARM					Supinators					FORE-ARM
					Pronators					
WRIST					Flexor—Radial deviation					WRIST
					Flexor—Ulnar deviation					
					Extensors—Radial deviation					
					Extensor—Ulnar deviation					
FINGERS					1 Flexor profundus digitorum 1					FINGERS
					2 Flexor profundus digitorum 2					
					3 Flexor profundus digitorum 3					
					4 Flexor profundus digitorum 4					
					1 Flexor sublimis digitorum 1					
					2 Flexor sublimis digitorum 2					
					3 Flexor sublimis digitorum 3					
					4 Flexor sublimis digitorum 4					
					1 Finger extensors 1					
					2 Finger extensors 2					
					3 Finger extensors 3					
					4 Finger extensors 4					
					1 Lumbricales 1					
					2 Lumbricales 2					
					3 Lumbricales 3					
					4 Lumbricales 4					
					Dorsal interossei					
					Palmar interossei					
THUMB					Opponens pollicis					THUMB
					Adductor pollicis					
					Abductor pollicis longus					
					Abductor pollicis brevis					
					Thumb extensors					
					Flexor pollicis longus					
					Flexor pollicis brevis					
					CONTRACTIONS AND DEFORMITIES					
					SHOULDER					
					ELBOW					
					FOREARM					
					WRIST					
					FINGERS					
					THUMB					

Date____________________ Therapist____________________

Fig. 11-11 cont'd Medical assessment for neurologically impaired.

CHART 2

NEW YORK UNIVERSITY MEDICAL CENTER
INSTITUTE OF REHABILITATION MEDICINE
PHYSICAL THERAPY

NAME________________ DATE________________

DIAGNOSIS________________ PATIENT STATUS______ IN____OUT______

DISABILITY________________________________

RANGE OF MOTION

1. Anatomical position is starting position. Range is measured with cauda as 0°, cranium as 180°. Rotating motions are from the midsagittal plane as 0° to lateral plane as 180°.
2. All ranges are expressed as passive range of motion. Check muscle chart attached for limitations caused by tightness, weakness, spasm, or contracture.
3. The scale is divided into units of 10°. Range of motion is recorded by filling in area of range directly on attached sketch with date and examiner's initial.
4. Use of same sheet for subsequent tests is recorded in same color and dated accordingly.
5. Retrogression is marked by diagonal lines over area of previous test and dated.
6. If position is other than in sketch, indicate S for supine, P for prone.

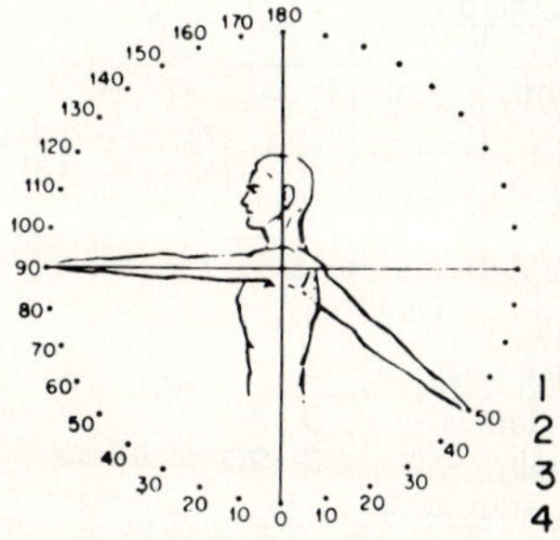

Shoulder

Flexion	0-90
Flexion and rotation of scapula	90-180
Extension and rotation of scapula	180-90
Extension	90-50

Limitations

	L		R	
	Fl.	Ext.	Fl.	Ext.
1				
2				
3				
4				

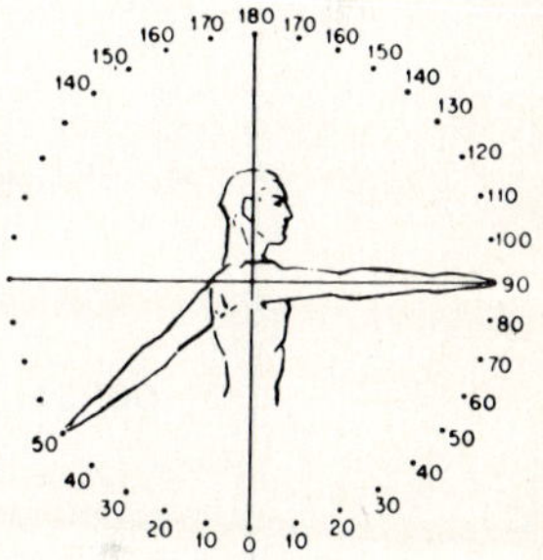

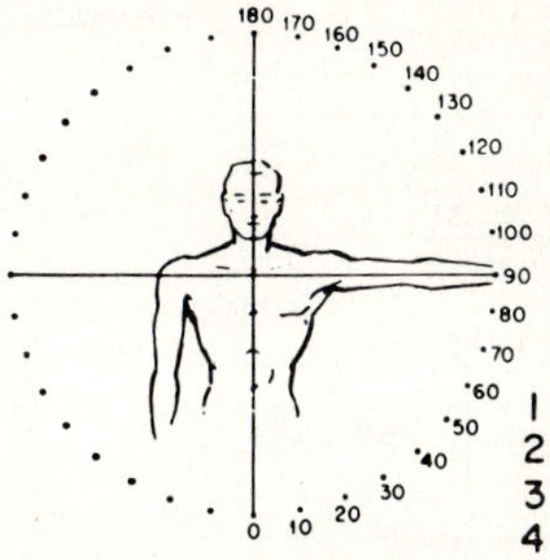

Shoulder

Abduction	0-90
Abduction and rotation of scapula	90-180
Adduction and rotation of scapula	180-90
Adduction	90-0

Limitations

	L		R	
	Abd.	Add.	Abd.	Add.
1				
2				
3				
4				

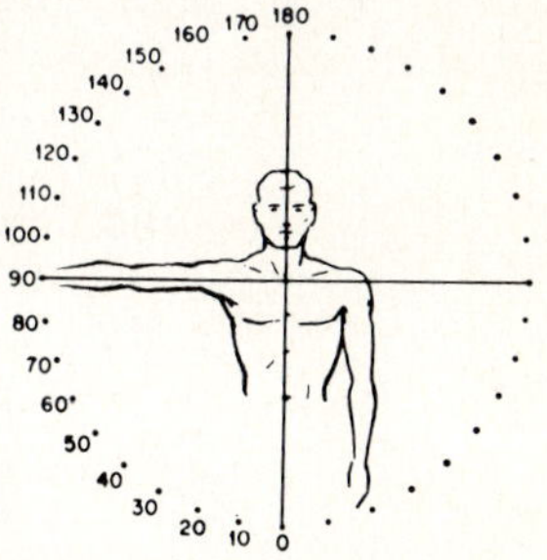

Continued.

Fig. 11-12 Chart to indicate the normal joint excursions numerically (range of motion). (From White, P.D., Rusk, H.A., Lee, P.R., and Williams, B.: Rehabilitation of the cardiovascular patient, New York, 1985, Blakiston Division, McGraw-Hill Book Co., Inc.)

CHART 2, cont'd

INT. EXT.

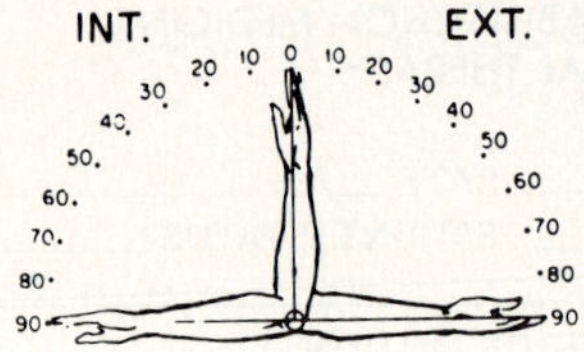

Shoulder Rotation

Elbow flexed 90°
Extension rotation 0–90
Internal rotation 0–90

Limitations

	L		R	
	Int.	Ext.	Int.	Ext.
1				
2				
3				
4				

EXT. INT.

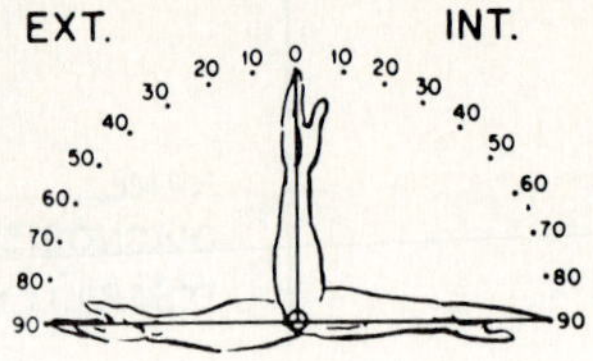

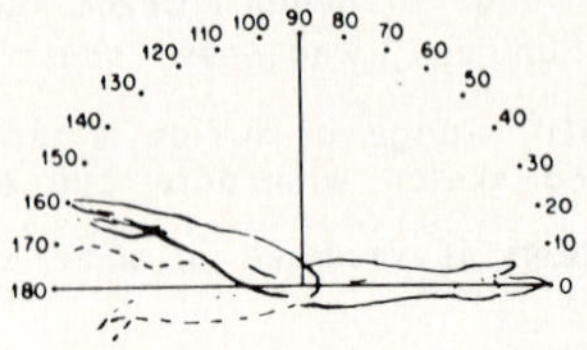

Elbow

Flexion 0-145-160
Extension 160-145- 0

Limitations

	L		R	
	Flex.	Ext.	Flex.	Ext.
1				
2				
3				
4				

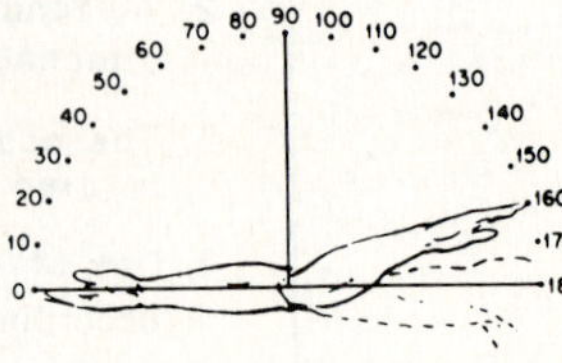

PRON. SUP.

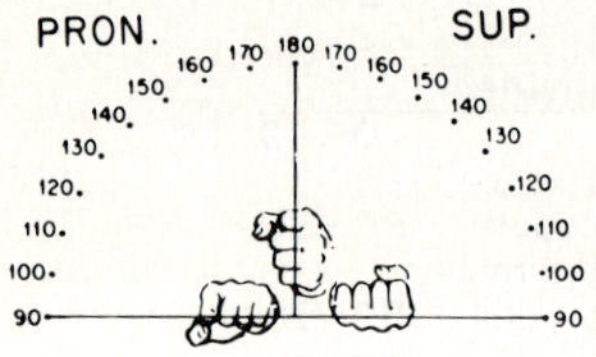

Radioulnar

Pronation 0–90
Supination 0–90

Limitations

	L		R	
	Sup.	Pron.	Sup.	Pron.
1				
2				
3				
4				

SUP. PRON.

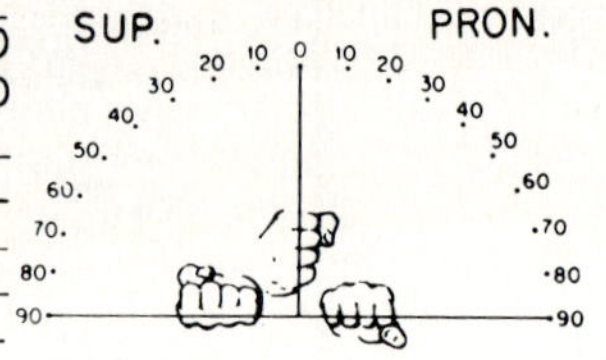

DORSAL VOLAR

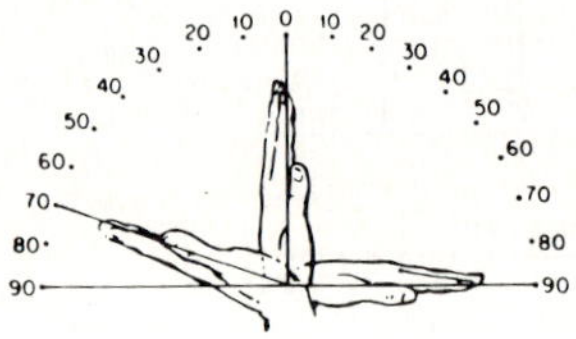

Wrist (flexion)

Dorsal flexion 0–70
Volar flexion 0–90

Limitations

	L		R	
	Dor.	Vol.	Dor.	Vol.
1				
2				
3				
4				

VOLAR DORSAL

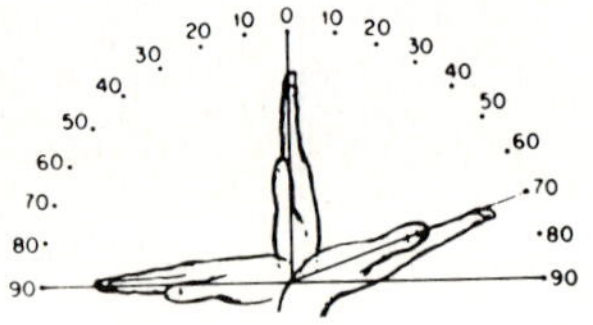

ABD. ADD.

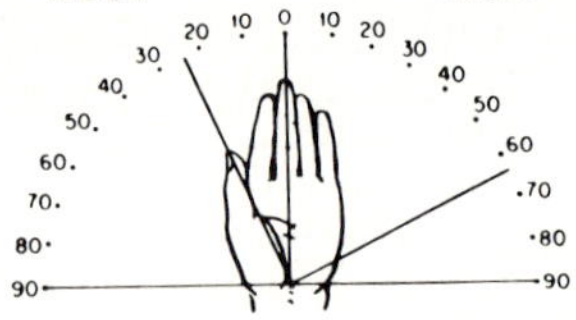

Wrist

Abduction 0–25
Adduction 0–55–65

Limitations

	L		R	
	Rad.	Uln.	Rad.	Uln.
1				
2				
3				
4				

ADD. ABD.

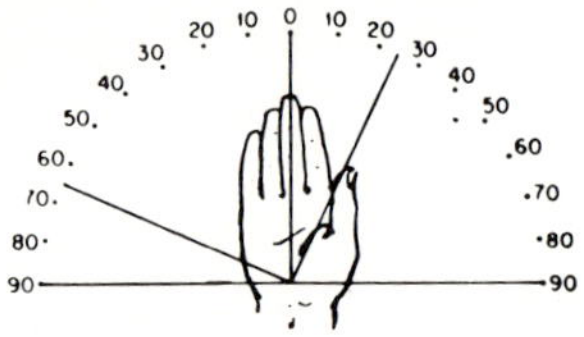

Fig. 11-12 cont'd Chart to indicate the normal joint excursions numerically (range of motion).

CHART 2, cont'd

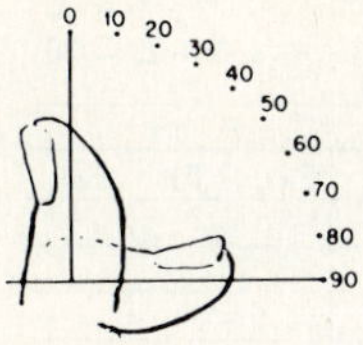

Thumb I P

Flexion	0–90
Extension	90– 0

Limitations

	L		R	
	Fl.	Ext.	Fl.	Ext.
1				
2				
3				
4				

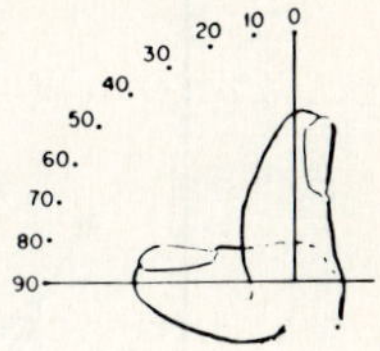

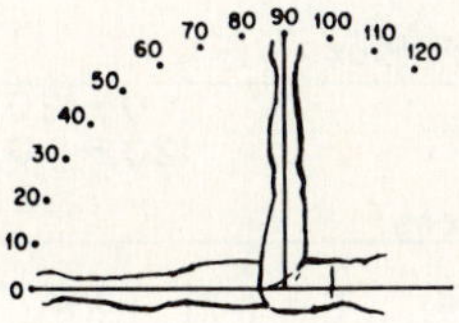

Hip

Flexion (straight knee)	0–90
Flexion (bent knee)	0–115–125
Extension	0– 10– 15
Extension and lumbar spine	0–15–45

Limitations

Flexion (straight knee)

	L		R	
	Fl.	Ext.	Fl.	Ext.
1				
2				
3				
4				

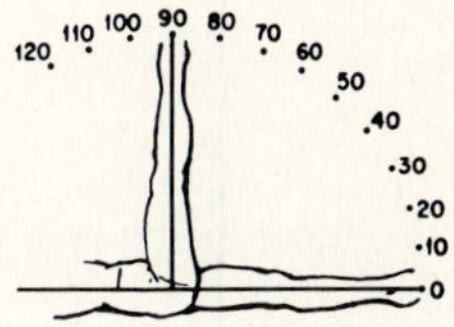

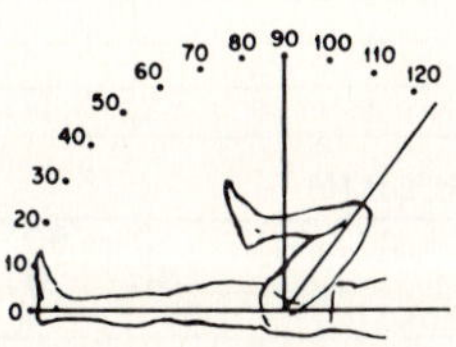

Flexion (bent knee)

	L		R	
	Fl.	Ext.	Fl.	Ext.
1				
2				
3				
4				

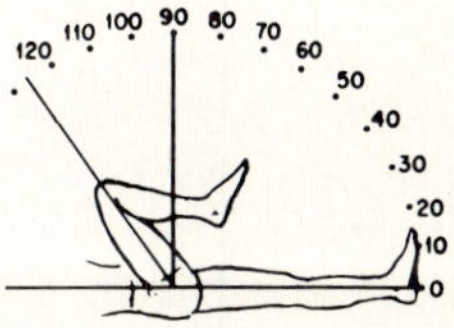

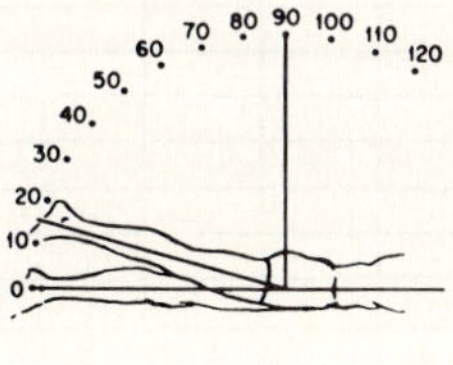

Extension

	L		R	
	Ext.	E&L	Ext.	E&L
1				
2				
3				
4				

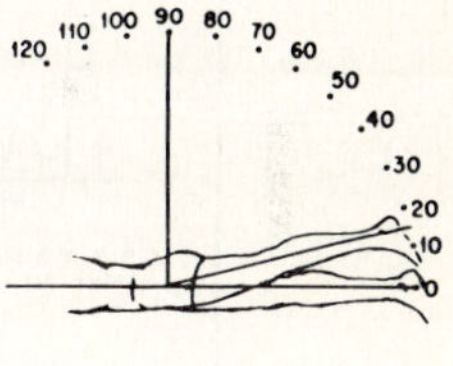

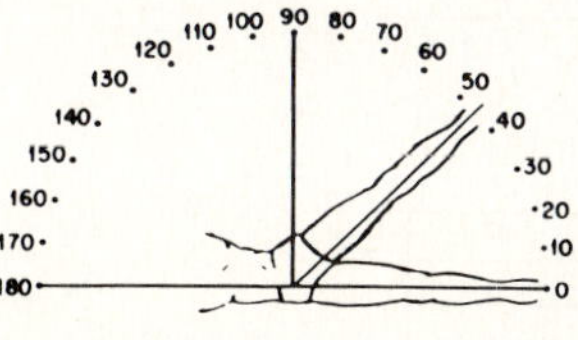

Hip

Abduction	0–45
Adduction	0–45

Limitations

	L		R	
	Abd.	Add.	Abd.	Add.
1				
2				
3				
4				

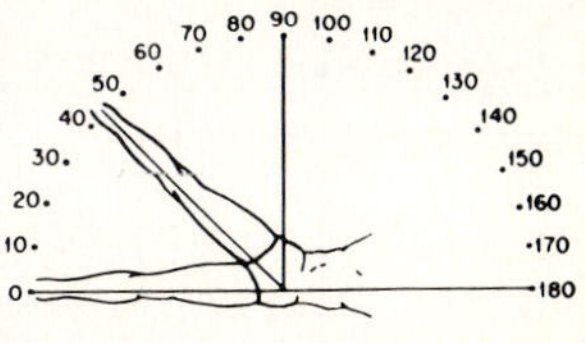

Continued.

Fig. 11-12 cont'd Chart to indicate the normal joint excursions numerically (range of motion).

CHART 2, cont'd

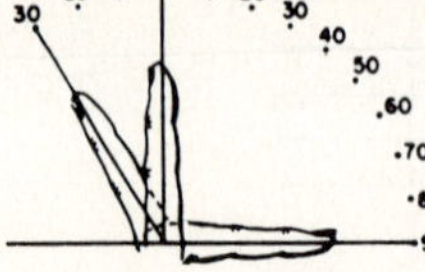

Fingers M P

Flexion	0 – 90
Extension	0 –20 – 30

Limitations

	L				R			
	Fl.	Ext.	Fl.	Ext.	Fl.	Ext.	Fl.	Ext.
1	II		III		II		III	
2								
3								
4								
1	IV		V		IV		V	
2								
3								
4								

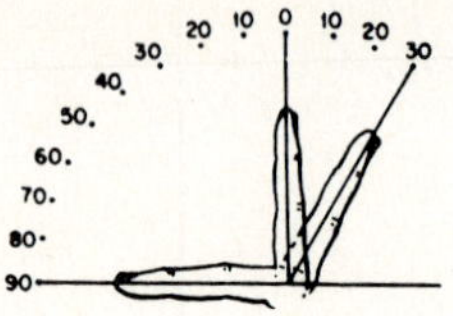

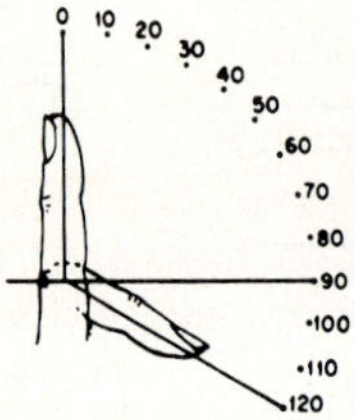

Fingers I P Prox

Flexion	0 – 120
Extension	120 – 0

Limitations

	L				R			
	Fl.	Ext	Fl.	Ext.	Fl.	Ext.	Fl.	Ext.
1	II		III		II		III	
2								
3								
4								
1	IV		V		IV		V	
2								
3								
4								

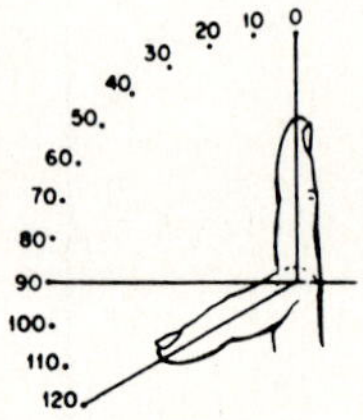

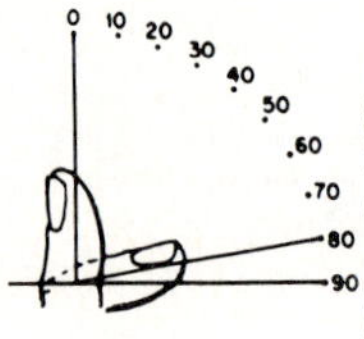

P.T.R.O.M.–NO. 3
5M-H.S.P.

Fingers I P Distal

Flexion	0 – 80
Extension	80 – 0

Limitations

	L				R			
	Fl.	Ext	Fl.	Ext.	Fl.	Ext.	Fl.	Ext.
1	II		III		II		III	
2								
3								
4								
1	IV		V		IV		V	
2								
3								
4								

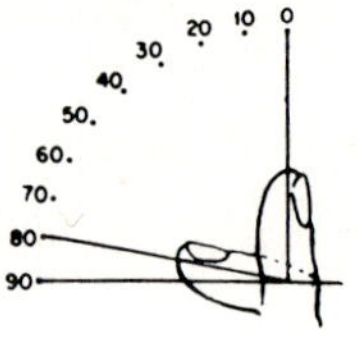

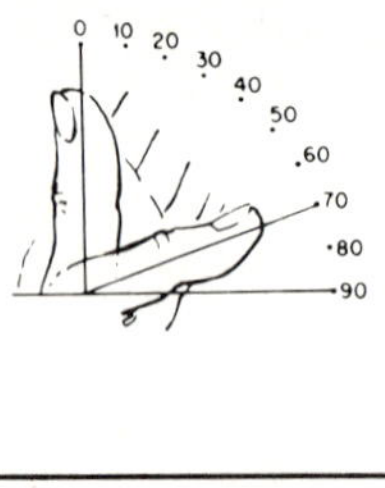

Thumb M P

Flexion	0 – 60 – 70
Extension	70 – 60 – 0

Limitations

	L		R	
	Fl.	Ext.	Fl.	Ext.
1				
2				
3				
4				

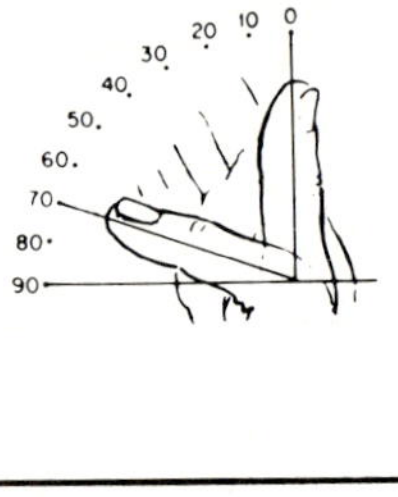

Fig. 11-12 cont'd Chart to indicate the normal joint excursions numerically (range of motion).

CHART 2, cont'd

INT. EXT.

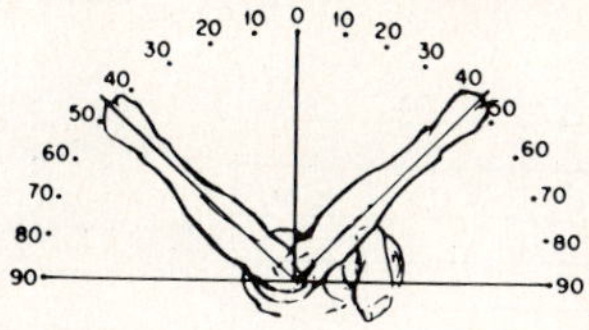

Hip (bent knee prone)

External rotation 0-45
Internal rotation 0-45

Limitations

	L		R	
	Int.	Ext.	Int.	Ext.
1				
2				
3				
4				

EXT. INT.

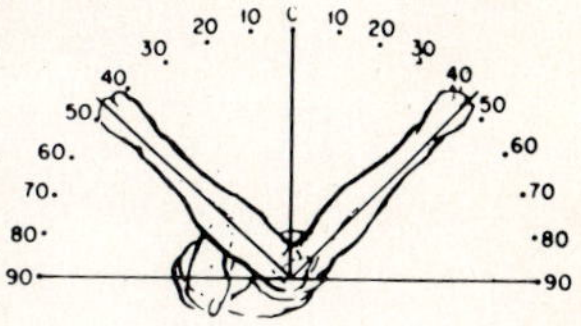

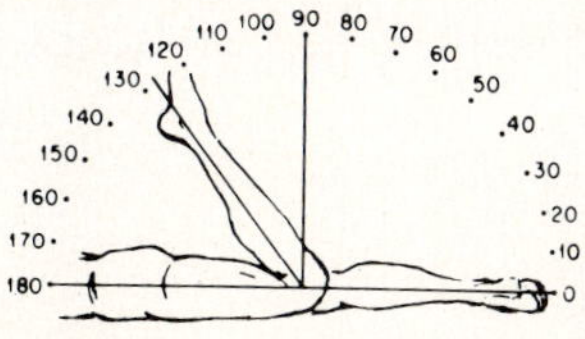

Knee

Flexion (prone) 0-120-130
Extension 130-120- 0

Limitations

	L		R	
	Fl.	Ext.	Fl.	Ext.
1				
2				
3				
4				

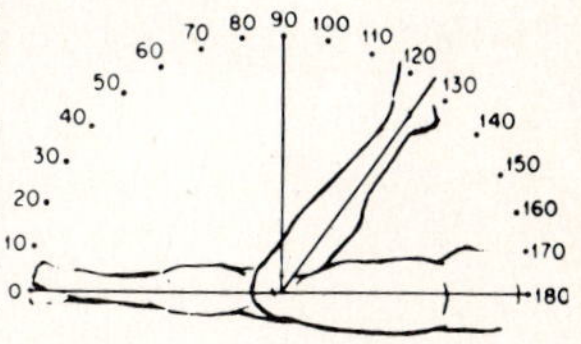

DORSAL PLANTAR

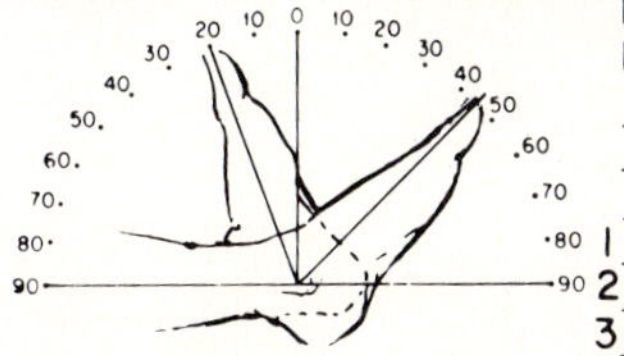

Ankle

Flexion 0-20
Extension 0-45

Limitations

	L		R	
	Fl.	Ext.	Fl.	Ext.
1				
2				
3				
4				

PLANTAR DORSAL

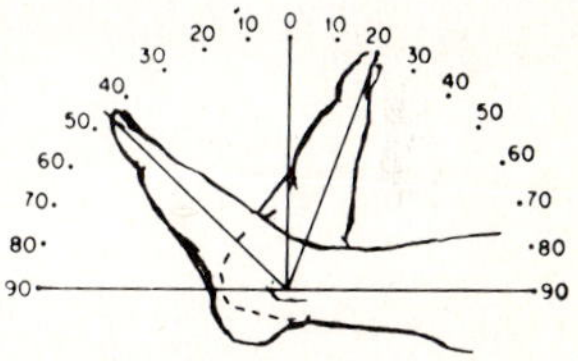

EV. INV.

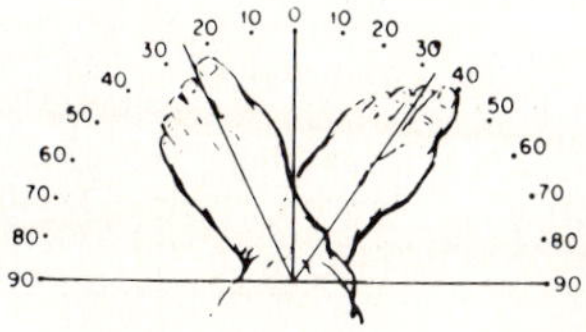

Foot

Eversion 0-25
Inversion 0-35

Limitations

	L		R	
	Ev.	Inv.	Ev.	Inv.
1				
2				
3				
4				

EV. INV.

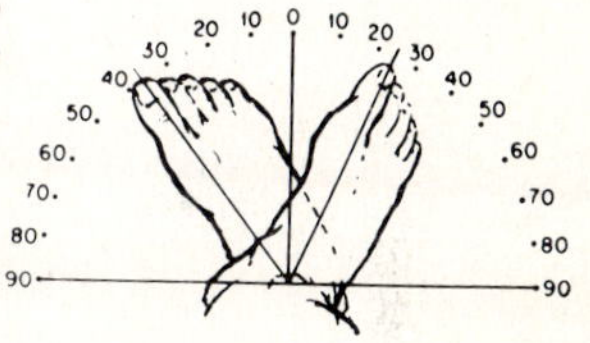

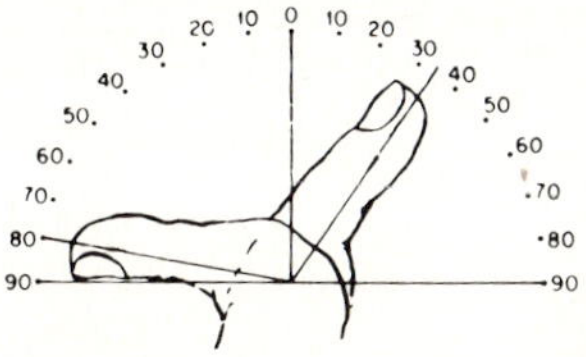

Toes M P

Flexion 0-25-35
Extension 0-80

Limitations

	L		R	
	Fl.	Ext.	Fl.	Ext.
1				
2				
3				
4				
5				

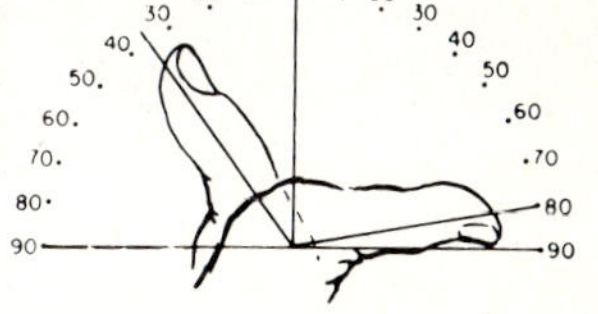

Continued.

Fig. 11-12 cont'd Chart to indicate the normal joint excursions numerically (range of motion).

CHART 2, cont'd

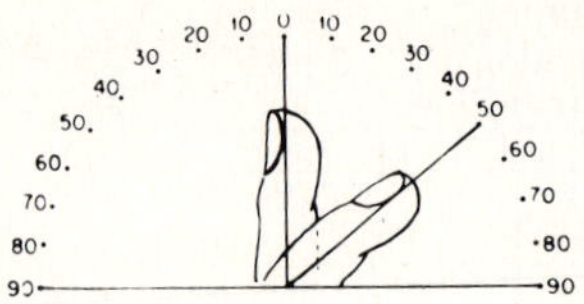

Toes I P

Flexion 0-50
Extension 50- 0

Limitations

	L		R	
	Fl.	Ext.	Fl.	Ext.
1				
2				
3				
4				

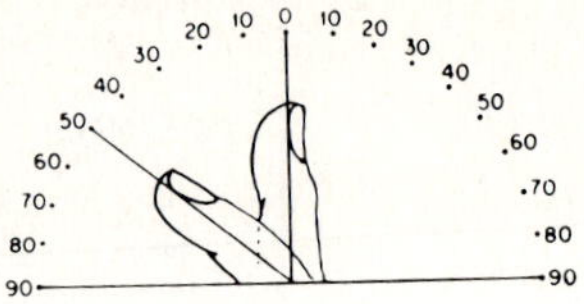

Fig. 11-12 cont'd Chart to indicate the normal joint excursions numerically (range of motion).

CHART 3

NEW YORK UNIVERSITY MEDICAL CENTER
INSTITUTE OF REHABILITATION MEDICINE

TEST
ACTIVITIES OF DAILY LIVING

Mr. Date of initial test ________ Patient: In ______ Out ______
Miss
Name Mrs. ________________________ Age ____ Room No. ______ M.D. ____________
last
Address ______________________________ Vocation ____________

Onset date ________ Lesion ________ flaccid ___ spastic ___ Admission date ________

Disability ____

Cause ____

Decubiti ____

Surgery ____

METHOD OF RECORDING TEST AND PROGRESS

Symbols for grade

✓ Patient can perform activity independently.
S Patient needs supervision.
A Patient needs assistance.
L Patient has to be lifted.
X Activity is not indicated.

1. *At initial testing* (use *blue pencil*):
   Enter grade symbol in column G/1 and your initials in column I. The initial date appears at top of page.

2. *Progress* is recorded with *red pencil*:
   Enter grade symbol in column G/2 and your initials in column I. Date in column "Date."

If there is more than one method or item listed with an activity, circle which indicated.

BED ACTIVITIES

	G/1	G/2	DATE	I
Moving in bed: lying, sitting				
Roll to right, to left				
Turn on abdomen				
Manage: pillows, blankets				
Sit up				
Reach objects on night table				
Operate signal light				

Continued.

Fig. 11-13 Chart to indicate activities of daily living. (From Rusk, H.A.: Rehabilitation medicine, ed. 4, St. Louis, 1977, The C.V. Mosby Co.)

CHART 3, cont'd

WHEELCHAIR ACTIVITIES

	G/1	G/2	DATE	I
Propel: forward, backward, turn				
Open, through, and close door				
Up, down ramp				
Bed to wheelchair				
Wheelchair to bed				
Wheelchair to straight chair				
Straight chair to wheelchair				
Wheelchair to easy chair, couch				
Easy chair, couch to wheelchair				
Wheelchair to toilet (high toilet seat, regular seat)				
Toilet to wheelchair				
Adjust clothing				
Wheelchair to tub				
Tub to wheelchair				
Wheelchair to shower (chair in stall shower, or tub)				
Shower to wheelchair				

Travel:

Wheelchair to car_____on curb				
Car to wheelchair____on curb				
Wheelchair to car____ no curb				
Car to wheelchair______no curb				
Place wheelchair in car_____on street				

SELF-CARE ACTIVITIES

HYGIENE (TOILET ACTIVITIES)	G/1	G/2	DATE	I
Comb, brush hair				
Brush teeth				
Shave (electric razor, safety razor), put on makeup				
Turn faucet				
Wash, dry hands and face				
Wash, dry body and extremities				
Take bath (wheelchair, walking)				
Take shower (wheelchair, walking)				
Use urinal, bedpan				

EATING ACTIVITIES	G/1	G/2	DATE	I
Eat with spoon				
Eat with fork				
Cut meat				
Handle: straw, cup, glass				

DRESSING ACTIVITIES	G/1	G/2	DATE	I
Undershirt; bra				
Shorts; panties				
Slipover garment				
Shirt; blouse				
Slacks; dress				
Tying necktie—bow				
Socks; stockings				
Shoes (laces, buckles, slip-on)				
Coat, jacket				
Braces, prosthesis, corset				

Fig. 11-13 cont'd Chart to indicate activities of daily living.

CHART 3, cont'd

MISCELLANEOUS HAND ACTIVITIES

	G/1	G/2	DATE	I
Write name and address				
Manage: watch				
match or cigarette lighter				
cigarette				
book, newspaper				
handkerchief				
lights: chain, switch, knob				
telephone: receiver, dial, coins				
handle: purse, coins, paper money				

WALKING ACTIVITIES

	G/1	G/2	DATE	I
Open, go through, and close door				
Walking outside				
Walking carrying				

STANDING UP AND SITTING DOWN

	G/1	G/2	DATE	I
Up from wheelchair				
Down on wheelchair				
Up from bed				
Down on bed				
Up from straight chair				
Down on straight chair				
Up from straight chair at table				
Down on straight chair at table				
Up from easy chair				
Down on easy chair				
Up from center of couch				
Down on center of couch				
Up from toilet				
Down on toilet				
Adjust clothing				
Into car, on curb, up curb				
Out of car				
Down on floor				
Up from floor				

CLIMBING AND TRAVELING ACTIVITIES

	G/1	G/2	DATE	I
Up flight of stairs (railing, no railing)				
Down flight of stairs (railing, no railing)				
Into and out of car, taxi				
Walk one block and back				
Down curb, cross street, on curb				
Into bus				
Sit down, get up from bus seat				
Out of bus				

Continued.

Fig. 11-13 cont'd Chart to indicate activities of daily living.

CHART 3, cont'd

HOME SITUATION

Note suggestions for adaptation next to each line or check when so indicated. In special instances, diagram of layout will be advisable.

Location: Urban_____ Suburban _____ Rural _____

APARTMENT: Floor _____ Rooms _____ Elevator _____ (self-service _____) None ___

Walk up _______

PRIVATE HOUSE: Floors _____ Rooms _____ Elevator _____ (self-service _____) None ___

ENTRANCE: Door _____ No. steps _____ Railing: right ___ left ___ none ___ Ramp _____

Note floor if in private home: Bedroom ____ Living room _____ Kitchen _____ Bathroom _______

BATHROOM: Door width ____ Tub ____ Shower over tub ____ Stall shower ________

Information uncertain (explain): ________________________

Information unavailable (explain): ________________________

APPLIANCES

Column 1—Initial Summary check blue; column 2—Discharge Summary check red.

WHEELCHAIR	1	2		1	2
8″ casters			Footrests: removable		
Wheels: knobs, tape			adjustable		
Pneumatic tires			stationary		
Cushion: seat _____ back			Armrests: removable		
Board: seat _____ back			desk		
Back: snap			stationary		
reclining			Brakes _____ extension		

BRACES	1	2	CRUTCHES	1	2	GAIT	1	2	DEVICES	1	2
Short leg			Axillary			Swing to					
double			Lofstrand			Swing through					
Long leg			Canes			4-point					
double			None			Other					
Pelvic band			Other			Hemi					
Knight spinal											

INITIAL SUMMARY ________________________

Fig. 11-13 cont'd Chart to indicate activities of daily living.

CHART 3, cont'd

DISCHARGE SUMMARY

RECOMMENDATIONS (circle)

Patient is independent

Patient needs: Supervision _____ Assistance _____ Lifting _____

Patient uses wheelchair: Exclusively_____ Partly_____

Patient is ambulatory: Exclusively_____ Partly_____

ENDURANCE AND SPEED

Endurance:

Propelling wheelchair: State number of feet_______________Time_______________
Walking: State number of feet_______________Time_______________
Climbing: State number of steps_______________Time_______________

Speed:

Propelling wheelchair: State time for 60 feet_______________
Walking: State time for 60 feet_______________
Climbing: State time for 10 steps_______________

ACTIVITIES

Grade in column G as follows: ✓, Independence; S, Supervision; A, Assistance; L, Lifting; time in column T (use red pencil).

	G	T
GETTING READY IN MORNING:_______________Total		
Toilet needs: From wheelchair		
Standing		
Complete dressing		
Eating: Breakfast		
Lunch		
GETTING OUT OF HOUSE: Stairs, ramp, entrance door_____Total		
TRAVEL TO WORK: Own car (hand controls), taxi_________Total		
Car: From wheelchair (including placing wheelchair)		
From standing		
Bus: Walk to station, cross street		

Date_______________ Signature_______________

Fig. 11-13 cont'd Chart to indicate activities of daily living.

Nursing care plan: **REHABILITATION OF THE NEUROLOGICALLY IMPAIRED INDIVIDUAL**

NURSING DIAGNOSIS	EXPECTED OUTCOMES	NURSING INTERVENTIONS
Impaired physical mobility	Patient has the ability to move with the maximum level of independence within the physical environment.	Prevent joint contractures and deformities by performing range-of-motion exercises or other exercises to increase muscle strength. Apply devices to prevent foot drop and hand, arm, and leg deformities. Pillows or commercial devices may be used. Position the patient to maintain hip and spine alignment with support to head, neck, shoulders, and extremities. Reposition the patient at least every 1 to 2 hours. Manual turning or mechanical beds are used. Early ambulation and weight-bearing are initiated and encouraged frequently. Teach the use of crutches and other devices. (See Figs. 11-14 to 11-16). Transport the patient with assistance or independently to wheelchair or chair (Fig. 11-17).
Potential impairment of skin integrity or potential skin breakdown	Skin is free of redness, ulceration, or breakdown.	Reposition the patient every 1 to 2 hours. Support bony prominences such as the elbows, heels, sacrum, ankles, shoulders, coccyx, occiput, and ears to protect them from prolonged pressure by using pillows, rolled towels, rubber donuts, foam pads and supports, egg shell foam, air or water mattresses, sheepskins. Remember that paralyzed patients are unable to feel pain from prolonged pressure or from changes in heat and cold sensation and that they must be repositioned often either manually or with mechanical device. Inspect the patient's skin frequently at sites of pressure or shearing. Avoid friction caused by dragging body parts across bed linens or bumping them on wheelchairs or other equipment during transfers and repositionings. Maintain a nutritionally balanced diet, high in protein. Keep the skin dry and clean and free from urine, feces, perspiration, vomitus, or moisture. Maintain a normal body temperature. Avoid extreme variances in environmental humidity. Avoid the use of constricting clothing or devices that may cause pressure or impair circulation. Report any sensation of pain or numbness expressed by a patient with a cast. Check capillary flow to fingertips and toes of patients with cast applications to their extremities or trunk.

Continued.

WALKING WITH SUPPORT

NOTE TO PRACTITIONER: Proper height of cane and crutch hand support. The height, when the support is placed on the floor, should allow patient's elbow to be bent slightly, as illustrated.

CAUTION: Do not let weak foot get ahead of cane or crutch.

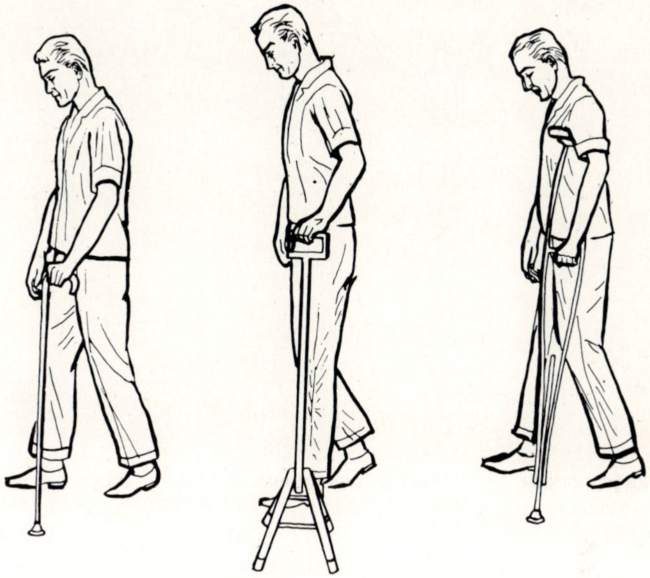

Cane

Place cane ahead of strong foot and slightly out to side. Step ahead with weak foot, placing it opposite cane. Take all of body weight on weak leg and the cane, and step ahead with strong foot. Repeat steps.

or

Start with both feet and cane in line, all slightly separated. Step ahead with cane and weak foot at the same time. Then taking body weight on weak leg and cane, step ahead with strong foot. Repeat steps.

Crutch for support

Be sure there is space under the arm between top of crutch and underarm. Be sure crutch has "Safe-T-Tip." Directions for walking with crutch are the same as for cane.

Wide-base cane

Place cane a few inches ahead of strong foot, then bring weak foot forward and place it opposite cane. Shift body weight to weak leg and cane, and step ahead with strong foot. Repeat steps.

NOTE TO PRACTITIONER: Usually short steps are easier than long steps. Try to keep the patient's steps uniform in size. Be sure cane is equipped with "Safe-T-Tip."

Fig. 11-14 Walking with support. (Reprinted with permission of the American Heart Association.)

CLIMBING STAIRS

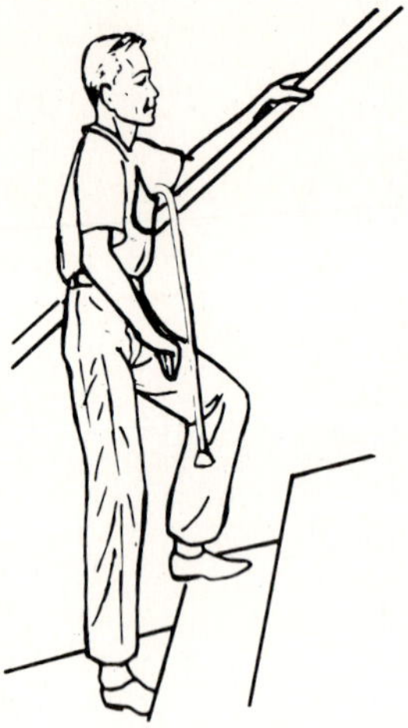

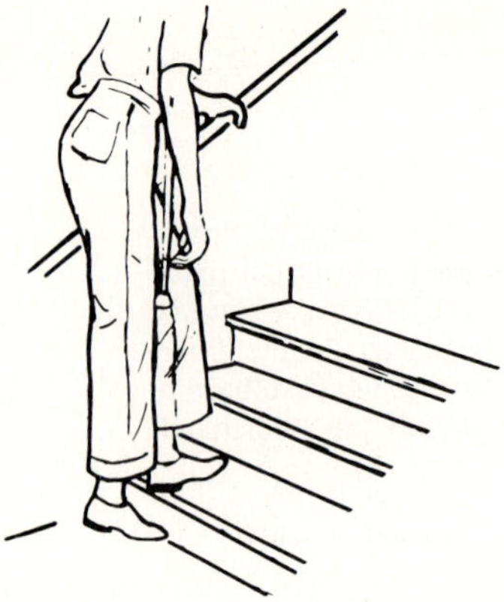

1. Hang cane in shirt pocket (or for women, other opening high on front of clothing). With strong hand, grasp rail. Place strong foot on step above.

2. Using strong hand on rail and strong leg for support, lean forward, straighten strong knee, and place weak foot beside strong foot on same step.

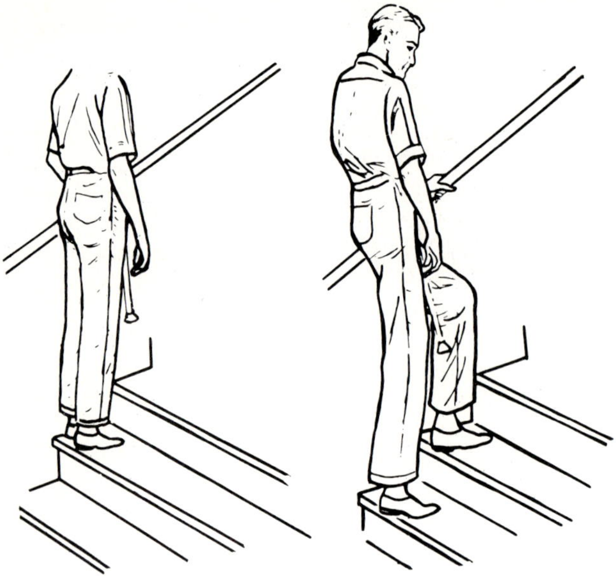

RULE: Go up with strong foot first. Bring weak foot to same step.

NOTE TO PRACTITIONER: It is not advisable for patient to go up and down stairs without a handrail unless he has nearly normal strength and balance. There should be a handrail down the center of the steps or one along each side. Going up and down stairs using a handrail can be done by a patient with a very weak leg provided he places his feet carefully and his weak knee is straight when he takes his weight on it.

3. Repeat steps 1 and 2, climbing one step at a time.

Fig. 11-15 Climbing stairs. (Reprinted with permission of the American Heart Association.)

DESCENDING STAIRS

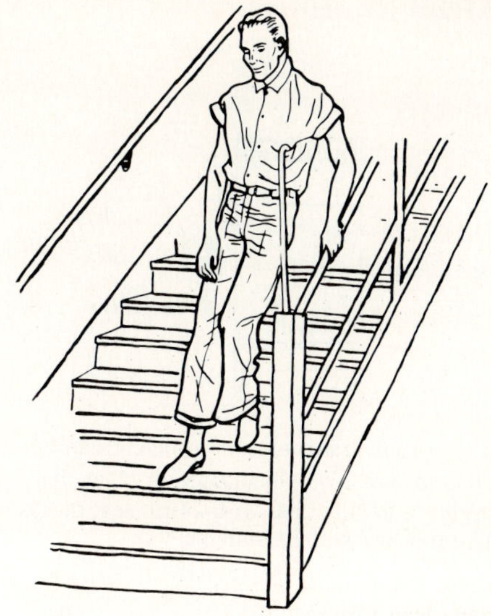

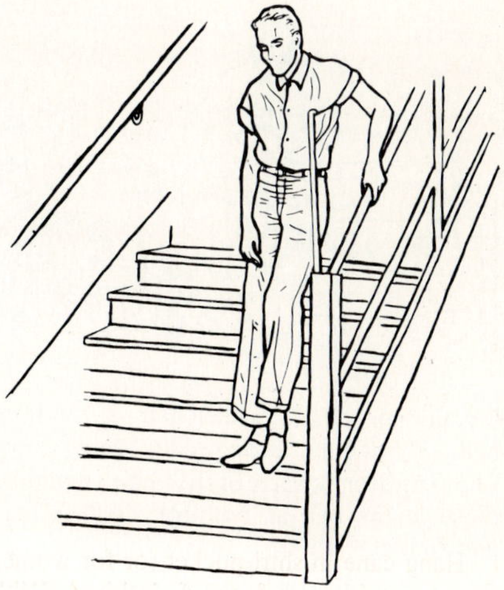

1. Make sure toes of strong foot overlap edge of step before starting down. Grasp handrail with strong hand. Place weak foot on next step below, bending strong knee as weak foot goes down.

2. When weak foot is firmly placed with knee straight and leg is able to support body weight, step down to same step with strong foot.

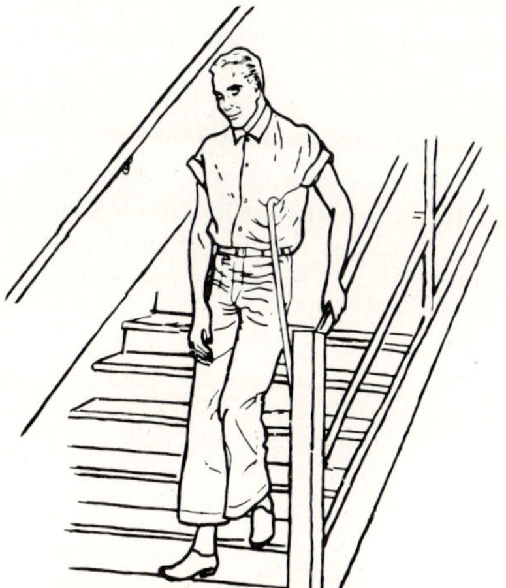

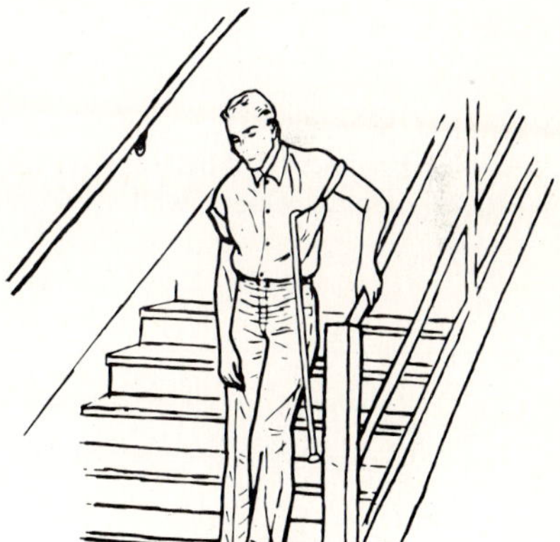

3. Repeat steps 1 and 2.

RULE: Go down stairs with weak foot first. Bring strong foot down to the same step.

Fig. 11-16 Descending stairs. (Reprinted with permission of the American Heart Association.)

MOVING INTO A WHEELCHAIR FROM THE BED

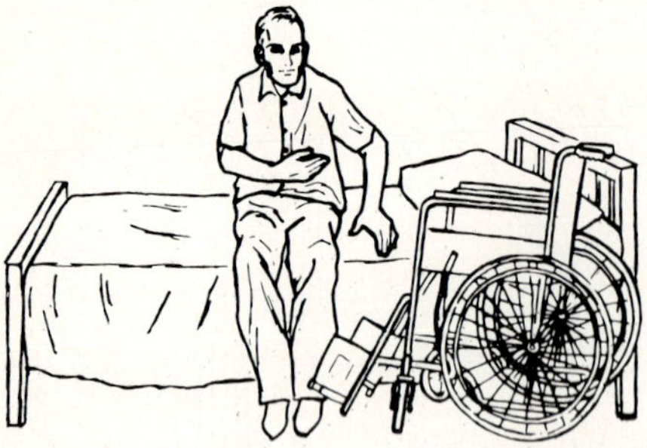

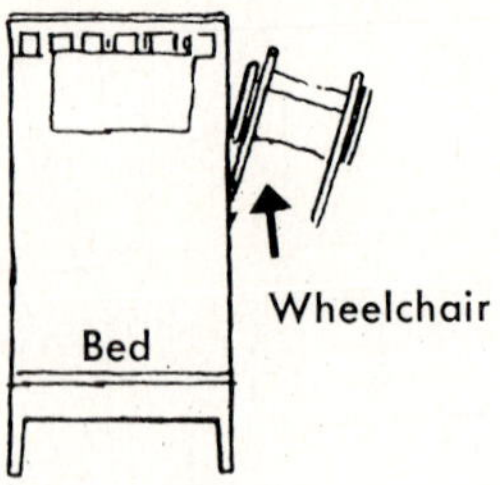

1. Practitioner places wheelchair at slight angle to bed, on patient's strong side, facing foot of bed. The right front corner of the chair should be kept as close to the bed as possible. Brakes are locked, and footrests are up.

NOTE TO PRACTITIONER: An armchair can be used by the bed instead of a wheelchair. A chair that is heavy enough not to slide and with a firm seat that is not too soft or too low will be suitable.

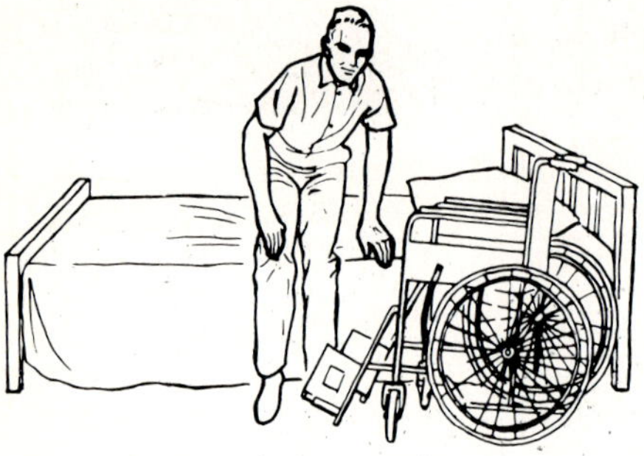

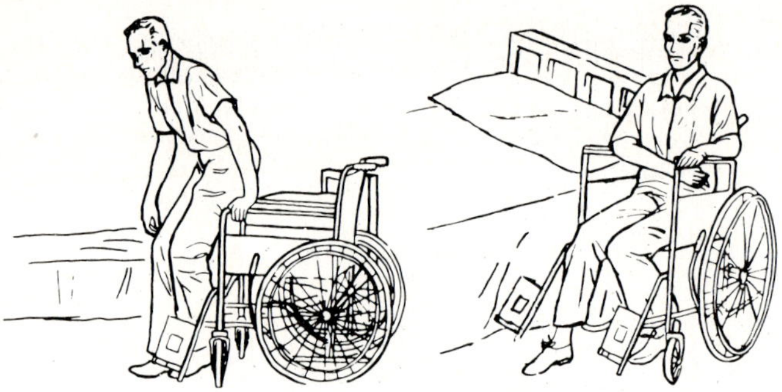

2. Keep feet beneath body, lean forward, placing strong hand near edge of bed, and push to standing position, keeping weight well over strong foot.

3. When standing position is steady enough for momentary release of support by strong hand, move strong hand to farther armrest of wheelchair. Keeping body weight well forward, turn on strong foot, and lower to sitting position.

Fig. 11-17 Moving into a wheelchair from the bed. (Reprinted with permission of the American Heart Association.)

Nursing care plan: REHABILITATION OF THE NEUROLOGICALLY IMPAIRED INDIVIDUAL—cont'd

NURSING DIAGNOSIS	EXPECTED OUTCOMES	NURSING INTERVENTIONS
Alteration in bowel elimination	Patient will be continent of stool and free from constipation or impaction.	Extablish a bowel program to provide the formation of a firm stool and to maintain adequate emptying of the rectum. Elements of a bowel program include: 1. Use of stool softeners and bulk-producing medications. 2. High-fiber diet. 3. Adequate fluid intake. 4. Encouragement of activity. 5. Establishment of a routine whereby defecation is done at the same time each day. 6. Administering local stimulation or Glycerine, Bisacodyl, or Vacuette suppositories digitally. 7. Administering the suppository at same hour each day. Transfer patient to the commode if patient is able to sit. If not, position patient on the left side and protect the bed with disposable underpads. A bowel program is done on a daily basis initially and is then advanced to every other or every third day. The use of bedpans is not recommended because of the increased chance of the development of pressure sores as a result of sensory deficits. 8. Stimulating peristalsis with hot liquids given 15 minutes before administration of the suppository. Scheduling the bowel program close to meal times is also effective in increasing peristalsis. Abdominal massage in the cecal area will also increase peristalsis. 9. Initiating digital stimulation for 15 to 30 minutes. Once a bowel program is established, this may be the only measure necessary to initiate defecation. 10. Placing the patient in the squatting position when on the commode by raising the feet on a stool and leaning the torso forward. 11. Stop stool softeners and readjust medications and diet to cause formation of a firm stool if diarrhea occurs. Check the patient for fecal impaction at the initial onset of diarrhea. 12. A bowel program takes time to establish. Documentation and evaluation are important to a successful one.

Continued.

Nursing care plan: REHABILITATION OF THE NEUROLOGICALLY IMPAIRED INDIVIDUAL—cont'd

NURSING DIAGNOSIS	EXPECTED OUTCOMES	NURSING INTERVENTIONS
Altered urinary elimination pattern	Patient is continent of urine and is free of overdistention, bladder and urinary tract infections, and urinary calculi, and normal kidney function is maintained.	Assess bladder function by determining voiding pattern, amount of residual urine after voiding, bladder capacity, amount of intact sensation (test gently with a pin or sharp object), type of urinary incontinence if voluntary control is present, methods used to stimulate micturition, presence of any infection, type of neurogenic bladder, and potential to cooperate in a bladder program. Determine a fluid intake-output profile for the patient by measuring the urine output ½ to 1 hour after the patient has been recumbent. Intermittently catheterize the patient to maintain bladder muscle tone, prevent overdistention, and prevent infection by ensuring complete emptying. (Indwelling catheters are not recommended because of the increased incidence of urinary tract infection.) Encourage fluid intake up to 3000 ml/day to keep urine dilute to prevent stasis, infection, and calculi. Restrict fluid intake to the waking hours to avoid interruption of sleep. Limit fluids to 1500-2000 ml per day when intermittent catheterization is used to prevent sudden overdistention. Keep urine acidic with ascorbic acid and an acid-ash diet that includes cereals, meat, poultry, fish. Encourage active exercise to increase calcium metabolism and prevent calculi. Antimicrobial agents may be ordered by the physician to prevent or control mild infections. Establish an individual bladder program for the patient according to the type of NGB he has. Provide patient education regarding the type of NBG the patient has and the procedures and techniques to be used in the program. For uninhibited NGB: 1. Provide stimulation to increase the patient's awareness of his body function in relation to the environment and take the patient to the bathroom or place him on the commode in a normal sitting position at scheduled times throughout the day. 2. Use stimulation and relaxation methods such as pouring warm water over the perineum and running the water faucet to stimulate voiding. For reflex NGB: 1. Have the patient void every 4 hours. 2. Instruct the patient to use cutaneous methods to stimulate voiding. These include pulling of pubic hair, abdominal massage, pinching, slapping, or stroking the skin, and digital rectal stimulation.

Nursing care plan: **REHABILITATION OF THE NEUROLOGICALLY IMPAIRED INDIVIDUAL—cont'd**

NURSING DIAGNOSIS	EXPECTED OUTCOMES	NURSING INTERVENTIONS
Altered urinary elimination pattern—cont'd		For autonomous bladder dysfunction: 1. Teach the patient to use the Crede maneuver and Valsalva maneuver to stimulate voiding. The Crede maneuver involves manual compression applied to the bladder to stimulate emptying. The Valsalva maneuver is any forced expiratory effort against a closed airway as observed during constipation when one tries to move the bowels. 2. Encourage the patient to do exercises to strengthen the abdominal muscles. 3. Instruct the patient to monitor fluid intake and urine output and to empty the bladder when a 350 ml capacity has been reached. For motor paralytic bladder: 1. Instruct the patient to use techniques similar to those used for autonomous bladder dysfunctions. 2. Along with the Crede and Valsalva maneuvers, the patient is instructed to do self-catheterization. Female patients are taught to use a mirror to perform self-catheterization. For sensory paralytic bladder: 1. Instruct the patient to empty the bladder frequently instead of waiting for a sensation of bladder fullness. Use catheterization in patients who have large residual amount of urine or bladder atonicity. Be alert to symptoms of autonomic dysreflexia or hyperreflexia during bladder conditioning. This is a complication common to patients with cervical or high thoracic lesions because the autonomic portions of the nervous system no longer function. A stimulus from a distended bladder or bowel will cause a hypertensive result in the parasympathetic or sympathetic reflexes. Signs to observe in the patient with autonomic dysreflexia are bradycardia, hypertension, headache, flushing of the face and neck, engorgement of temporal and neck vessels, and nasal congestion. Seizures may also occur. This is an acute situation and can lead to myocardial infarction and cardiac arrest or to intracranial or retinal hemorrhage. Care to relieve the problem includes: 1. Placing the patient in a sitting or reverse Trendelenburg position. 2. Removing the source of stimulation such as by emptying a distended bladder. A distended bowel should not be evacuated until the blood pressure is lowered. 3. Check blood pressure and pulse every 3 to 5 minutes until lowered.

Continued.

Nursing care plan: REHABILITATION OF THE NEUROLOGICALLY IMPAIRED INDIVIDUAL—cont'd

NURSING DIAGNOSIS	EXPECTED OUTCOMES	NURSING INTERVENTIONS
Sexual dysfunction	Patient will achieve role identity to ensure sexual satisfaction and positive relationship with significant other.	Understand the cause of altered body structure or function. Recognize each individual's basic need for love. Assess the patient's pre-injury sexual activity. Provide an open environment in which sex counseling can be done, beginning when the patient is ready. The practitioner should be well informed about the subject before initiating sex counseling with the patient. Furnish the patient with information via referral to sex counselors or literature on the topic of sex. Use educational films to show the spinal-cord injured patient about adaptations for sex, illustrating attitudes, positions, props and aids to use, and fantasies. Instruct the patient to know himself through self-exploration activities such as masturbation to discover erogenous zones, areas of hypersensation, and internal sensations. Teach the patient or significant other to remove clothing. Encourage communication between partners to allow each to express feelings, relate what is pleasurable and what is painful, and express the idea that a lack of ejaculation is not unfulfilling. Be aware that a role change may occur between partners. For instance, the one who was passive before the injury may now need to take the assertive role and vice versa. Establish rapport with the patient and significant other to create open lines of communication. Assess the attitudes of the patient and significant other about the disability and effects on sexual function. (Persons with a good feeling about their own sexuality before the injury will adjust better during the rehabilitation phase [Bullard and Knight, 1981]). Respect the family's right to privacy and provide private areas in the hospital where the patient and family may be allowed to reestablish their relationships. Some hospitals have motel facilities adjacent to or within the hospital building to facilitate achievement of this goal. Encourage touching, feeling, and togetherness. A neuropsychiatric evaluation is necessary to understand the cognitive and physical deficits of the patient before a retraining program can be established. Work with mental health departments, community-based programs, or other sexuality-related services to promote coping mechanisms to develop social skills and educate patients about their sexual identities. Promote research on sexuality and illness to make more information on the subject available.

Nursing care plan: **REHABILITATION OF THE NEUROLOGICALLY IMPAIRED INDIVIDUAL—cont'd**

NURSING DIAGNOSIS	EXPECTED OUTCOMES	NURSING INTERVENTIONS
Body image disturbance	The patient will have an integrated perception of body function characteristics and limits.	Trauma or illness changes body structure and function. The nurse must assist the patient to overcome guilt, fear, and negative feelings about altered function, appearance, and limits of body parts. Encourage verbalization and interaction with others to relieve anxiety. Accept the patient and let him know that you care about his personal problems. Be a good listener. Use crisis intervention to assist the patient to adapt to the new environment. Encourage independent behavior.
Impaired verbal communication	Patient will be able to express self utilizing modified techniques of verbalization.	Identify verbal, written, gestural, and perceptual problems that interfere with the patient's ability to communicate. Use short, direct questions that require simple, short answers. Encourage the use of writing, gestures, and drawing as alternate methods of communication. Keep directions and explanations simple and short. Rephrase questions to clarify meaning to enable the patient to reply. Give the patient time to answer a question. Impatience and continuous repetitions may increase the patient's frustration. Establish a thorough understanding of the patient and his signs of frustration. Provide the patient with materials to promote his ability to express himself. Collaborate with the communicologist to assist the patient with his communication-retraining program.
Total self-care deficit **Self-bathing deficit** **Self-dressing deficit** **Self-toileting deficit** **Self-feeding deficit** **Self-ambulation deficit**	Patient is independent in performance of ADL: bathing, dressing, toileting, eating, ambulation.	The patient learns to bathe self, feed self, dress self, transfer techniques, and homemaking skills by activities in the occupational therapy department (Figs. 11-18 to 11-19). Observe safety measures during transfer from bed to ensure locked wheels, avoid skin trauma, and so on. Apply assistive devices for eating and dressing, and braces and supports for ambulation. Allow the patient to be independent within his limits. Teach the patient how to perform ADL with the use of devices and how to modify them according to his functional deficit or deformity. Example: the use of stretch fabrics without buttons and zipper openings for clothing (Figs. 11-20 to 11-24). Collaborate with the occupational and physical therapist to provide continuity in the patient's plan of care. Plan the patient's care to ensure that the patient arrives on time to scheduled therapy sessions.

Continued.

PUTTING ON TROUSERS

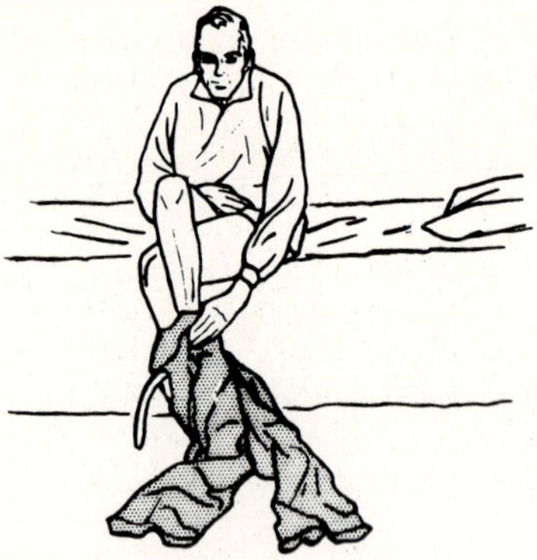

1. Sitting on side of bed, with strong hand across weak leg, pull right pant leg over weak foot.

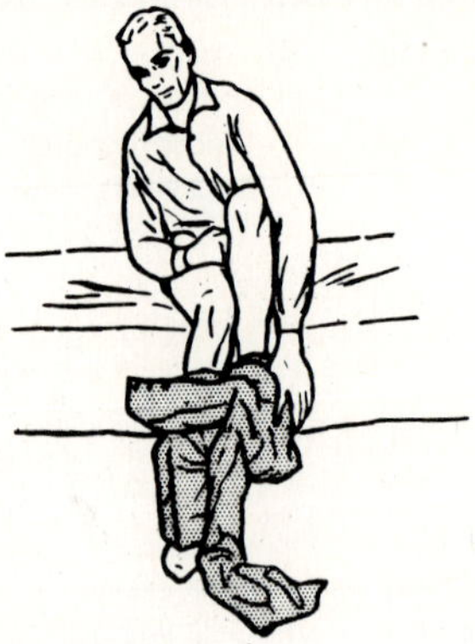

2. Place strong foot in left pant leg, and pull pants up as far as possible.
   - If unable to stand without support, lie down and proceed as illustrated in steps 3 and 4.
   - If able to stand without support, proceed to step 2a.

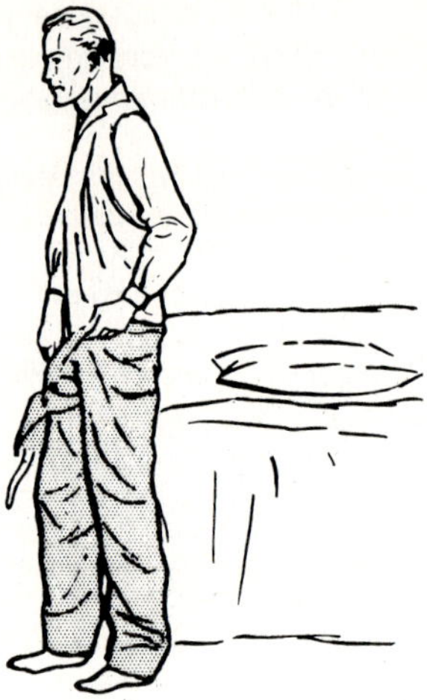

2a. If standing balance against bed without support of strong hand is possible, stand leaning against bed for support and pull pants up with strong hand.

NOTE TO PRACTITIONER: If patient cannot cross legs, he can rest his weak foot on a small stool to assist in this activity.

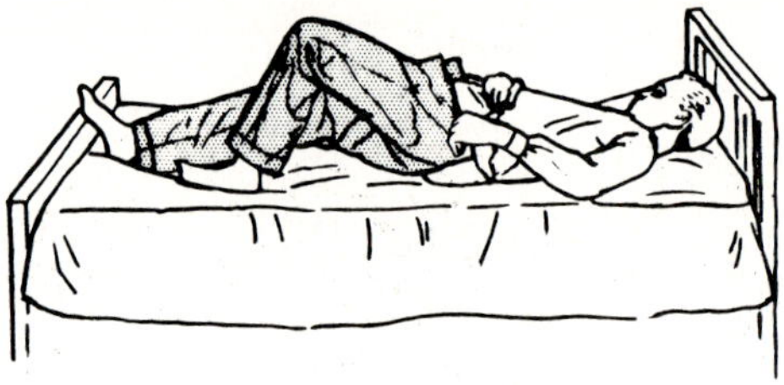

3. Lie down; bend strong knee and hip, pushing strong foot against bed to raise hips. Pull pants up over hips.

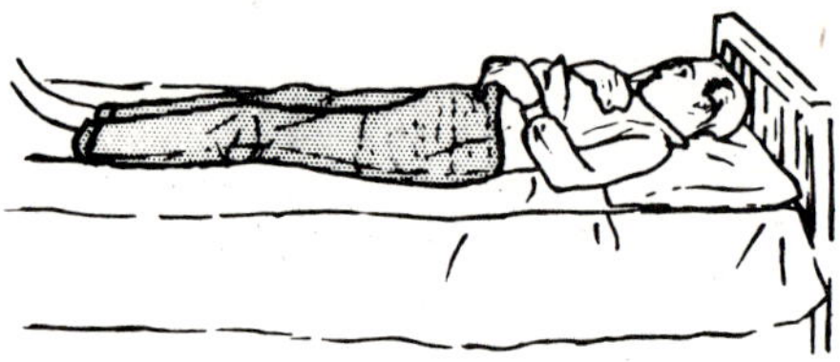

4. Fasten front of pants.

Fig. 11-18 Putting on trousers. (Reprinted with permission of the American Heart Association.)

PUTTING ON A SHIRT OR DRESS

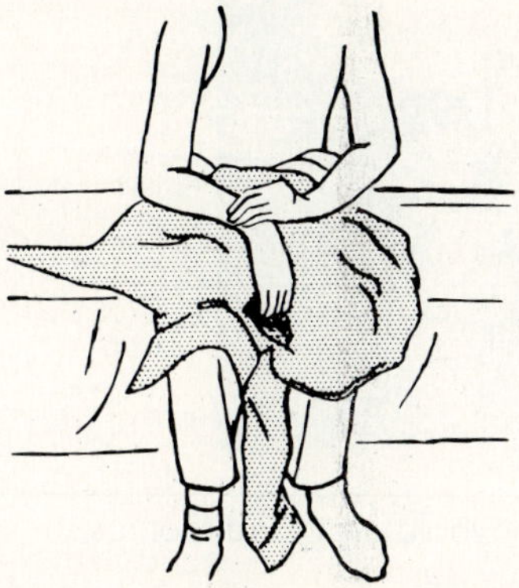

1. Spread shirt on lap inside up and collar away from body.

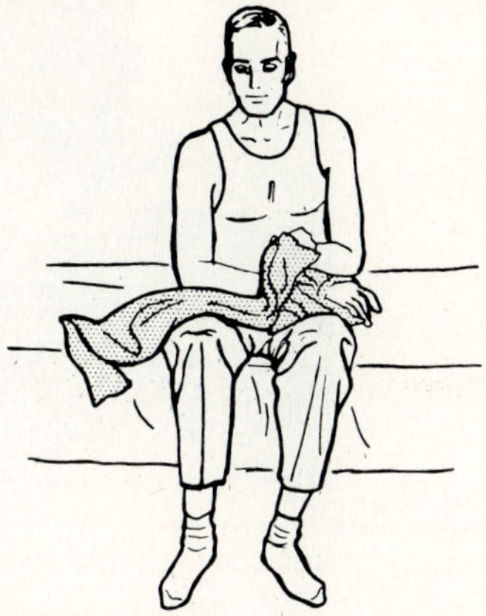

2. Using strong hand, place weak hand in right armhole and pull sleeve up weak arm.

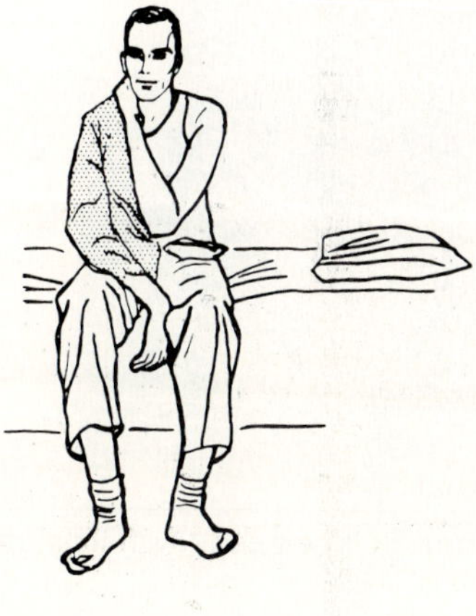

3. Throw rest of garment behind body, and pull right sleeve all the way up.

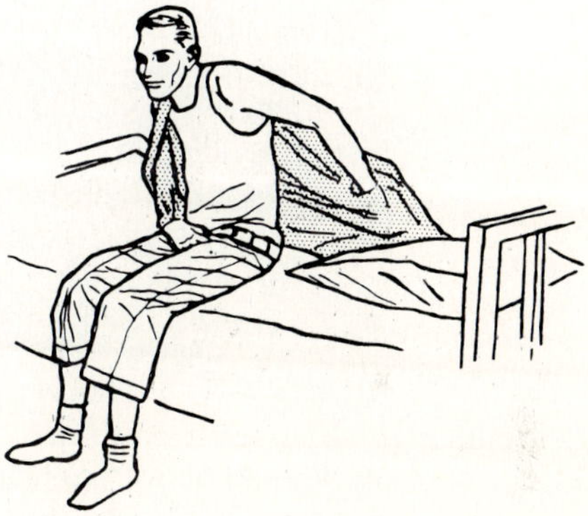

4. Reach behind with strong hand, and place it in left armhole. Work sleeve into position.

NOTE TO PRACTITIONER: Dressing while sitting on side of bed is easier than in wheelchair if balance is good. If balance is poor, have patient sit in wheelchair or heavy armchair to dress.

An open-down-the-front dress, sweater, or coat is put on the same way as a shirt, but it is necessary to stand up and straighten the skirt before it can be fastened.

Large buttons are easier to fasten than snaps.

Fig. 11-19 Putting on a shirt or dress. (Reprinted with permission of the American Heart Association.)

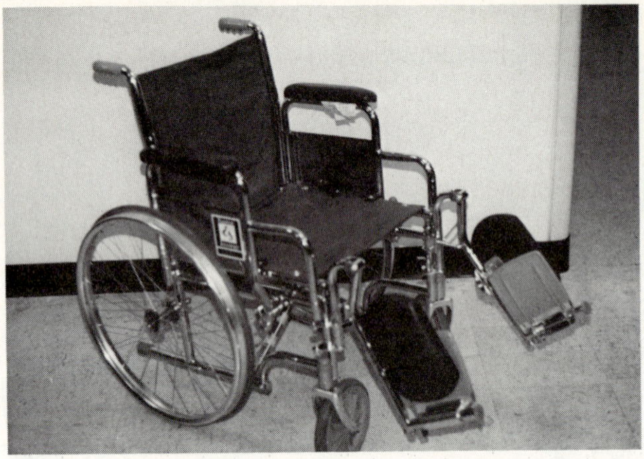

Fig. 11-20 Standard collapsible wheelchair with removable arms and foot rests.

A

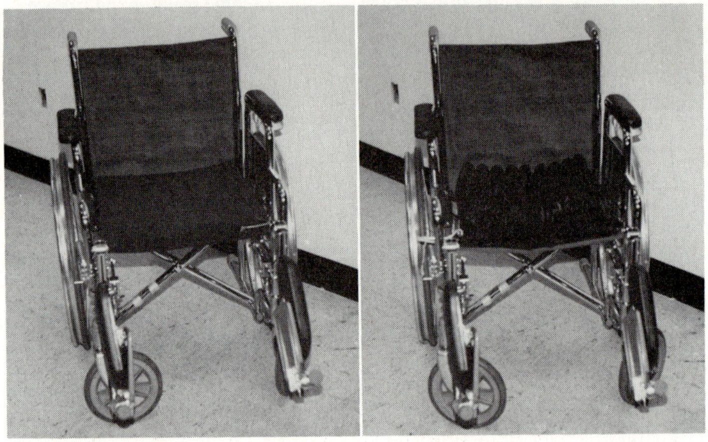

B

Fig. 11-21 **A**, Wheelchair with cushion of silicone foam. **B**, Wheelchair with inflatable cushion.

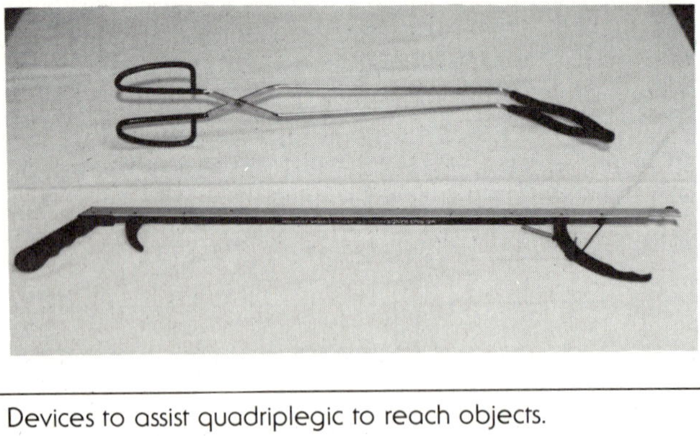

Fig. 11-22 Devices to assist quadriplegic to reach objects.

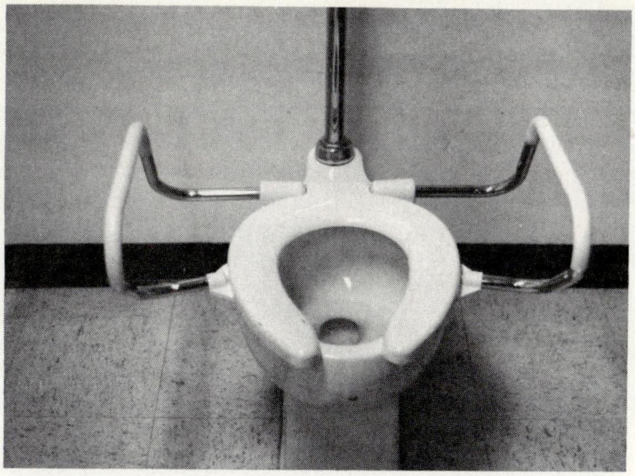

Fig. 11-23 Grab bars added to home toilet.

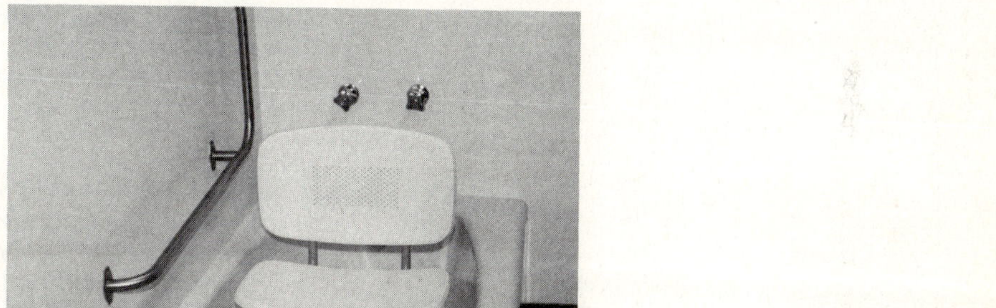

A

B

C

Fig. 11-24 **A,** Shower/tub chair. **B,** Shower chair that attaches to side of tub. **C,** Shower chair with wheels that can be used to transport person from bed or chair to shower room.

Nursing care plan: REHABILITATION OF THE NEUROLOGICALLY IMPAIRED INDIVIDUAL—cont'd

NURSING DIAGNOSIS	EXPECTED OUTCOMES	NURSING INTERVENTIONS
Impaired home maintenance management	Patient will maintain a safe and growth-promoting home environment.	Plan with the patient and family for adaptations to facilitate his functioning in the home. Assess financial needs of the family and refer to financial assistance agencies. Evaluate architectural features of the home and make recommendations for adaptations. Assess stairs, ramps, entrance size, rails, door sills (to be eliminated), door size (36 inches wide is desirable, sliding doors are best), elevators, curbs. Refer the patient and family to agencies such as extension services, utility and food companies, editors of home magazines, architects, home builders, carpenters, plumbers, electricians, engineers, friends, and neighbors to help with home adaptations. Teach the patient and family factors about home management. These include nonskid floors and elimination of mats and carpets, washable surface walls, casement windows to facilitate opening, bay windows to provide a view for those confined to indoors, wall switches 24 to 36 inches from the floor (so they can be reached easily from a wheelchair), having light switches near the door or entrance to rooms, and adequate heating and ventilation to maintain a comfortable environment. Evaluate bedrooms, bathrooms, kitchen, and living areas to ensure accessibility and convenience for work and performance of ADL. (Note that occupational therapy is responsible for teaching standard guidelines and techniques to meet this goal.) Focus the training program for independence on the home situation while the patient is hospitalized. This will facilitate meeting the goals of the discharge plan that was established at the beginning of the rehabilitation program. Collaborate with the social service worker to assist the patient and family reach goals for a home maintenance program.

Suggested readings

Baxter, R.T.: Sex counseling and the SCI patient, Nursing **8**(9):46-52, Sept., 1978.

Bullard, D.G., and Knight, S.E.: Sexuality and physical disability, St. Louis, 1981, The C.V. Mosby Co.

Butts, P.: Assessing urinary incontinence in women, Nursing **9**(3):72, March 1979.

Cameron, G.: Pressure sores: what to do when prevention fails, Nursing **9**(1):46-47, Jan. 1979.

Conway-Rutkowski, B.L.: Carini and Owens' neurological and neurosurgical nursing, St. Louis, 1982, The C.V. Mosby Co.

Dudar, S., and King, R.: Rehabilitation of patients with spinal cord injury, Nurs. Clin. North Am. **15**(2):228-239, June 1980.

Gordon, M.: Manual of nursing diagnosis, New York, 1982, McGraw-Hill Book Co.

Hirschberg, G.G.: Rehabilitation, a manual for the care of the disabled and elderly, Philadelphia, 1964, J.B. Lippincott Co.

Johnson, J.: Symposium on rehabilitation nursing, rehabilitators aspects of neurologic bladder dysfunction, Nurs. Clin. North Am. **15**(2):293-307, June 1980.

Lazure, L.L.: Defining the dangers of autonomic dysreflexia, Nursing (Horsham) **10**(9):52-53, Sept. 1980.

Meer, R.M.: Skin destruction: overcoming the myths, Life Support Nurs. **11**(5):5-15, Sept.-Oct. 1981.

Olson, E.V.: The hazards of immobility, Am. J. Nurs. **67**(4):779-797, April 1967.

Piotrowski, M.: Programmed instruction: functioning of the normal and neurogenic bladder, ARN, **10**(2):13-20, March-April 1980.

Power, D.J.: Two approaches to bladder training in the elderly with uninhibited neurogenic bladders, Appendixes H and I. Unpublished Masters thesis, University of Washington, 1981.

Rusk, H.A.: Rehabilitation medicine, St. Louis, 1977, The C.V. Mosby Co.

Sine, R.D., and others: Basic rehabilitation techniques—a self-instructional guide, Rockville, Md., 1981, Aspen Systems Corporation.

Stryker, R.: Rehabilitative aspects of acute and chronic nursing care, Philadelphia, 1977, W.B. Saunders Co.

Sullivan, N.: Kinetic nursing: treating the immobilized patient, 1-15, Kinetic Concepts, San Antonio, Tex., 1981.

Tecklin, J.S.: Positioning, percussing, and vibrating patients for effective bronchial drainage, Nursing **9**(3):65, March 1979.

VanHook, D.: Lapidus and capillary pressure, Health Care Devices, 1972.

Watson, P.G.: Rehabilitation legislation of the seventies and the severely disabled, ARN **9**(3):4-11, May-June 1979.

Young, C.: Exercise, how to use it to decrease complications in immobilized patients, Nursing **5**(3): 81-82, March, 1975.

Other resources

Access Living of Metropolitan Chicago, Illinois Department of Rehabilitation Services, Chicago, IL 60610.

Center for Decubitus Ulcer Research Information, 408 N.E. Alde Avenue, Jensen Beach, FL 33457.

Kinetic Concepts, 3417 Steen Drive, San Antonio, TX 78219.

"Lotus" Flotation Systems for the Prevention and Healing of Decubitus Ulcers, 1981, Lotus Health Care Products, Naugatuck, CT 06770.

Rehabilitation Institute of Chicago, 345 East Superior Street, Chicago, IL 60611.

Span-America, Inc. P.O. Box 5231, Greenville, SC 29606.

Stryker Corporation, Kalamazoo, MI 49001.

CHAPTER 12

Paresis and paresthesias

A paresis is an incomplete paralysis or weakness of an extremity. Paresthesias are abnormal sensations, which can range from a numbness and tingling to a heightened sensitivity (hyperesthesia). A person may experience either a paresis or paresthesia from a variety of causes. These include spinal cord injuries or injury to the nerve roots secondary to traumatic injuries, compressing tumors, and herniated discs. A demyelinating disease such as multiple sclerosis will also cause a paresis or paresthesia. Additional disorders in which a paresis will result include myasthenia gravis, which affects the neuromuscular junction, and muscular dystrophy, which directly affects the muscle. The care of patients with traumatic spinal cord injuries and compressing tumors have been discussed in Chapters 9 and 8, respectively.

HERNIATED INTERVERTEBRAL DISC

Etiology

The causes of a herniated intervertebral disc may be divided into two categories:

Degeneration of the posterior ligaments along the spinal cord and the fibers surrounding the vertebral body.

Trauma to the spinal cord resulting from falls, automobile accidents, lifting strains, and repeated minor stresses. There may also be an underlying degenerative disease present.

The most frequent sites of a herniated disc are the lower lumbar and lumbosacral regions (L4, L5 to the sacrum). These herniations tend to occur secondary to trauma and affect the younger individual. The cervical disc herniate less frequently, and these herniations tend to occur because of degeneration, affecting mainly the older individual. Rarely do the thoracic discs herniate (Taylor, 1980).

Pathophysiology

When an intervertebral disc herniates, there is a posterior protrusion of the nucleus pulposus creating either direct pressure upon the cord (central) or pressure upon one or two spinal roots (lateral). Pressure upon a spinal root occurs more frequently than pressure on the spinal cord. There may also be a rupture of the annulus fibrosus or it may remain intact.

Nursing assessment

Subjective assessment data

History of accident, trauma, falls, and so on

Pain: location, onset, type, duration, radiation, aggravations (such as sneezing, coughing, lifting)

Restricted movements

Abnormal sensations along the distribution of the affected nerve

Weakness in an extremity

Objective assessment data

Nonverbal behavior (facial expressions, guarding)

Weak extremity

Muscle spasms

Restricted mobility of the spine

Limited straightening of the leg when the thigh is flexed (lumbar herniation)

Depressed deep tendon reflexes

Refer to Table 12-1 for signs and symptoms of a herniated disc in relationship to its location.

Table 12-1 Signs and symptoms of a herniated disc in relationship to its location

Herniated disc	Signs and symptoms
Cervical	Stiffness of neck
	Local shoulder pain that radiates down the arm to the fingers
	Parasthesias of hand
	Arm reflexes may be decreased
Lumbar	Lower back pain that radiates down one of the legs
	Movement of back is restricted
	Walking is painful
	Muscle spasms
	Aggravation of pain by straining (coughing, defecation, bending, lifting)
	Depressed deep tendon reflexes
	Hyperesthesia in distribution of affected nerve root

Nursing care plan: **HERNIATED INTERVERTEBRAL DISC**

NURSING DIAGNOSIS	EXPECTED OUTCOMES	NURSING INTERVENTIONS
Impaired physical mobility	Soft tissue is healed No additional changes in sensory and motor impulses No further cord trauma	In the initial phase of an intervertebral disc herniation conservative treatment is usually tried first. This allows the disc to be free from stress. Assess the motor and sensory impulses every 2 to 4 hours. Encourage the patient to remain in bed. Apply traction, corsets, and braces as per physician orders. Refer to Chapter 9 for additional interventions Place a bedboard under the mattress for extra support. Keep the body in proper straight alignment. When the patient is in traction, he should lie supine on a flat bed. When he is not in traction: Encourage the patient to log-roll. Assist the patient with positioning as allowed. Comfortable positions include (a) having the backrest elevated 20 to 30 degrees with the knees slightly flexed, (b) lying supine with 1 to 2 pillows under the legs, (c) a side position with a pillow behind the back and a folded bath blanket between the knees. Trapezes may be contraindicated. Fracture bedpans should be used. The patient should never sleep in the prone position because it hyperextends the spine. Patients with cervical herniations should not prop their heads up.
Total self-care deficit	Patient has a balanced intake and output Patient's electrolytes are within normal limits No weight loss or gain Normal urinary and fecal elimination patterns Intact skin with good turgor Clean skin, oral mucosa, and teeth	The herniated disc patient for whom bed rest has been prescribed is prone to potential disturbances in these areas. Refer to Chapter 11 for interventions dealing with the care of the bedridden patient and adapt them as necessary.
Potential alteration in comfort **Sensory and motor deficits**	Patient complains of minimal pain Patient has no more changes in sensory or motor impulses	Refer to Total self-care deficit. Assess pain and muscle spasms every 2 to 4 hours. This may need to be done more frequently depending upon the patient's condition. Administer prescribed muscle relaxants, anti-inflammatory medications, analgesics, and sedatives. Observe for potential side effects of medications. Utilize heat and massage. NOTE: Prolonged heat application may be contraindicated because it increases congestion. Utilize diversional activities such as radio and television.

Nursing care plan: HERNIATED INTERVERTEBRAL DISC—cont'd

NURSING DIAGNOSIS	EXPECTED OUTCOMES	NURSING INTERVENTIONS
Knowledge deficit: exercises and proper lifting techniques	Patient and family understand the importance of exercises Patient can demonstrate exercises and proper lifting techniques	After the acute symptoms subside, most patients are started on a back-strengthening exercise program. Teach the patient the exercises (William's exercises). Encourage the patient to start gently and gradually. Instruct the patient to stop exercises if pain worsens. Refer the patient for physical therapy. Instruct the patient about correct posture. Instruct the patient and family on correct stooping and lifting techniques.
Knowledge deficit: diagnostic procedures	Patient verbalizes fears and concerns Patient cooperates with procedures	See Chapter 2 for a detailed description of each procedure and specific nursing interventions. NOTE: Following a complete history and physical examination conducted by the physician, the following studies may be conducted to confirm the diagnosis: spinal x-rays, myelogram, and lumbar puncture.
Knowledge deficit: surgical procedures	Patient and family verbalize fears and concerns Patient and family verbalize understanding of the procedure Patient appears relaxed and comfortable	NOTE: If conservative treatment is ineffective or neurological deficits are increasing, surgical treatment is performed. This consists of a laminectomy, which may or may not be followed by a spinal fusion. A laminectomy is the removal of the lamina to expose the spinal cord. The portion of the protruding nucleus pulposus is also removed. A spinal fusion is the removal of a piece of bone from another part of the body (usually the iliac crest) and then the grafting of the bone onto the vertebrae to fuse the spinous processes. This then stabilizes the area. A spinal fusion will cause an area of permanent stiffness that limits mobility somewhat. This limitation is greatest when the fusion is done in the cervical spine. Preoperative and postoperative nursing care of spinal cord surgery patients is discussed in Chapter 10.
Knowledge deficit: home care measures	Patient functions as independently as possible Patient feels comfortable and knowledgeable enough to take care of himself at home Appropriate referrals are utilized for both physical and psychological support	Identify the physical limitations and strengths of the patient. Discuss these limitations and strengths with the patient and family. NOTE: Normal activities can be resumed on a gradual basis, but patients should be advised to refrain from specific strenuous activities until they are permitted to do them by the physician. Refer the patient for physical therapy. See also Knowledge deficit: exercises and proper lifting exercises.

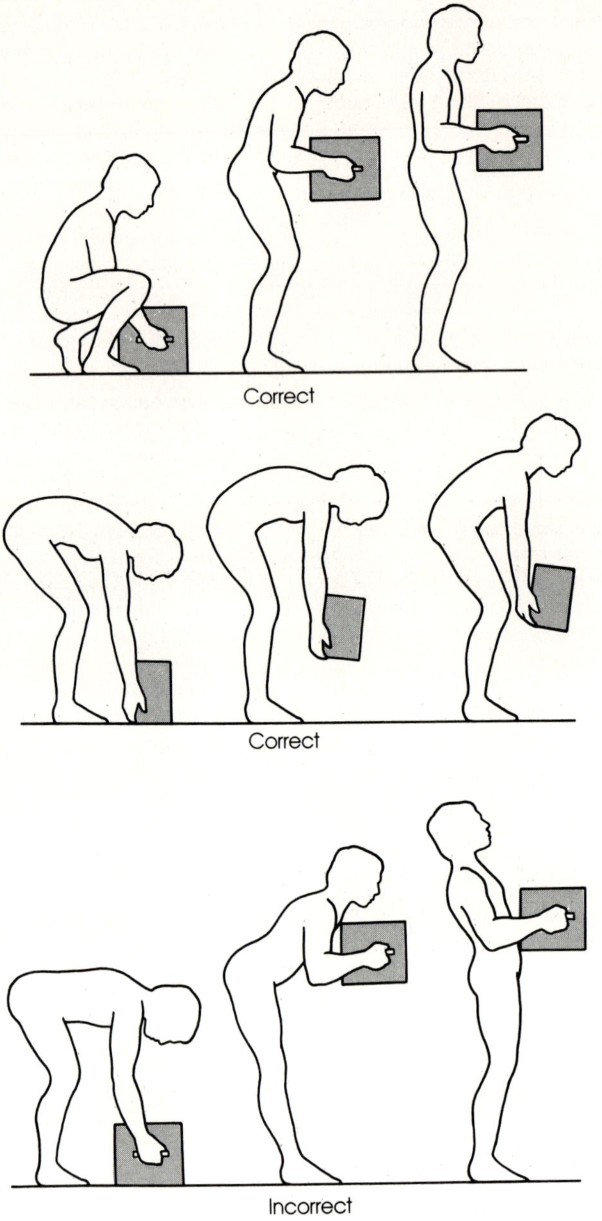

Fig. 12-1 Correct and incorrect stooping and lifting techniques. (From Rudy, E.B.: Advanced neurological and neurosurgical nursing, St. Louis, 1984, The C.V. Mosby Co.)

MYASTHENIA GRAVIS

Etiology

Research indicates that myasthenia gravis is caused by an autoimmune disturbance affecting the neuromuscular junction. It is estimated that about 50,000 persons in the United States have myasthenia gravis. The peak age of onset is between 20 and 30 years. Women are affected more frequently when young and men more often when over the age of 40. Myasthenia gravis is not considered to be hereditary (Conway-Rutkowski, 1982, Taylor, 1980).

Pathophysiology

The autoimmune disturbance affecting the neuromuscular junction has been localized to the skeletal muscle motor endplates. The changes in the postsynaptic membranes (endplates) are thought to result from the presence of humoral antibodies that bind to the nicotinic acetylcholine receptors, thus reducing the number of available receptor sites for acetylcholine. These antibodies can be detected in the serum of most patients with myasthenia gravis (Elias, 1979).

The weakness that is manifested in this condition affects the skeletal muscles. There is no evidence of central or peripheral nervous system involvement. The most frequently affected muscles are those that control eye movements, chewing, swallowing, speech, breathing, and head control.

The role of the thymus is not clear. However, approximately 80% of myasthenia gravis patients have cellular changes in the thymus gland. Thymectomy increases the rate of remission among patients with myasthenia gravis and it results in clinical improvements in many patients.

Nursing assessment

Subjective assessment data

Onset: is usually insidious and progresses slowly

Weakness of muscles: Weakness increases as muscles are used. With rest muscles usually regain power rapidly. Note affected muscle groups and any loss of the ability to do activities of daily living (ADL)

Extraocular muscle involvement: Note any diplopia. Involvement of ocular muscles is the most common initial symptom

Inability to chew or swallow: Note if there is any choking and the kind of diet the patient can eat

Weakness of voice

Breathing difficulties

Difficulty in holding the head up

Difficulty in brushing teeth, shaving, and combing hair

In advanced cases loss of bowel and bladder control

Paresthesias and aching of weakened muscles

Objective assessment data

Ptosis: one or both eyes affected

Difficulty in smiling

Expressionless appearance: In addition to ptosis and difficulty in smiling, patient has smoothed features and a tendency of the mouth to hang open
Nystagmus
Nasal and dysarthric speech
Aphonia: loss of the voice
Need to hold the head up with the hand
Mild atrophy of affected muscles
Hypotonia
Decreased tidal volume and vital capacity

Nursing care plan: MYASTHENIA GRAVIS

NURSING DIAGNOSIS	EXPECTED OUTCOMES	NURSING INTERVENTIONS
Potential ineffective airway clearance	Tidal volume and vital capacity within normal limits for the patient Lung sounds clear No complaints of dyspnea	NOTE: Because of the involvement of the respiratory muscles, these individuals have an increased susceptibility to pulmonary infections. Instruct the patient to deep breath and cough at least every 2 hours. Instruct the patient that strenuous activity is contraindicated. Instruct the patient to avoid exposure to persons with upper respiratory tract infections. Assist with percussion and postural drainage. Assist with obtaining tidal volume and vital capacity measurements every 4 hours. Observe the patient for signs of respiratory embarrassment. Maintain emergency respiratory equipment nearby: Endotracheal tube Ambu bag Suction machine Oxygen setup Notify the physician immediately about any complaints of dyspnea or any significant decrease in tidal volume and vital capacity.
Potential for alteration in nutrition **Potential fluid volume deficit** **Potential electrolyte disturbance**	No or minimal weight loss No aspiration of food or liquids Precautions are taken to minimize nausea, diarrhea, constipation, and abdominal cramping	NOTE: Muscle weakness may make it difficult for the patient to receive an adequate nutritional intake. Give anticholinesterase medications 45 minutes to 1 hour before meals to provide optimum strength.

Nursing care plan: MYASTHENIA GRAVIS—cont'd

NURSING DIAGNOSIS	EXPECTED OUTCOMES	NURSING INTERVENTIONS
Potential for altered urinary elimination pattern Potential for altered bowel elimination		Allow the patient to eat slowly. Give small frequent meals to avoid abdominal distention and prevent nausea, diarrhea, constipation, and abdominal cramps. Administer antiemetics as ordered. Administer anti-diarrhea agents as ordered. (Diphenoxylate [Lomotil] should not be given because of its atropine effects.) Keep a call light, emesis basin, and bedpan nearby. Mechanical soft diets may be required. Discuss the fluid preferences with the patient. Encourage fluids up to 3000 ml a day to prevent constipation. Administer mild cathartics or suppositories as ordered. Be aware that these medications may make the patient weaker. Observe the patient for choking, nasal regurgitation, and aspiration. Suction the patient as necessary. Notify the physician of problems with eating. Prepare to initiate tube feedings and intravenous solutions per physician's orders.
Altered visual function	Eyes are moist and free of corneal abrasions Patient is free from injury Patient is relaxed and comfortable	NOTE: Because of the weakness of the ocular muscles, the patient may have diplopia and ptosis, which will result in limited vision. Alternatively patch the eyes every 2 to 3 hours while the patient is awake. Apply lid crutches to minimize ptosis. Apply normal tear solution every hour to the eyes. Utilize eye shields if necessary in severe cases. Assist with ADL when necessary. Ambulate the patient with assistance when necessary. Explain all procedures to the patient and also the possible need for assistance to allay fears of increasing dependency. Refer to Ineffective patient and family coping.
Impaired verbal communication	Nurse understands patient Patient's needs are understood by staff Patient's frustration level is low	NOTE: These patients are often very difficult to understand because of their dysarthric and nasal speech. Take time to listen to the patient and repeat information to verify it. Instruct the patient to speak slowly and read the patient's lips. Keep the call bell within patient's reach. Depending upon the patient's strength, the following may be used: Flash cards Magic slates Notebook and pencil Develop appropriate hand signals. Make a referral for speech therapy.

Continued.

Nursing care plan: **MYASTHENIA GRAVIS—cont'd**

NURSING DIAGNOSIS	EXPECTED OUTCOMES	NURSING INTERVENTIONS
Decreased activity tolerance **Sleep pattern disturbance**	Patient plans daily activities with the nurse. This plan includes periods of relaxation No verbal complaints of being overtired Patient performs own care when able to do so Patient sleeps 8 to 10 hours a night depending on need	NOTE: These individuals become very weak after exertion and at the end of the day. Activities must be planned carefully to conserve energy. Muscle strength usually improves after rest. However, in some cases it may not improve and in others the muscles may become weak even without exercise. Individualize patient care. Plan the day's activities with the patient. Include frequent rest periods. Assist the patient with ADL as necessary. Observe muscle strength in relation to drug therapy. Provide the patient with as much uninterrupted sleep at night as possible. Make a referral for physical therapy. Instruct the patient on range-of-motion exercises.
Ineffective patient and family coping	Patient is relaxed and comfortable Patient's and family's questions are answered	Spend time with the patient and family to develop a trusting relationship. Discuss their fears. Answer questions regarding the disease. See Knowledge needs and Discharge planning. Offer positive suggestions regarding changes that need to be made in the patient's life-style. Be honest. Demonstrate acceptance.
Knowledge deficit: diagnostic procedures	Patient verbalizes fears and concerns Cooperates with procedures	NOTE: Diagnosis is determined by the history, clinical manifestations, and observing the individual's response to neostigmine (Prostigmin) or edrophonium (Tensilon). Each of these anticholinesterase drugs causes a dramatic improvement in muscle strength in the myasthenia gravis patient. Neostigmine is given orally, IM, or IV. Its peak effect is 30 to 60 minutes after injection and it persists for several hours. Neostigmine is very valuable in evaluating the motor function of the extremities. Tensilon is injected IV. A positive response can be seen in 1 minute with improvement lasting up to 5 minutes. Tensilon is very valuable in evaluating the oropharyngeal and ocular muscles. Keep atrophine sulfate available to counteract potential cardiac arrhythmias. Monitor for bradycardia. NOTE: If edrophonium and neostigmine are not effective, minute doses of curare may be used. Curare will cause an immediate increase in weakness. Assess respiratory status. Prepare to give respiratory assistance. Refer to Chapter 2 for other diagnostic procedures such as electrical stimulation and electromyography.

Nursing care plan: MYASTHENIA GRAVIS—cont'd

NURSING DIAGNOSIS	EXPECTED OUTCOMES	NURSING INTERVENTIONS
Knowledge deficit: medications	Patient does not experience any crisis Patient demonstrates knowledge of medications, side effects, actions, and dosage	NOTE: Anticholinesterase drugs increase the response of muscles to nerve impulses, thereby improving strength. The common anticholinesterase drugs are neostigmine bromide (Prostigmin), pyridostigmine bromide (Mestinon), and ambenonium chloride (Mytelase). Drug dosages may vary from day to day because of fluctuating symptoms. Give medication at precise times to maintain blood levels. Administer medication at the same times each day. These cannot vary because of the drug's half-life. Meals should be eaten 45 minutes to 1 hour after administration of medication. Small amounts of food may be given with medication to alleviate gastrointestinal effects. Observe for positive effects of medication. Observe for side effects and toxicity of medication. Instruct the patient on anticholinesterase drugs. Do not administer magnesium sulfate, morphine or its derivatives curare, quinine, quinidine, or procainamide because these increase the weakness. NOTE: Prednisone may also be used in the treatment of myasthenia gravis because of its immunosuppressive effect. The drug is administered in high doses on alternate days. Worsening of symptoms may be noted followed by improvement. Myasthenia gravis patients may also receive potassium supplements, antacids, and a diet low in sodium and carbohydrates. Observe for untoward effects of prednisone. These include adrenocortical insufficiency, electrolyte imbalances, glucosuria, and Cushing's syndrome. Instruct the patient to avoid large crowds and people with upper respiratory infections. Instruct the patient to call the physician if he develops a prolonged illness. Administer antacids to relieve gastrointestinal upset. Observe stools for bleeding. Instruct the patient to notify the physician if there is blood in the stool or if hematemesis or epigastric pain occurs 1 to 3 hours after a meal. Instruct the patient to notify the physician about any large weight gain or signs of edema. Monitor blood pressure frequently. Tell the patient that appetite may be increased and not to overeat. Instruct the patient on good skin care since prednisone may cause acne.

Continued.

Nursing care plan: MYASTHENIA GRAVIS—cont'd

NURSING DIAGNOSIS	EXPECTED OUTCOMES	NURSING INTERVENTIONS
Knowledge deficit: surgical treatment	Patient and family verbalize fears and concerns Verbalize understanding of procedures Patient appears relaxed and comfortable	NOTE: Thymectomy does not always work immediately and it may take several years before a remission occurs or it may not occur at all. The most marked improvement occurs in those patients who have the surgery within 2 years of the onset of myasthenia gravis. One of two approaches may be used. These are transcervical and the sternal split. The transcervical approach takes less time and there is decreased postoperative discomfort. However, paresis of the laryngeal nerve can occur. The sternal split approach decreases the risk of incomplete removal of the thymus. With the transcervical approach, the patient may return to the general floor with only a small dressing and an intravenous as compared to the patient with a sternal split approach who may be admitted to the intensive care unit (ICU) intubated. Instruct the patient preoperatively on appropriate postoperative procedures: deep breathing, coughing, the ICU and the equipment that may be used, wound care, and intravneous infusions. Postoperatively observe for signs of respiratory obstruction, pneumothorax, and infection.
Knowledge deficit: plasmapheresis **Proper care before, during, and after plasmapheresis**	Patient verbalizes fears and concerns Verbalizes understanding of the procedure Patient appears relaxed and comfortable Patient does not experience any complications	NOTE: Plasmapheresis is a method by which autoantibodies are removed from the plasma. Adjunct therapy includes the administration of immunosuppressive drugs to inactivate the cells that produce the antibodies. The procedure takes 2 to 5 hours to complete. An antecubital vein or shunt may be used. Instruct the patient on the procedure. Instruct the patient to eat a good meal before the procedure. Weigh the patient before the procedure. Instruct the patient that blood studies will be drawn before the procedure. Administer proper care to shunt. Check for bruits every 2 to 4 hours. Maintain shunt patency. Keep double bulldog clamps at bedside. Observe the puncture site for signs of bleeding or ecchymosis. Observe for side effects of anticholinesterase medications since the patient may not need as much medication. Allow the patient to rest.

Nursing care plan: MYASTHENIA GRAVIS—cont'd

NURSING DIAGNOSIS	EXPECTED OUTCOMES	NURSING INTERVENTIONS
Knowledge deficit: proper care during a crisis	No hazards of immobility Clear lung sounds Intact skin Adequate nutrition, fluids, and electrolytes Minimal fear, anxiety, and apprehension	NOTE: Two types of crises may occur. These are a cholinergic crisis caused by an overdose of anticholinesterase drugs, and a myasthenia crisis resulting from an exacerbation of the disease. Signs of a myasthenia crisis include a dramatic increase in myasthenic symptoms, nausea, vomiting, sweating, bradycardia, muscular tightness, general weakness, dysphagia, and respiratory distress. Generally these patients are intubated and placed in the ICU. A crisis may last for weeks. A cholinergic crisis is often difficult to distinguish from a myasthenia crisis because the symptoms are the same. Edrophonium (Tensilon) is usually used first to make the diagnosis. Atropine sulfate, 1 mg IV, is used in a cholinergic crisis to control symptoms. For interventions refer to the previous sections of the Nursing care plan: myasthenia gravis. Refer to Chapter 11 for interventions for immobility.
Knowledge deficit: self and home care measures	Patient demonstrates adequate understanding of disease process Patient is able to recognize important changes in condition Patient is able to function as independently as possible The family feels comfortable and demonstrates knowledge in assisting with management of the patient. Appropriate referrals and community resources have been utilized for both physical and psychological support.	Instruct the patient and family on the disease process. Provide emotional support. Encourage the patient and family to ask questions. Instruct the patient and family on adequate oxygenation, food, fluids, electrolytes, proper elimination, eye care, speech interventions, adequate exercise, rest, sleep, and medications. Instruct the patient on signs of an exacerbation. These include increased weakness, increased diplopia, ptosis, and problems with chewing and swallowing. Instruct the patient and family on factors that predispose the patient to an exacerbation. These include infection, stress, surgery, hard physical exercise, sedatives, enemas, strong cathartics. Instruct the patient to notify the physician before taking common cold preparations and antibiotics. Some cold preparations contain quinine. The mycins and tetracyclines can cause neuromuscular blockage. Advise the patient to wear a Medic Alert bracelet. Advise the patient about the Myasthenia Gravis Foundation. The foundation works with education and research and assists with financial aid. (Address: 15 East 26th Street, New York, NY 10010.)

MUSCULAR DYSTROPHIES

The muscular dystrophies are a group of chronic diseases that have two main characteristics in common. These include their hereditary nature and the involvement of voluntary muscles.

Etiology

The exact cause of the muscular dystrophies is not known. Although several theories have been tested, the data is not conclusive. The incidence of muscular dystrophies depends upon and varies with each specific type. Approximately 200,000 individuals in the United States are afflicted with the disease.

Pathophysiology

The involved voluntary muscles progressively degenerate and are ultimately replaced by fat and connective tissue. As a rule there are no disturbances of the peripheral and central nervous systems.

Classifications

In the literature there are several methods for classifying the muscular dystrophies. For the purposes of this manual only the four most prevalent types will be discussed. All of the muscular dystrophies are characterized by muscular weakness, are insidious in onset, and are continuously progressive, but the age of onset of symptoms and the rate of progression vary greatly from one type to another (Gardner-Medwin, 1980; Ketenjian, 1978).

- Duchenne
  - X-linked recessive.
  - Prevalence: about 3/100,000 in the general population.
  - Occurs mainly in males or in females with Turner's syndrome. Females are carriers and may show a slow progression of weakness over 5 or more decades.
  - Onset in childhood (ages 3-10).
  - Progresses rapidly (between the ages of 7 to 14 the patient may develop the inability to walk).
  - Symptoms: initially, weakness and hypertrophy of muscles (abnormal walk or run, swayback, waddling gait), no facial involvement, eventually weakness and atrophy of arms and hands, contracture formation, and finally confinement to a wheelchair.
  - Intellectual retardation is common (cause not known).
  - Death may result from respiratory infection or aspiration and possibly from cardiac failure. Most patients die before the age of 20.
- Myotonic
  - Autosomal dominant.
  - Prevalence: about 5/100,000 in the general population.
  - Occurs in both sexes.
  - Onset is usually detected before the age of 20 and often before 10.
  - Progresses slowly (most patients are significantly handicapped within 20 years).

Symptoms: involves weakness of forearms, hands, legs; facial, masticatory, and sternocleidomastoid muscles; ptosis; cataracts; voice changes; myotonia (inability to relax a muscle when stimulation is withdrawn). Other abnormalities include heart conduction defects, early baldness, syncope, pulmonary hypoventilation, dysphagia, aspiration pneumonitis, constipation, testicular atrophy.

Mental retardation may be present especially if the disease is present at birth.

Death may result from anesthetic difficulties, pulmonary aspiration, cardiac arrhythmias.

Becker

X-linked recessive.

Prevalence: about 1/100,000 in the general population.

As with Duchenne muscular dystrophy, occurs mainly in males and in females with Turner's syndrome

Onset occurs mainly between 5 and 15 years of age.

Progresses slowly (most patients are significantly handicapped in their twenties).

Symptoms: same as with Duchenne muscular dystrophy. Most patients notice difficulties with school sports. Muscle cramps are common

Mental retardation may occur; however, this is rare.

Same causes of death as Duchenne muscular dystrophy. Patients may live into their fourth decade.

Facioscapulohumeral

Autosomal dominant.

Prevalence: about 0.2-0.5/100,000 in the general population.

Occurs in both sexes.

Onset is mainly during adolescence or early adulthood (ages 10 to 25).

Progresses slowly (many can walk beyond middle age).

Symptoms: initially, facial and shoulder weakness (difficulty closing the eyes or lips, winging of the shoulders); weakness gradually spreads to other voluntary muscles.

Intellect is never affected.

Life expectancy is almost normal. The heart is rarely involved.

Nursing assessment

Subjective assessment data

Complaints of muscle or generalized weakness

Problems with walking

- Difficulty in climbing up and down stairs
- Muscle cramps
- Difficulty in raising arms over the head or lifting objects
- Frequently falls and then has trouble getting up
- Syncope

Difficulty chewing and swallowing
Constipation
Difficulty in closing eyes or lips

Objective assessment data. Signs and symptoms are dependent upon the type of muscular dystrophy.

- May be mentally slow
- Masklike expression with prominent lips. Facial movements may be diminished or absent
- Symmetrical involvement of musculature
- Dystrophy of muscles
- Hypertrophic muscles feel firm and rubbery
- Pseudohypertrophy of muscles
- Atrophy of muscles
- Atonia
- Steppage waddling gait; toe walking
- Lumbar lordosis
- Movements of arm may be accompanied by winging of scapula
- Gower's sign (when in the supine position the person first has to turn over onto the abdomen and then he raises the trunk to the crawling position. He then places the feet firmly on the ground with his hands and gradually elevates the upper part of the body by ''climbing up his own trunk'' with the arms
- Normal sensations
- Deep tendon reflexes may be lost
- Normal cutaneous reflexes
- Early baldness
- Testicular atrophy
- Ptosis and cataracts

Nursing care plan: **MUSCULAR DYSTROPHIES**

NURSING DIAGNOSIS	EXPECTED OUTCOMES	NURSING INTERVENTIONS
Potential ineffective airway clearance **Potential ineffective breathing patterns**	Tidal volume and vital capacity within normal limits for the patient Lung sounds clear No complaints of dyspnea Respiration rate normal Is afebrile	NOTE: In the early stage of these disease the patients usually do not have any problems with oxygenation. However, in advanced stages pneumonia may occur secondary to aspiration or to decreased pulmonary function. Teach the patient how to do disphragmatic breathing exercises. Encourage the patient to deep breathe and cough every 1 to 2 hours. Keep the patient as active as possible. Instruct the patient on respiratory aids such as the incentive spirometer. Turn the patient every 1 to 2 hours. Assist with percussion and postural drainage. Utilize and make referrals to respiratory therapy. Suction as necessary.
Potential for alteration in nutrition **Potential fluid volume deficit** **Potential electrolyte disturbance** **Potential for altered urinary elimination pattern** **Potential for altered bowel elimination**	Minimal weight loss or gain No aspiration Electrolytes within normal limits No signs of urinary statis, urinary infection, or constipation	NOTE: As long as these individuals are able to remain as active as possible, no problems should be encountered except for those with myotonic dystrophy who may have dysphagia. In the later stages of the disease, problems may be encountered because of immobility and confinement to a wheelchair. Obesity hastens functional disability and creates problems with such tasks as transferring and bathing. Wheelchair-confined patients may reduce their fluid intake and allow the bladder to fill and retain urine as long as possible because they are reluctant to ask for assistance. Encourage a well-balanced diet with calories and proportions sufficient for age and weight. Encourage the patient to eat fruits and vegetables instead of high-calorie snacks. Encourage high-fiber foods and those that lower urine pH (meats, cereals, poultry, fish, cranberry juice). Instruct the patient to drink between 2000-3000 ml of fluids a day. (If cardiac problems are evident, reduce as necessary.) Instruct patients on the need to use the toliet as soon as they have the urge. Observe dysphagic patients closely. Instruct the dysphagic patient to sit upright, eat slowly, and eat soft and pureed foods.
Altered visual function	Eyes are moist and free of corneal abrasions Patient is free from injury	NOTE: Patients with myotonic dystrophy may have ptosis and cataracts, and patients with facioscapulohumeral dystrophy may not be able to close their eyelids completely. Special precautions may be needed to keep their eyes moist. Apply lid crutches to minimize ptosis. Apply normal tear solution to the eyes every to 4 hours depending on the patient's condition. Assist with ADL when necessary. Ambulate the patient with assistance if necessary.

Continued.

NURSING DIAGNOSIS	EXPECTED OUTCOMES	NURSING INTERVENTIONS
Impaired verbal communication	Nurse understands patient Patient's needs are understood by staff Patient's frustration level is low	NOTE: Because of enlargement of the tongue, changes in the jaw, weakness of facial muscles, decreased vocal intensity, and decreased breath support, these patients may be difficult to understand. Take time to listen to the patient and repeat information to verify it. Instruct the patient to speak slowly and read the patient's lips. Keep the call bell within the patient's reach. Depending on the patient's strength, the following may be used: Flash cards Magic slate Notebook and pencil Make a referral for speech therapy.
Decreased tolerance for activity Sleep pattern disturbance	Patient plans dailiy activities with the nurse Patient is as independent as possible Contractures are minimized No verbal complaints of being overtired	Individualize patient care. Plan the day's activities with the patient. Include frequent rest periods. Assist the patient with ADLs as necessary. Make a referral for physical therapy. Assist the patient with exercises. Refer to Chapter 11 for additional interventions dealing with the patient who has an impairment of mobility.
Ineffective patient and family coping	Patient is relaxed and comfortable Patient and family's questions are answered	Spend time with the patient and family to develop a trusting relationship. Discuss their fears. Answer their questions regarding the disease. Refer to Knowledge deficits and Discharge planning. Offer positive suggestions in regards to changes that need to be made in the patient's life-style. Be honest. Demonstrate acceptance. Assist the family in establishing realistic goals with their child. Make a referral for psychiatric counseling for the patient and family if necessary. Make a referral for genetic counseling for both the parents and female siblings. Make a referral for group therapy. NOTE: Children with muscular dystrophy will encounter many problems. These include problems of body image, family adjustment, peer interaction, sexuality, and establishment of emotional independence from parents.
Knowledge deficit: diagnostic procedures	Patient and family verbalize fears and concerns Patient cooperates with procedures	NOTE: Diagnosis is determined by the history, clinical manifestations, elevated serum levels of creatinine phosphokinase, characteristic changes on an electromyogram, and muscle biopsy. Refer to Chapter 2 for nursing interventions dealing with the electromyogram and muscle biopsy.

Nursing care plan: MUSCULAR DYSTROPHIES—cont'd

NURSING DIAGNOSIS	EXPECTED OUTCOMES	NURSING INTERVENTIONS
Knowledge deficit: surgical procedures	Patient and family verbalize fears and concerns Verbalize understanding of procedures Patient appears relaxed and comfortable	NOTE: Surgical procedures may be done to stretch contractures and lengthen tendons. (Refer to an orthopedic surgery textbook for a discussion of such surgery.) A spinal fusion and Harrington rod fixation may also be performed to stabilize scoliosis and improve body image and to enhance the cardiac and respiratory functions and relieve discomfort. Refer to Chapter 10 for nursing interventions. Refer to page 323 for a discussion of spinal fusion.
Impaired physical mobility due to confinement to a wheelchair	Paralytic scoliosis of the spine is retarded. No cardiopulmonary difficulties. No dependent edema. Minimal contractures. No urinary stasis. Skin is intact.	Refer to Chapter 11 for nursing interventions dealing with an impairment of mobility.
Knowledge deficit: self and home care measures	Patient demonstrates adequate understanding of the disease according to age Patient functioning as independently as possible Patient and family are able to recognize important changes in condition The family feels comfortable and demonstrates knowledge in assisting with management of patient Appropriate referrals and community resources have been utilized for both physical and psychological support	Instruct the patient and family on the disease process. Provide emotional support. Encourage the patient and family to ask questions. Instruct the patient and family on how to care for the nursing diagnoses mentioned previously. Advise the patient and family about local and national Muscular Dystrophy Associations. The national association's main area is research while the local chapters deal with diagnostic services, special equipments, physical therapy, transportation, educational and recreational programs, and orthopedic appliances, which are provided or arranged for on request without cost.

MULTIPLE SCLEROSIS

Etiology

The definite cause of multiple sclerosis is not known. Several factors have been cited as possible causes. These include viral agents, environmental agents, metabolic disturbances, allergic reactions, and nutritional deficiencies. At present the most popular theory is that multiple sclerosis is an autoimmune reaction. (Lewis, 1979).

Multiple sclerosis has been reported in all parts of the world. However the incidence is much higher in the colder and temperate climate areas. The disease is very rare in children. Generally the onset occurs between the ages of 20 and 40 years. Women are affected almost twice as often as men (Stater, 1980; Swift, 1979; Brance, 1980).

Pathophysiology

Multiple sclerosis is an inflammatory disorder of the protective myelin sheath surrounding the nerve axons. The inflammation occurs in unpredictable and patchy areas within the central nervous system, with no involvement of peripheral nerves. The individual experiences periods of remissions and exacerbations. Initially, the clinical manifestations of exacerbations may be totally reversible, reflecting the inflammatory depression of neurotransmission without total destruction of the myelin. However, with repeated and more severe attacks it appears that the myelin becomes totally disrupted and the nerve fiber involved in those particular areas degenerates, resulting in irreversible or only partial improvement of the clinical manifestations. The disease process is considered to be a progressive one and clinical manifestations will vary from one person to another.

Nursing assessment

Initial signs and symptoms are highly variable, depending upon the location and extent of the lesions.

Subjective assessment data

Patient history reflecting periods of remissions and exacerbations
Blurring or loss of vision in one or both eyes
Numbness or tingling sensations
Weakness of a limb on one side of the body
Difficulty with speech
Difficulty with walking
Difficulty swallowing
Dizziness
Fatigue

Objective assessment data

Sensory dysfunction (for example, decreased perception to pain, touch, temperature, position sense, and vibration sense; also Lhermitte's sign, which involves shock-like sensations that run down the back when the head is flexed)

Visual disturbances (for example, optic neuritis, which may result in blurred vision or may progress to complete blindness, diplopia, nystagmus, temporal pallor of the disks)

Motor dysfunction (for example, intention tremor, ataxia, weakness or paralysis of extremities, scanning speech, dysphagia)

Abnormal reflexes: usually a late sign (for example, hyperreflexia, absent reflexes, positive Babinski and Hoffman signs)

Emotional and mental changes: early (for example, apathy, euphoria, depression); late (for example, confusion, memory deficit)

Bladder and bowel disturbances (for example, urgency, frequency, retention, incontinence)

Nursing care plan: **MULTIPLE SCLEROSIS**

NURSING DIAGNOSIS	EXPECTED OUTCOMES	NURSING INTERVENTIONS
Potential ineffective airway clearance	Tidal volume and vital capacity within normal limits for the patient Lung sounds clear Respiration rate normal Is afebrile	NOTE: This may be a problem during severe exacerations or when patients are so debilitated that they are confined to a bed or wheelchair. Aspiration pneumonia may also be a problem in these patients. Instruct on diaphragmatic breathing exercises. Encourage the patient to deep breath and cough every 1 to 2 hours. Keep the patient as active as possible. Develop a turning schedule based on the patient's needs but no less than every 2 hours. Instruct the patient on the use of respiratory aides such as the incentive spirometer. Make a referral to respiratory therapy. Refer to Potential for alteration in nutrition to prevent possible aspiration.
Altered visual function	Maximal visual function is maintained Is free from injury	Assess visual acuity every shift. Notify the physician of any changes in visual function. Instruct the patient on the use of an eye patch. Alternate eyes every 4 hours. Instruct the patient to rest the eyes when fatigue is noticed. Use large-type materials and talking books if necessary. Inform the patient that blindness is unusual in multiple sclerosis and that the visual symptoms usually improve after the exacerbation.
Sensory deficits	Is free from injury Maximum level of function is maintained	Assess sensory impairments and observe for changes in sensory levels every shift. Instruct the patient in proper safety measures: 1. Testing bath water and dishwater with an unaffected extremity or a thermometer. 2. When cooking do not get in contact with steam or touch hot utensils. Use pot holders. 3. Dress warmly in cold weather. Wear gloves. 4. Do not sit or lean against hot or extremely cold materials. Instruct the patient to examine the skin every day. Instruct the patient to become mentally aware of where the extremities are when performing activities. Watch the hands and feet.
Potential for altered urinary elimination patterns	Urinates every 4 hours or less often Continence is maintained Nocturia is absent Residual volume is below 100 ml Identifies signs and symptoms of urinary tract infection Frequency and severity of urinary tract infections are reduced Social and vocational functions are not limited	Identify with the patient those symptoms that interfere with daily functioning. Identify with the patient those symptoms that may be harmful to his health. Assist the physician in determining the patient's basic parameter of bladder function. Administer prescribed medications. These include: Vitamin C to acidify the urine and decrease bacterial growth. Adrenergic blocking agents to restore urethral function. Cholinergic and anticholinergic drugs to rehabilitate the detrusor reflex. Encourage the patient to drink cranberry juice or prune juice to acidify the urine and supply vitamin C.

Continued.

Nursing care plan: MULTIPLE SCLEROSIS—cont'd

NURSING DIAGNOSIS	EXPECTED OUTCOMES	NURSING INTERVENTIONS
Potential for altered urinary elimination patterns—cont'd		Encourage the patient to drink at least 2000 to 3000 ml a day. Record the patient's intake and output daily. Instruct the patient to eliminate fluids after dinner if nocturia is a problem. Instruct the patient on appropriate mechanical assistance to aid in urination: Credè maneuver Valsalva maneuver Digital stimulation Lower abdominal pressure Intermittent catheterization Instruct the patient on symptoms of urinary tract infections.
Potential for alteration in nutrition	Weight normal for age and height No aspiration Patient understands importance of eating foods high in fiber	NOTE: In addition to potential dysphagia, diarrhea, or constipation, the patient may be obese. Obesity adds additional strain on weak muscles and impairs circulation. Instruct the patient on a reducing diet if necessary. Encourage the patient to eat slowly and chew foods thoroughly. Instruct the patient on eating semisolid or blenderized foods if swallowing is difficult. Instruct the patient on the use of an upright position while eating. Refer to Altered bowel elimination for additional interventions. Weight the patient every other day if necessary.
Knowledge deficit: diagnostic procedures	Patient verbalizes fears and concerns Cooperates with procedures	NOTE: There is no specific diagnostic test for multiple sclerosis. A history of remissions and exacerbations with the resulting signs and symptoms are clues to its diagnosis. A myelogram may be used to rule out lesions of the spinal cord. A CAT scan may reveal plaques. The cerebrospinal fluid may contain a slightly elevated total protein and often an elevated gamma globulin level. Therefore a lumbar puncture is performed. Refer to Chapter 2 for specific nursing interventions.
Impaired physical mobility	Verbalizes and demonstrates safety measures Is free of injury Maximum level of function is maintained	Assess mobility level every shift. Encourage the patient to stay as active as possible but to avoid fatigue. Instruct the patient in proper safety measures: Use of assistive ambulatory equipment. Use of a wheelchair. Instruct on the use of active and passive exercises. Make appropriate referrals to physical therapy and occupational therapy. Discuss individual needs for the use of assistive ambulatory equipment in different situations. Refer to Chapter 11 for nursing interventions dealing with an impairment of mobility.

Nursing care plan: **MULTIPLE SCLEROSIS—cont'd**

NURSING DIAGNOSIS	EXPECTED OUTCOMES	NURSING INTERVENTIONS
Sexual dysfunction	Expresses satisfaction of sexual needs by partner and self	Discuss their sexual history with the patient and partner when appropriate. Discuss their expectations and what may occur. Discuss alternate methods. Encourage the patient to identify other erotic areas. Encourage verbalization regarding attitudes toward alternate sexual methods. Encourage the use of visual aids for additional stimulation. Discuss the importance of an open and loving relationship. Discuss the effects fatigue and such medications as antidepressants and tranquilizers have upon sexual activity. Make referrals for sexual counseling as appropriate.
Knowledge deficit: medications	Patient demonstrates knowledge of medications, side effects, actions, and dosage Verbalizes willingness to follow prescribed regimens	NOTE: Adrenocorticotropic hormone (ACTH) and other corticosteroids are used during exacerbations of the disease to reduce the inflammatory process. A remission seems to occur more rapidly with the use of these medications. Their use is not indicated during a remission. Discuss the treatment plan with the patient and family, including effects of medications Refer to p. 387 for a detailed discussion of untoward effects and nursing interventions for corticosteroids. NOTE: Baclofen (Lioresal) and diazepam (Valium) may be ordered to decrease the spasticity of skeletal muscles.
Inadequate knowledge to prevent or decrease frequency of exacerbations	Verbalizes knowledge of potential precipitation factors Exacerbations occur infrequently and are mild	NOTE: Several factors are considered as possible precipitating or aggravating causes of an exacerbation. These include infectious process, physical trauma, emotional stress, excessive exertion or undue fatigue, pregnancy, and a lowered state of health. Instruct the patient and family on potential precipitating factors for an exacerbation.
Ineffective patient and family coping	Patient is relaxed and comfortable Patient and family's questions are answered	Spend time with the patient and family to develop a trusting relationship. Discuss their fears. Answer questions regarding the disease. Refer to Knowledge deficits and Discharge planning. Offer positive suggestions with regard to changes that need to be made in the patient's life-style. Be honest. Demonstrate acceptance. Assist the patient and family in establilshing realistic goals. Make a referral for psychiatric counseling if necessary. NOTE: The family should understand the need for multiple sclerosis patients to maintain maximum physical condition and also that the patient must make many decisions for himself and be responsible for implementing his own care if possible.

Continued.

Nursing care plan: MULTIPLE SCLEROSIS—cont'd

NURSING DIAGNOSIS	EXPECTED OUTCOMES	NURSING INTERVENTIONS
Knowledge deficit: disease process	Verbalizes understanding of multiple sclerosis Verbalizes fears and concerns	Give an explanation appropriate to the patient's and family's level of comprehension and emotional state. Give encouragement and the opportunity to ask questions. Be honest. NOTE: The disease process progresses at varying rates from individual to individual. The disease must be kept in prospective for the sake of all involved.
Knowledge deficit: self and home care measures	Patient demonstrates adequate understanding of disease according to age Patient is functioning as independently as possible Patient and family are able to recognize important changes in condition The family feels comfortable and demonstrates knowledge in assisting with management of patient Appropriate referrals and community resources have been utilized for both physical and psychological support	Instruct the patient and family on the disease process. Provide emotional support. Encourage the patient and family to ask questions. Instruct the patient and family on how to care for the nursing diagnoses mentioned previously. Consider appropriate referrals to a social worker, psychologist, or psychiatrist to determine possible organic brain involvement or when sensory maladaptive behaviors or abnormal thought patterns are identified. Also make referrals to a rehabilitation counselor. Refer the patient to the National Multiple Sclerosis Society. There are 140 chapters. The national headquarters is at 205 East 42nd Street, New York, NY 10017.

Suggested readings

Adams, R.C., and Victor, M.: Principles of neurology, ed. 2, New York, 1981, McGraw-Hill Book Co.

Brand, K.P.: Multiple sclerosis, adrenocorticotropic hormone, and nursing implications, J. Neurosurg. Nurs. **12**(2):62-65, June 1980.

Conway-Rutkowski, B.L.: Carini and Owens' neurological and neurosurgical nursing, ed. 8, St. Louis, 1982, The C.V. Mosby Co.

Elias, S.B., and Appel, S.H.: Current concepts of pathogenesis and treatment of myasthenia gravis, Med. Clin. North Am. **63**(4):745-755, July 1979.

Gardner-Medwin, D.: Clinical features and classifications of muscular dystrophies, Br. Med. Bull. **36**(2):109-115, 1980.

Hrovath, M.: Myasthenia gravis; a nursing approach, J. Neurosurg. Nurs. **14**(1):7-12, Feb. 1982.

Hunter, S.: The heart in muscular dystrophy, Br. Med. Bull. **36**(2):133-134, 1980.

Ketenjian, A.: Muscular dystrophy: diagnosis and treatment, Orthop. Clin. North Am. **9**:25-42, 1978.

Lewis, S.M., and Lewis, V.H.: Multiple sclerosis: does the mystery remain? J. Neurosurg. Nurs. **11**(3):176-182, Sept. 1979.

McDonnell, M., and others: M.S. problem oriented nursing care plans, Am. J. Nurs. **80**:292-297, Feb. 1980.

Merritt, H.H.: Textbook of neurology, ed. 6, Philadelphia, 1979, Lea & Febiger.

Newsom-Davis, J.: The respiratory system in muscular dystrophy, Br. Med. Bull. **36**(2):135-138, 1980.

Pennington, R.J.T.: Clinical biochemistry of muscular dystrophy, Br. Med. Bull. **36**(2):123-126, 1980.

Rodnitzky, R., and Goeken, J.: Complications of plasma exchange in neurological patients, Arch. Neurol. **39**:350-354, June 1982.

Rubin, J.W., and others: Thymectomy in myasthenia gravis: the timing of surgery and significance of thymic pathology, Am. Surg. **47**:152-156, April 1981.

Siegal, I.M.: The management of muscular dystrophy: a clinical review, Muscle Nerve **1**:453-460, 1978.

Siegel, I.M.: Muscular dystrophy; multidisciplinary approach to management, Postgrad. Med. **69**(2):124-133, Feb. 1981.

Slater, R.J., and Yearwood, A.C.: M.S. facts, faith, and hope, Am. J. Nurs. **80**:276-281, Feb. 1980.

Sneddon, J.: Myasthenia gravis—the difficult diagnosis, Br. J. Psychiatry **136**:92-93, 1980.

Swift, N.: Why the M.S. patient needs your help, Nursing79 **9**:57-61, Sept. 1979.

Taylor, J.W., and Ballenger, S.: Neurological dysfunctions and nursing intervention, New York, 1980, McGraw-Hill Book Co.

CHAPTER 13 Cerebrovascular dysfunctions

Cerebrovascular dysfunctions (cerebrovascular accidents, cerebrovascular infarctions, strokes) affect approximately 2 million Americans per year. Of this number about 200,000 people die yearly according to the U.S. Vital Statistics.

A cerebrovascular accident occurs in response to an interruption of oxygen (blood) supply to the brain. The resulting neurological deficits are very devastating to the patient because they may alter the patient's ability to function independently in the activities of daily living (ADL). Prevention is the best treatment for a cerebrovascular accident and a very important aspect of nursing care. Everyone should be aware of the risk factors and how life-styles play an important role in this dysfunction.

ETIOLOGY

The three main causes of cerebrovascular accidents are thrombus, embolism, and hemorrhage. Other causes or precipitating factors may include cerebral tumors, cerebrovasospasm, aneurysm, atherosclerosis, and arteriovenous malformations. Factors that increase the risk of cerebrovascular accidents include hypertension, diabetes, high serum cholesterol, cardiac disease, obesity, cigarette smoking, stress, and the use of oral contraceptives. The individual who has a multiple combination of these factors is at greater risk for a cerebrovascular accident.

PATHOPHYSIOLOGY

A thrombus may be caused by atherosclerosis or by an inflammation within the vessel wall itself. As atherosclerotic plaques form on the lumen of the cerebral vessels, blood flow is progressively occluded (Fig. 13-1). A transient ischemic attack (TIA) is a focal disturbance of the cerebral circulation as a result of a temporary occlusion or decrease in cerebral blood flow. TIAs are brief in duration; they may last 10 to 20 mintues up to a maximum duration of 24 hours (Russell, 1976). An example is transient arm numbness that is eventually totally resolved. Collateral circulation may prevent full ischemia initially, but as the occlusion worsens so does the ischemia. The most common site is in the carotid sinus at the point where the internal carotid artery arises from the common carotid (Merritt, 1979). TIAs may be indicative of an impending stroke, but there is no way to identify which persons will have a stroke if no treatment is given for TIAs.

An embolism is a portion of a thrombus that has broken loose and has become lodged in a smaller cerebral vessel. The embolism may have originated within the cerebral vessels or in the heart. Emboli from the heart may break loose during atrial fibrillation following a myocardial infarction.

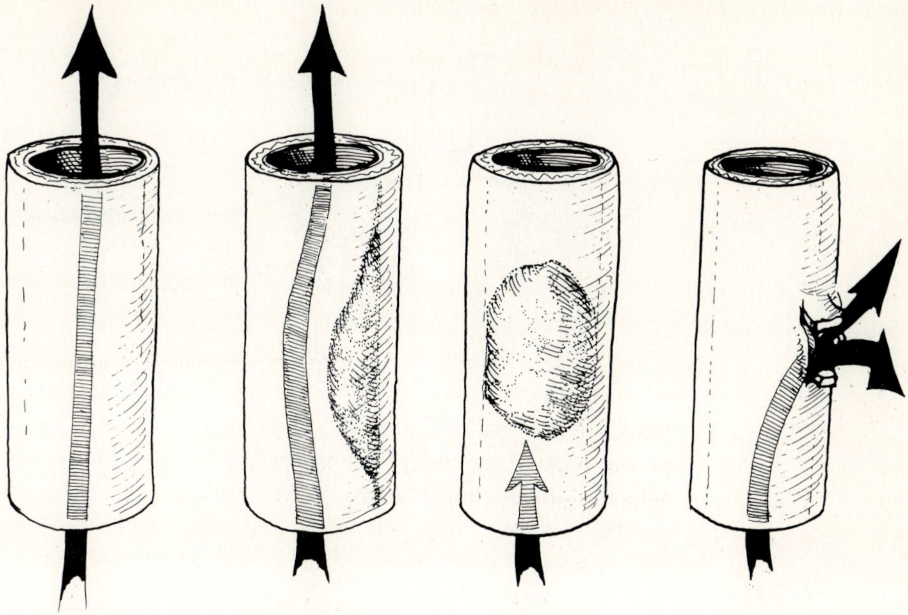

Fig. 13-1 Vascular changes preventing blood flow.

A cerebral hemorrhage occurs when there is a rupture of a cerebral vessel. The rupture may occur anywhere within the brain, resulting in intracerebral bleeding or in bleeding into the subarachnoid space.

An aneurysm results from a weakness in the arterial wall that is thought to be caused by a developmental defect in the muscular layer of the vessel. When the elastic layer of the vessel is not present, an outpouching or sac forms on the cerebral arteries. The common aneurysm sites, such as the bifurcations, are shown in Fig. 13-2.

Arteriovenous malformations (AVM) occur primarily in the parietal and occipital lobes, the brainstem, or the spinal cord. AVMs are a result of congenital developmental defects of the intracerebral arteries and veins. In AVMs blood is shunted into the malformation as a result of arterial dilatation because of decreased resistance to blood flow. The malformation cannot supply blood to the brain tissue because there are no capillaries, and the blood flow moves into the venous system (Fig. 13-3).

A cerebral vasospasm (CVS) may occur following a subarachnoid hemorrhage. CVS is a constriction of some cerebral vessels; consequently cerebral blood flow is decreased because of diminished size in the diameter of the artery. Ischemia and changes in cerebral tissue metabolism can result from CVS.

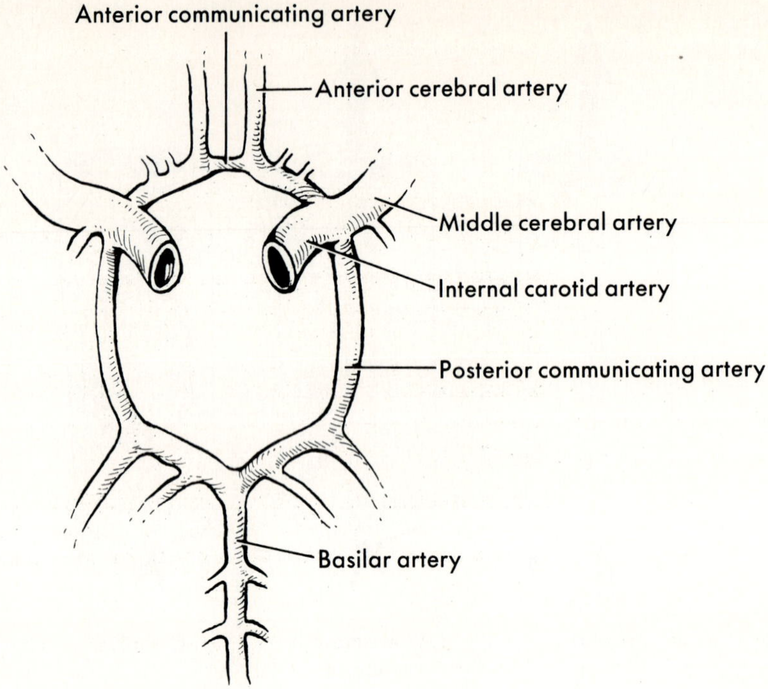

Fig. 13-2 Common aneurysm sites.

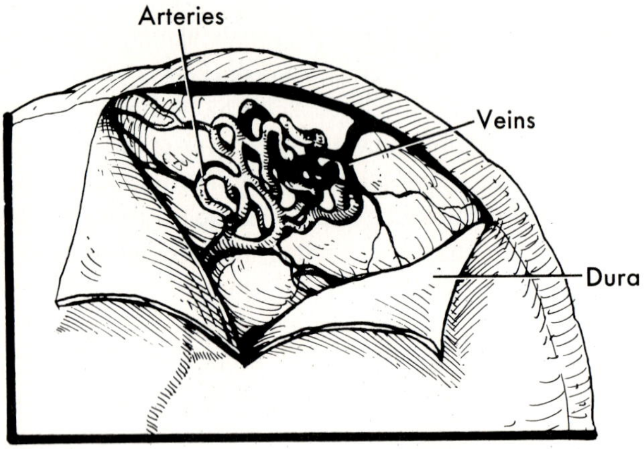

Fig. 13-3 Arteriovenous malformation

Hypertension may be a precipitating factor for cerebrovascular dysfunctions and it is a strong contributor to the risk of cerebral ischemia. Aneurysms frequently rupture as a result of hypertension. Tumors are space-occupying and may also cause cerebrovascular dysfunctions. Refer to Chapter 8.

CLASSIFICATIONS

Cerebrovascular dysfunctions are usually classified according to their etiology. Refer to the discussion of etiology.

NURSING ASSESSMENT

For a more detailed explanation of and for signs and symptoms of increased intracranial pressure (ICP), refer to Chapter 9.

Subjective assessment data

General clinical manifestations (result of increased ICP, obstruction of cerebrospinal fluid)
- Headache (presence, location, severity, onset)
- Nausea/vomiting (nausea may or may not occur; it may be projectile; not related to food ingestion; often associated with headache)
- Dizziness and vertigo
- Mental changes (for example, lethargy, drowsiness, confusion, irritability, apathy, memory failure, inappropriate behavior)
- Seizures (focal or tonic-clonic)

Localized clinical manifestations (presenting signs depend upon the location and extent of the cerebrovascular accident)
- Visual changes (for example; hemianopsia, nystagmus, diplopia, blindness, signs of papilledema)
- Speech changes (for example, aphasia)
- Sensory changes (for example, loss of sensation, pain, sensory hallucinations)
- Motor changes (for example, ataxia, falls, head tilt, weakness, paralysis)
- Bowel/bladder changes (for example, incontinence, urinary retention, constipation)
- Hearing changes (for example, tinnitus, deafness)
- Sexual changes (for example, impotence, delay of secondary sexual characteristics, infertility)

Objective assessment data. Objective data are gathered by conducting a complete neurological examination that includes an evaluation of the patient's:
- Mental status
- Cranial status
- Sensory status
- Cerebellar function
- Motor system
- Vital signs

For a detailed description of the neurological examination refer to Chapter 1.

Nursing care plan: CEREBROVASCULAR DYSFUNCTIONS

NURSING DIAGNOSIS	EXPECTED OUTCOMES	NURSING INTERVENTIONS
Ineffective airway clearance Ineffective self-oral hygiene Nutritional deficit Potential impairment of skin integrity Alteration in bowel and bladder elimination Potential for thrombophlebitus	Minimal complications have occurred Refer to Chapters 5 and 11	The care of the bedridden or comatose patient centers around proper respiratory care, oral hygiene, nutrition, skin care, bladder and bowel management, and prevention of thrombophlebitus. Refer to Chapters 5 and 11 for specific nursing interventions.
Potential injury due to a seizure Impaired verbal communication Impaired memory and intellect Visual field deficits Impaired sensory perception Sexual dysfunction Emotional disturbance	Patient is functioning as independently as possible Dignity and self-esteem are maintained Patient and family have worked through the feelings of anger and guilt Refer to Chapters 5, 6, and 11	The common neurological disturbances resulting from increased ICP include seizures, aphasia, impaired memory and intellect, visual field defects (such as hemianopsia), hemiparesis, diplopia, dysphagia, paraplegia, and impaired sexual functions. Specific nursing interventions may be found in Chapters 5 and 11 for all the above stated disturbances except for seizures, which are discussed in Chapter 6.
Knowledge deficit: diagnostic procedures	Verbalizes understanding of procedures Verbalizes fears and concerns Cooperates with procedures	Give an explanation appropriate to the patient's and family's level of comprehension and emotional state. Give encouragement and the opportunity to ask questions. Provide psychological support. Make appropriate referrals, (such as to a psychiatric nurse). Refer to Chapter 2 for detailed descriptions of each procedure and specific nursing interventions. NOTE: Following a complete history and physical examination conducted by the physician, the following studies may be conducted to confirm the diagnosis: skull x-rays, computerized axial tomogram (CAT-scan), brain scan, electroencephalogram (EEG), echoencephalogram, cerebral angiogram, oculoplethysmography, and chest x-ray. A lumbar puncture may also be performed; however it may be contraindicated if there is the possibility of brainstem herniation because of increased ICP. Pneumoencephalograms are infrequently done since the development of the CAT scan. Diagnostic procedures for specific tumors include audiometric studies, electronystagmogram, caloric tests, cisternograms, and endocrine evaluation studies.
Knowledge deficit: surgery	Verbalizes understanding of surgery Verbalizes fears and concerns	Refer to Chapter 10 for a description of the preoperative and postoperative nursing care for the patient having a craniotomy.

Nursing care plan: CEREBROVASCULAR DYSFUNCTIONS—cont'd

NURSING DIAGNOSIS	EXPECTED OUTCOMES	NURSING INTERVENTIONS
Knowledge deficit: symptomatic medications **Potential complications of symptomatic medications**	Cerebral edema is minimal Seizure activity is decreased or under control Early recognition and treatment of untoward effects of symptomatic pharmacotherapy Verbalizes understanding of dosage, administration, and possible untoward effects of drug therapy	Cerebrovascular dysfunctions create edema in the surrounding tissue. Medications may be administered to decrease the increased ICP. The more common of these drugs include dexamethasone (Decadron), mannitol, or urea. Nursing interventions are as follows: Monitor intake, output, and electrolytes. Closely monitor blood pressure. Weigh patient daily. Urea is contraindicated in patients with severely impaired renal or hepatic functions. Mannitol is contraindicated in patients with severely impaired renal function and congestive heart failure. Dexamethasone is contraindicated in the presence of active or healed tuberculosis and ocular herpes simplex. Observe for signs of untoward effects of dexamethasone. These may include adrenocortical insufficiency, electrolyte imbalances, and Cushing's syndrome. Observe for signs of infections because dexamethasone may mask usual symptoms. Refer to a pharmacology text for detailed discussions of dosages and administration routes.
Knowledge deficit: home care	Patient is functioning as independently as possible Family and patient feel comfortable and are knowledgeable enough to take care of the patient at home if they so desire Appropriate referrals and community resources are utilized for both physical and psychological support	Identify the physical limitations and strengths of the patient. Discuss these limitations and strengths with the patient and family. Include the patient and family in the coordination and delivery of care. Encourage the patient to do as much as possible. Identify appropriate referrals. These may include a (1) nutritionist to discuss ways to maintain nutritional intake and approaches to deal with problems such as stomatitis, diarrhea, and constipation; (2) physical therapist to discuss and demonstrate proper body mechanics, range-of-motion, and transfer techniques; (3) occupational therapist to discuss ways of maintaining the patient's activity level and independence; (4) social worker to discuss community resources such as visiting nurses, financial resources, equipment support groups, and information or other services that can be found by contacting the American Cancer Society. Encourage the patient and family to continue socialization outside the home (such as by maintaining work status if possible or attending clubs and church groups).

Suggested readings

Adams, R.O., and Victor, M.: Principles of neurology, New York, 1981, McGraw-Hill Book Co.

Asaka, K.: Prolonged vasospasm produced by the breakdown products of erythrocytes, J. Neurosurg. **47:**403-411, Sept. 1977.

Bouvette, J.M.: Preoperative and postoperative care of patients with cerebral aneurysms, Nurs. Clin. North Am. **9:**655-666, 1974.

Conway-Rutkowski, B.L.: Carini and Owens' neurological and neurosurgical nursing, ed. 8, St. Louis, 1982, The C.V. Mosby Co.

Heros, R., Zervas, N.T., and Negors, M.: Cerebral vasospasm, Surg. Neurol. **15:**354-362, June 1976.

Johanson, B.C., and others: Standards for critical care, St. Louis, 1981, The C.V. Mosby Co.

Lewis, R.R., Beasley, M.G., and Gosling, R.C.: Disease at the carotid bi-furcation: diagnosis by doppler ultrasound imaging, Gerontology **25:**291-298, 1979.

Merrit, H.: A textbook of neurology, Philadelphia, 1979, Lea & Febiger.

Nursing Skillbook Series, Nursing 80, Coping with neurologic problems proficiently, Horsham, P., 1980, Intermed Communications.

Redelman, K.: Neurological injuries, Crit. Care Q., Germantown, Md., June 1979, Aspen Systems Corporation.

Russell, R.W., and Ross, M.: Cerebral arterial disease, London and New York, 1976, Churchill Livingstone.

Samuels, M.A.: Manual of neurologic therapeutics, Boston, 1978, Little, Brown & Co.

Snyder, M., and Jackle, M.: Neurologic problems, Bowie, Md., 1982, Robert J. Brady Co.

Sundt, T.M.: Management of ischemic complications after subarachnoid hemorrhage, J. Neurosurg. **43:**418-425, Oct. 1975.

Taylor, J.W., and Ballenger, S.: Neurological dysfunctions and nursing intervention, New York, 1980, McGraw-Hill Book Co.

Toole, J.F., and others: Transcient ischemic attacks due to atherosclerosis, Arch. Neurol. **32:**5-12, 1975.

CHAPTER 14

Chronic neurological impairments

Chronic neurological problems affect intellectual functioning including memory, abstract thinking, judgment and personality, sensory, motor, and refined motor functions. These problems occur with enough severity that they also interfere with a person's social and occupational functioning. Patience and understanding are qualities to be possessed by those caring for patients who suffer from intellectual and behavioral dysfunction.

ETIOLOGY

The brain, nerve pathways, muscles, and extrapyramidal tracts are involved in chronic dysfunctional disorders of the nervous system. Causes for these disorders include alcoholism, head trauma, atherosclerosis and other vascular disorders, metabolic and nutritional disorders, hypoxia or anoxia, intracranial space-occupying lesions, epilepsy, infections, drugs, and toxic substances such as poisons and heavy metals.

PATHOPHYSIOLOGY

Many chronic neurological dysfunctions are presently incurable. Abnormal tissue changes occur in the involved anatomy, and general symptoms arise for each disorder. Heredity plays a significant part in the occurrence of a few of these conditions.

CLASSIFICATIONS

The categories of dementia, decreased motor and sensory function, degenerative disorders, and associated health problems will be used to discuss the various chronic disorders that affect the nervous system.

Dementia

Senile dementia is falsely thought to occur in all persons as a result of old age. Actually, only 1,000,000 Americans over 65 suffer from dementia, and 65% of these have Alzheimer's disease (Kaplan, 1981). Dementia frequently occurs after age 60 and the onset is gradual except in the event of head trauma, cardiac arrest, or encephalitis.

Organic dementias. Wernicke-Korsakoff is a condition made up of two syndromes that occur together in chronic alcoholism. The pathophysiology of these two conditions is not fully understood and research on the problems in the next decade will hopefully provide a resolution to the problem.

Pathophysiology. Wernicke's encephalopathy is a cerebral disorder that is caused by thiamine deficiency. It is characterized by a triad of symptoms including memory defects, ophthalmoplegia causing diplopia, and ataxia. Other symptoms found are nystagmus, peripheral nerve disease, and cardiovascular dysfunction including postural hypotension, sudden death following mild exertion, drowsiness, stupor, coma, and even death. The onset of this syndrome is acute and with prompt treatment the symptoms will generally clear within a few days.

It appears that Wernicke's encephalopathy is precipitated in thiamine-deficient persons and that carbohydrate metabolism enhances the assimilation of thiamine. The physiological mechanism of thiamine in carbohydrate metabolism is not completely researched. It is known that when glucose is administered to a thiamine-deficient person, full-blown Wernicke's encephalopathy symptoms occur. Therefore when glucose infusions are administered to any alcoholic or any undiagnosed comatose patient, it is recommended that thiamine also be given. It is known that glucose precipitates the need for thiamine and that dextrose needs thiamine to complete the process of oxidation.

The pathophysiology of Wernicke's encephalopathy has been narrowed to three concepts: metabolic disturbance, neurophysiological disturbance, and genetic abnormalities. All of these concepts are related to the enzyme activity that is dependent on the thiamine pentose phosphate pathway utilizing the coenzymes of transketolase, pyruvate decarboxylase, and alpha-ketoglutorate decarboxylase. Many hypothesis have been formulated about the effect of the pentose phosphate cycle in thiamine deficiency and its relationship to neurological signs. The exact cause of the impairment has not been proven. There is believed to be a correlation between cerebral energy metabolism and synthesis of acetylcholine and the generation of neurotransmitters in brain myelin components to maintain neuronal integrity and propagation. Research has been done to understand neurological changes in Wernicke's syndrome and much more will need to be done to describe the pathogenesis of this disorder.

Korsakoff's syndrome is also a result of thiamine deficiency in chronic alcoholics. It is characterized by memory loss, especially for current events, confusion, disorientation, and confabulation. The person will have difficulty learning new information. Korsakoff's psychosis may be caused by other disorders such as by a ruptured anterior communicating artery aneurysm, encephalitis, posterior cerebral artery strokes, and head trauma. Korsakoff's psychosis is not curable when associated with chronic alcoholism because the deficit in higher cortical function associated with the ability to form new memories is impaired further than the other functions.

Nursing assessment. Clinically the alcoholic shows the following signs and symptoms:

Flushed face
Bloodshot eyes
Decreased visual acuity
Spider angiomas of the upper extremities, chest, back, and face
Hepatomegaly and abdominal tenderness
Dry skin

Redness/swelling of the lips and tongue
Gums that bleed easily
Pale, red, or dry conjunctiva and corneas
Scaling or flakiness around the nose or mouth

Other assessment tools include a complete neurological and physical assessment to determine orientation, sensation, and muscle tone. (See Chapter 1 for information on the neurological examination.) Diagnostic laboratory studies to determine serum levels of thiamine and pyruvate may be helpful in making a conclusive diagnosis.

Organic hallucinosis. These are recurrent or persistent hallucinations that occur during full wakefulness. This condition is associated with chronic alcoholism or may result as a side effect of Levodopa (Dopar).

Organic delusional syndrome. The presence of delusions in a state of full wakefulness is known as organic delusional syndrome. This syndrome exists with amphetamine intoxication and paranoid psychosis.

Organic affective syndrome. This syndrome is characterized by a depressive or manic mood disorder. Its cause is attributed to organic conditions, drugs, (namely, reserpine, corticosteroids, methyldopa, levodopa, cycloserine, ethinonomide, oral contraceptives, amphetamines, hallucinogens), endocrine diseases (Cushing's and Addison's diseases, hypothyroidism and hyperthyroidism), infections (influenza, infectious mononucleosis, infectious hepatitis, viral pneumonia), pernicious anemia, cancer of the pancreas, brain tumor, systemic lupus erythematosus, parkinsonism, carcoroid syndrome, and neurosyphilis.

Organic personality syndrome. This syndrome involves a change in personality traits or style that is manifested by an impaired control of behavioral expression and impulses. Head trauma and subarachnoid hemorrhage of the anterior communicating artery are significant causes.

Substance-induced organic mental disorders and chemical or environmental disorders. These disorders are related to the organic syndromes. Major causes of these include barbiturates, tranquilizers, amphetamines, belladonna alkaloids and synthetic anticholinergics, anorectics, psychotropic drugs, anticonvulsants, levodopa, cardiovascular agents, anesthetics, hormones, salicylates in high doses, anti-ulcer drugs, anti-inflammatory drugs, anti-infectives (antibiotics, antivirus agents, antiparasitic and antifungal drugs), disulfiram, antineoplastic agents, poisons, gases, noxious vapors, solvents, heavy metals, and insecticides.

Other disease conditions. Other conditions that may involve chronic neurological deficits include the following: confusion after cardiac surgery, transient global amnesia (inability to recall recent events), acute intermittent porphyria (autosomal inherited trait), intracranial neoplasms, muscular dystrophy, multiple sclerosis, and nutritional disorders.

Degenerative disorders

Degenerative disorders are discussed in Table 14-1.

Decreased motor and sensory function

Nutritional polyneuropathy (neuropathic beriberi). This neurological disorder generally occurs as a result of a thiamine deficiency, but other vitamins may be involved. It occurs in alcoholics who are nutritionally deficient.

The pathology of the disorder involves degeneration of the axons with demyelination. Changes occur in the distal parts of long fibers. The course of the condition begins in the distal parts of the feet and legs and then involves the fingers and arms.

Signs and symptoms involve a mixture of sensory and motor function impairments. Symptoms include loss of reflexes, flaccid paralysis with wasting, and impairments of the vibrating sense, proprioception, pain, and temperature sensation in a "stocking-glove" distribution. Dysethesias are common and are experienced as severe burning, cramping, or shooting pains in the feet and hands. Stimulation may increase the pain. The autonomic system may be involved and may cause abnormal sweating of the affected areas or hypotension. The progression of the disease is gradual and slow. Recovery may take a year or more and may not be complete.

Treatment for neurological impairments resulting from alcohol include thiamine 50-100 mg administered intramuscularly for 3 consecutive days along with a well-balanced diet with other vitamin supplements if necessary. Mild analgesics for the pain of polyneuropathy may be ordered. Physical therapy may be ordered to prevent deformities and to improve the function of involved extremities.

Polyneuritis. This is an inflammation of peripheral nerves that results from impaired nutrition and vascular supply. These deficiencies in vascularity and nutrition lead to degeneration of multiple peripheral nerves. Polyneuritis can be caused by inhalation, ingestion, or absorption of exogenous toxic substances or by endogenous dysfunctions. In the United States, the most common form of polyneuritis is that caused by vitamin deficiencies secondary to alcoholism and malnutrition.

As a result of exogenous or endogenous poisoning, the peripheral nerve becomes inflammed and edematous. The vascular supply and hence the nutritional support for peripheral nerve function is diminished, causing degeneration and fragmentation of the protective, nutritive myelin. Lacking adequate nutrients and oxygen, the peripheral axon degenerates (Merritt, 1979).

The classification of polyneuritis is derived from the causation.

Toxic:

- Heavy metals
- Chemicals

Text continued on p. 419.

Table 14-1 Degenerative disorders of the nervous system

Disease	Symptoms and behavior	Treatment	Prognosis
Alzheimer's disease			
A degenerative disease causing senility as a result of decreasing numbers of cortical neurons. It occurs before or after age 65.	Memory loss, spatial disorientation. As the disease progresses, signs of frontal lobe dysfunction appear including loss of social inhibitions, incontinence, and loss of spontaneity. Aphasia and/or apraxia may occur at any time in the progression of the disease. Patients are inappropriate in language and actions and frequently embarrass family members. They are incontinent of urine and feces, confused, agitated, and may wander away from home and get lost. Depression is a common problem. Motor dysfunctions appear late in the course of the disease, which presents problems with ADL.	There is no available treatment for the disease itself. Interventions are designed to assist the patient and family to adjust physically and psychologically to the disease, to improve living arrangements and environment, and to provide supportive care.	There is a progression of symptoms until patient is completely incapacitated; death results 4-10 years after onset as a result of complications of immobility.
Pick's lobar atrophy			
Cause is unknown. It occurs in middle age and more frequently in females.	Symptoms are related to frontal and temporal lobes. Receptive aphasia is a dominant problem. Other symptoms are similar to those of Alzheimer's disease. Patient has a light-hearted, anxious personality. There is an eventual loss of speech.	Same as Alzheimer's disease	This is a progressive disease over a 5-year period with death resulting.

Continued.

Table 14-1 Degenerative disorders of the nervous system—cont'd

Disease	Symptoms and behavior	Treatment	Prognosis
Parkinson's disease			
Commonly referred to as the "shaking palsy." A deficiency of dopamine in the nigrostriatal complex is the cause of Parkinson's. Onset occurs after age 50. The administration of phenochlorpromazine and haloperidol used to treat psychiatric disorders may produce symptoms of parkinsonism. Onset is insidious and the disease is progressive. Parkinson's disease is a disorder of the basal ganglion.	The triad of tremor, rigidity, and dyskinesia are characteristics of Parkinson's. Dementia accompanies the disease, but is difficult to correlate directly with Parkinson's because Alzheimer's disease occurs in the same age group and because the extreme disorders of movement make it difficult to assess intellectual function since the patients are slow to respond. Resting tremor is most prevelant in the fingers (pill-rolling movement). Emotional stress, fatigue, and cold exaggerate the tremor during purposeful activity. Posture, gait, ambulation, and mobility are affected by rigidity. Short steps taken rapidly with the body leaning forward is a classic symptom of Parkinson's disease. Other symptoms include loss of reflex activity for blinking and facial mobility (masked facies and fixed gaze), salivation caused by infrequent swallowing, and drooling. Writing, speaking, chewing, eating, and swallowing are impaired as the disease progresses.	Palliative measures. Antiparkinsonian drugs: levodopa (L-dopa, Sinemet). Anticholinegic drugs: trihexyphenidyl (Artane) or cycrimine (Pagitane). Stop drugs that produce Parkinson's. Physical therapy. Psychotherapy.	No cure. Disease progresses and death results from failure of a major body system, such as respiratory, cardiovascular, renal system. Proper treatment, however, can produce a good prognosis.

Huntington's chorea			
A rare, familial, progressive degenerative disease of adults occurring in the 30- to 50-year age group. It is a congenital disease involving a dominant gene and is passed from generation to generation.	Depression and temper outbursts. Choreiform movements: gradual progression from slight to severe restlessness; facial grimacing; arm movements—appearance of a salute; irregular leg movements; trunk movements of a twisting, turning, and shrugging nature; tongue and finger movements. Personality changes: irritability, paranoia, demanding, memory loss, decreased intellectual function, and dementia. Psychosis is seen in the last stages. Person is in constant motion in the end stages.	Drugs used include chlordiazepoxide (Librium), haloperidol (Haldol), fluphenazine (Prolixen), chlorpromazine (Thorazine), and imipramine (Tofranil). Drugs reduce some of the movements and subdue behavior changes. Provide supportive care.	No cure. Disease progresses until patient is completely helpless and speechless.
Amyotrophic lateral sclerosis (ALS, also known as Lou Gehrig's disease).			
A progressive deteriorating asymmetrical muscular atrophy. Cell body death from the degeneration of the axon and second demyelination of the upper and lower motor neurons occurs in the fibers that innervate striated muscle. Cause is unknown.	Signs and symptoms are those of motor neuron lesions. Twitching; weakness in extremities that progresses to trunk. The spread is variable and may result in paraparesis, hemiparesis, dysphagia, or dysphasia.	No cure. Supportive care.	Life expectancy is 3-5 years. Death usually results from malnutrition, paralysis of the accessory respiratory muscles or aspiration pneumonia (Merritt, 1979).

Continued.

Table 14-1 Degenerative disorders of the nervous system—cont'd

Disease	Symptoms and behavior	Treatment	Prognosis
Rare neurological deficit syndromes			
Creutzfeldt-Jakob disease and kuru are believed to be viral in nature with the causative organisms being subacute spongiform virus. There is degeneration of the nerve cells of the cerebral and cerebellar cortex.	Rapidly progressive dementia similar to Alzheimer's disease. Myoclonus, rigidity and weakness, ataxia.	None. Nursing care: same as for demented and immobile patients. Practice precautions to prevent transmission of the disease as indicated in wound care and other isolation procedures.	Rapid deterioration to eventual coma. Fatal within a few months to a few years.
Familial dementia with spastic paraparesis caused by a demyelination of pyramidal tracts in the spinal cord and corpus callosum.	Muscle atrophy; speech and visual defect; loss of intellectual function that increases in severity; spastic paresis; no sensory loss; increase in reflexes and extensor plantar responses.	None. Supportive nursing care.	No cure.
Cortical basal ganglionic syndrome results from atrophy of the parietal cortex; degeneration of the substantia nigra, and neuronal and medullated fiber loss in all layers.	Ridigity and inability to move extremities on one side or both; apraxia, ataxia, tremors; mental deterioration in late stages.	Supportive care.	Eventual incapacity to all of the side or both sides of body; late mental deterioration.
Vertigo			
Vestibular neuronitis (acute labyrinthitis) is believed to be caused by a virus; is usually associated with an upper respiratory condition; affects adults aged 20 to 60.	Sudden and severe vertigo, nausea, vomiting, spontaneous nystagmus with the rapid response toward the affected ear. Tinnitus or a full feeling occurs in the affected ear. Hearing is impaired. Normal audiological examination. No neurological signs.	Drugs to suppress the symptoms: antihistamines, belladonna alkaloids, phenothiazines, antiemetics. Other measures include fixing one's gaze on a nearby object instead of lying down with eyes closed; mental relaxation. The patient should avoid turning and tilting the head.	Vertigo resolves spontaneously in a period of a few days to several weeks, and recovery is complete.

Benign positional nystagmus and vertigo (Barany's vertigo) is a condition that occurs in a variety of disorders including brainstem disorders, multiple sclerosis, infarct, tumors, and barbiturate and alcohol intoxications. Cause is unknown.	Vertigo, nausea, vomiting, ataxia	Symptomatic treatment. Anti-motion sickness drugs may be used. A soft cervical collar may be prescribed to limit head and neck motion.	Condition is not life threatening and removal of other conditions leads to resolution.
Posttraumatic vertigo results from a trauma to the head and neck that injures the labyrinth.	Vertigo, nausea, and vomiting, spontaneous nystagmus with the rapid movement away from the affected side, loss of balance.	Anti-motion sickness drugs. Symptoms improve within a few days.	In some instances the symptoms may be present for 6 months. If they do not subside within 2 years, the condition may become permanent.
Meniere's disease usually occurs in persons 30 to 40 years of age. Cause is not known definitely. Theories suggest that there is a degeneration of the cochlear hair cells of the labyrinth.	Typical signs include episodes of nausea, incapacitating vertigo, tinnitus, feeling of fullness or pressure in the ear, and fluctuating hearing loss. Deafness may occur after repeated episodes.	Antihistamines in the acute phase; also bed rest, a low salt diet, ammonium chloride, diuretics, fluid restrictions, antiemetic drugs; mild sedatives. Surgery may be done by dividing the vestibular portion of the acoustic nerve intracranially. A relatively new surgical procedure, developed by James, is done with an ultrasonic beam to destroy the vestibular apparatus without damage to the cochlear division.	Attacks are recurrent several times a week with periods of remission lasting several years.
Brainstem origin vertigo (ischemia, central vertigo) results from vascular neoplastic or demyelinative diseases of the brainstem. Strokes that occur in the vertebral-basilar artery will cause vertigo, nausea, and vomiting.	Vertigo, dysarthria, facial numbness, ataxia, hemiparesis, diplopia, and visual disturbances are the symptoms.	Anticonvulsants, salicylates, aminoglycosides, anticoagulants.	Prolonged and continuous symptoms.

Continued.

Table 14-1 Degenerative disorders of the nervous system—cont'd

Disease	Symptoms and behavior	Treatment	Prognosis
Vertigo—cont'd			
Hyperventilation syndrome and psychogenic disease result from anxiety	Light-headedness resulting from decreased cerebral flow, hypocapnia, and increased cerebovascular resistance will bring on the symptoms of an "anxiety attack." Symptoms are accompanied by perspiration, shakiness, palpitations, shortness of breath, paresthesias of the fingers, and fear.	Breathing into a paper bag or an oxygen-rebreathing mask; mild tranquilizers. Encourage verbalization about anxiety-producing situations.	Condition is not physically detrimental.

Metabolic

- Vitamin/nutritional deficiencies: beriberi
- Wasting diseases: cancer, tuberculosis
- Endocrine or electrolyte disturbances
- Kidney/liver disease
- Chronic infectious diseases

Nursing assessment. Signs and symptoms of these cerebral and peripheral nerve disorders are similar. A complete history to determine ingestion of any toxic substances, drug profile, occupation, and a complete neurological, physical, and psychiatric evaluation should be done to determine the cause of the disorder.

Nursing care plan: CHRONIC NEUROLOGICAL IMPAIRMENTS

NURSING DIAGNOSIS	EXPECTED OUTCOMES	NURSING INTERVENTIONS
Alteration in nutrition **Fluid and electrolyte deficit**	Weight gain Serum electrolytes and vitamin levels within normal limits Patient free of weakness and deformities	Establish a set schedule for meals and fluids for a 24-hour period and see that the patient adheres to it. Recognize hunger and thirst. Provide a well-balanced diet high in protein, carbohydrates, vitamins, and nutrients. Include foods high in vitamin B content: whole grains, vegetables, lean meat (especially liver), nuts, eggs, milk. Have the nutritionist visit the patient and family. Have the patient eliminate alcohol and drugs. Encourage the patient to feed self. In the event of a physical disability, feed the patient. Administer prescribed vitamin supplements. Record intake and output. Weigh the patient daily. Remind the patient to eat since mental confusion may cause the patient to forget how to chew or swallow. Feed small portions at a time, since feeding is time consuming because of lack of dentures, drooling, loss of muscle tone. Tube feedings may be necessary.
Potential for poisoning	No arsenic, lead, or toxins in system	Remove agent with use of gastric lavage, administration of prescribed laxatives, or enemas. Milk is given to precipitate lead from the system.

Continued.

Nursing care plan: CHRONIC NEUROLOGICAL IMPAIRMENT—cont'd

NURSING DIAGNOSIS	EXPECTED OUTCOMES	NURSING INTERVENTIONS
Potential for physical injury	Patient is free from physical harm and reasonably psychologically comforted	Observe for signs and symptoms of restlessness, increased confusion, seizures, auditory and visual hallucinations. Maintain an environment free of stimuli for the patient undergoing alcohol or drug detoxification. Place siderails on bed and a pad if necessary. Use soft restraints for extremities and trunk as necessary. Have things the patient will need to use within easy reach to avoid the need to get out of bed. Administer prescribed tranquilizers and anticonvulsants when indicated. NOTE: The restlessness and agitation associated with brain damage are not readily controlled with sedatives and tranquilizers. Be aware of the location of confused patients at all times because they may wander off and get lost. Make sure that all hospitalized and institutionalized patients have identification bands. Prevent falls and injuries during transfers. Provide assistive devices for ambulation: canes, walkers, wheelchairs.
Knowledge deficit Short-term memory deficit Impaired thought processes Sensory-perceptual alterations	Knowledge of disease and self-care Family support	Test cognitive function, memory, and awareness. Keep the patient oriented to present. Identify yourself to patient on each encounter. Keep a clock and calendar near the patient. Modify education procedures and give short, simple explanations at the time events are to happen. Provide environmental and sensory stimulation to the elderly and chronically ill who are institutionalized. Use television, radio, books, magazines, place the patient near a window or take him outdoors, provide recreational and occupational programs. Initiate patient/family teacing about nutrition, safety, prevention of complications of immobility, and avoidance of alcohol, toxins, poisons. Refer the patient to community agencies as appropriate: Alcoholics Anonymous, social welfare, community food pantries, National organizations such as for multiple sclerosis, Alzheimer's or Huntington's disease, or other federal and local foundations.
Sleep-pattern disturbance	Ability to sleep without disturbance	Brain-damaged patients are believed to have less rapid-eye-movement (REM) sleep. At night they become agitated and confused (sundowning). A quiet peaceful environment, reassurance, and provision of physical comfort measures are beneficial.

Nursing care plan: **CHRONIC NEUROLOGICAL IMPAIRMENTS—cont'd**

NURSING DIAGNOSIS	EXPECTED OUTCOMES	NURSING INTERVENTIONS
Impaired physical mobility Alteration in bowel and bladder elimination Impaired skin integrity Total self-care deficit Impaired verbal communication		Refer to Chapter 11 for nursing care of immobility.
Self-esteem disturbance	Positive feeling about self-concept	Set realistic goals for patient/family to cope with dysfunction. Assist the patient and family to accept the behavior of the chronic brain-damaged. Identify phases of the guilt process and assist the patient and family to work through these. Respect the individual as a person of worth. Work with the patient and family to develop a trust relationship. Encourage the presence of children and young adults around the elderly. Provide resources and make agency referrals to help the family manage the patient in the home or to make an appropriate placement. Be a good listener. Teach about medications and care procedures. Provide emotional support by including a mental health professional.

Suggested readings

Berman, M.O.: Neuropsychological consequences: long-term chronic alcoholism, Am. Sci. **68:**410-419, 1980.

Charatan, F.B.: Therapeutic supports for the patient with OBS, Geriatrics **10**(9):100-102, Sept. 1980.

Conway-Rutkowski, B.L.: Carini and Owens' neurological and neurosurgical nursing, St. Louis, 1982, The C.V. Mosby Co.

Cutting, J.: Differential impairment of memory in Korsakoff's syndrome, Cortex **15:**501-506, 1979.

Czank, J.Z., Zweig, J.P.: Relative mortality of chronically ill geriatric patients with organic brain damage, before and after relocation, J. Am. Geriatr. Soc. **28:**76-82, Feb. 1980.

Hylands, J.: The Wernicke-Korsakoff syndrome, Nursing79 **9**(7):26-29, July 1979.

Jones, D.A., Dunbar, C.F., and Jirovec, M.M.: Medical-surgical nursing, a conceptual approach, 1978, New York, McGraw-Hill Book Co.

Kaplan, H.I., and Sadlock, B.J.: Modern synopsis of psychiatry, ed. 3, Baltimore, 1981, The Williams & Wilkins Co.

Merritt, H.H.: A textbook of neurology, Philadelphia, 1979, Lea & Febiger.

Power, D.J., and Craven, R.F.: National Institute of Mental Health, Senile dementia (Alzheimer's disease), Fact Sheet: DHEW Pub. No. (ADM) 80-929-1980, Rockville, Md. 1980.

Power, D.J., and Craven, R.F.: Al's and aging: a case study in autonomy and control, Image: J. Nurs. Scholarship **15**(1):22-25, Winter 1983.

Russell, R.M.: Vitamin A and zinc metabolism in alcoholism, Am. J. Clin. Nutr. **33:**2741-2748, Dec. 1980.

Samuels, M.A.: Manual of neurologic therapeutics, Boston, 1978, Little, Brown & Co.

Schenker, S., and others: Hepatic and Werniche's encephalopathies: current concepts of pathogenesis, Am. J. Clin. Nutr. **33:**2719-2726, Dec. 1980.

Spitzer, J., and Ventry, I.M.: Central auditory dysfunction among chronic alcoholics, Arch. Otolaryngol. **106:**224-229, April 1980.

Taylor, J.W., and Ballenger, S.: Neurological dysfunctions and nursing interventions, 1980, New York, McGraw-Hill Book Co.

U.S. Department of Health and Human Services, Alzheimer's disease, a scientific guide for health practitioners, NIH Pub. No. 81-2251, Bethesda, Md., Nov. 1980.

U.S. Department of Health, Education, and Welfare, Huntington's disease, hope through research, NIH Pub. No. 80-49, Bethesda, Md., Oct. 1979.

Wood, F.: Effects of alcohol in the body, Healthcare Horizons **5**(2):71, Jan. 24, 1982.

Index

O

P